Current and Future Trends in Otorhinolaryngology–Head and Neck Surgery

Current and Future Trends in Otorhinolaryngology–Head and Neck Surgery

Guest Editor

Konstantinos Chaidas

MDPI

Basel • Beijing • Wuhan • Barcelona • Belgrade • Novi Sad • Cluj • Manchester

Guest Editor
Konstantinos Chaidas
Ear, Nose, and Throat Department
Democritus University of Thrace
Alexandroupolis
Greece

Editorial Office
MDPI AG
Grosspeteranlage 5
4052 Basel, Switzerland

This is a reprint of the Special Issue, published open access by the journal *Journal of Clinical Medicine* (ISSN 2077-0383), freely accessible at: https://www.mdpi.com/journal/jcm/special_issues/HUR1369TMG.

For citation purposes, cite each article independently as indicated on the article page online and as indicated below:

Lastname, A.A.; Lastname, B.B. Article Title. *Journal Name* **Year**, *Volume Number*, Page Range.

ISBN 978-3-7258-7314-2 (Hbk)
ISBN 978-3-7258-7315-9 (PDF)
https://doi.org/10.3390/books978-3-7258-7315-9

Contents

About the Editor

Konstantinos Chaidas

Konstantinos Chaidas, MD, PhD, FRCS(ORL-HNS) is an Assistant Professor in ENT at Democritus University of Thrace School of Medicine, Alexandroupolis, Greece, and an Honorary ENT Consultant at the Imperial College Healthcare NHS Trust, London, UK. Professor Chaidas graduated from the Medical School of Aristotle University in Greece in 2005. After the completion of his higher surgical training, he undertook a two-year fellowship, training in robotic ENT (thyroid/parathyroid and sleep apnea) surgery at St Mary's Hospital in London. He had been a Consultant ENT surgeon at John Radcliffe Hospital—Oxford University Hospitals NHS Foundation Trust in Oxford (2015-2022). Since 2022, he has been an Assistant Professor in ENT at Democritus University of Thrace School of Medicine in Alexandroupolis, Greece. He has also been an Honorary ENT Consultant at the Imperial College Healthcare NHS Trust in London, UK. He is a fellow of the Royal College of Surgeons of England. Professor Chaidas has an active interest in research and teaching. He was awarded a PhD in 2010. He has published widely, with over 60 peer-reviewed publications and book chapters.

Journal of
Clinical Medicine

MDPI

Editorial

Current and Future Trends in Otorhinolaryngology–Head and Neck Surgery

Konstantinos Chaidas [1,2]

[1] Ear, Nose, and Throat Department, University Hospital of Alexandroupolis, School of Medicine, Democritus University of Thrace, 68100 Alexandroupolis, Greece; konchaidas@gmail.com

[2] Ear, Nose, and Throat Department, Imperial College Healthcare NHS Trust, London W2 1NY, UK

Over the past decade, there has been a significant increase in available knowledge in the specialty of otorhinolaryngology–head and neck surgery with a remarkable development in diagnostic and therapeutic modalities. As a result of continuous advances in digital technologies, their integration into clinical practice has become a notable trend. Telemedicine proved to be an effective tool in ENT clinics, especially during the COVID-19 pandemic due to associated restrictions in face-to-face consultations [1]. Furthermore, machine learning algorithms are increasingly being used for data and image analysis with the aim to improve diagnostic accuracy and outcome prediction [2–4]. At the same time, the adoption of minimally invasive and function-preserving techniques continues to improve patient safety and recovery times while maintaining excellent results. Namely, thermal ablation is currently used not only for the management of benign thyroid nodules, but also for patients with papillary thyroid microcarcinoma with satisfactory outcomes [5]. Likewise, the role of transoral robotic surgery in selected patients with obstructive sleep apnea or head and neck cancer has been established. The use of a surgical robot provides better surgical access and dexterity, satisfactory outcomes, and reduced postoperative morbidity [6,7]. Of course, a multidisciplinary patient-centered approach is vital to ensuring the provision of high-quality care for all patients.

Our Special Issue, "Current and Future Trends in Otorhinolaryngology–Head and Neck Surgery", aims to provide readers with the latest developments in the field of otorhinolaryngology–head and neck surgery and underscore current and future trends. The included contributions cover a wide range of topics reflecting both clinical innovation and translational research.

The COVID-19 pandemic has significantly affected medical practice in general and ENT specialty in particular, as demonstrated in this Special Issue (Contributions 1–3). Some of the studies evaluated the use of new diagnostic methods for patients with nasal dysfunction (Contributions 4, 5). Moreover, innovative treatment strategies were explored, with a number of articles assessing the efficacy of new techniques or the current role of traditionally used techniques (Contributions 6–9). In addition, the valuable experience of certain institutions in the management of challenging clinical problems was shared (Contributions 10–14), with the role of diagnostic biomarkers also investigated (Contributions 15, 16). Finally, the evolving trends and future demands in ENT procedures were reported (Contribution 17).

In summary, this Special Issue highlights the innovation of the global community of otorhinolaryngology–head and neck surgery, illustrating how technological advancements, increasing scientific knowledge, and clinical excellence converge to shape the future of our specialty. Ultimately, continuous collaboration between researchers and clinicians is essential for improving patient care.

Conflicts of Interest: The author declares no conflicts of interest.

List of Contributions:

1. Lee, M.L.; Finegersh, A.; Chen, M.M. Impact of the COVID-19 Pandemic on the Treatment of Head and Neck Cancers. *J. Clin. Med.* **2025**, *14*, 1424. https://doi.org/10.3390/jcm14051424.
2. Patel, D.; Devivo, A.; Leibner, E.; Shittu, A.; Govindarajulu, U.; Tandon, P.; Lee, D.; Owen, R.; Fernandez-Ranvier, G.; Hiensch, R.; et al. The COVID-19 Tracheostomy Experience at a Large Academic Medical Center in New York during the First Year. *J. Clin. Med.* **2024**, *13*, 2130. https://doi.org/10.3390/jcm13072130.
3. Valajärvi, V.-E.; Lamminmäki, S.; Lundberg, M.; Hafrén, L. Ten-Year Trends in Otolaryngological Surgery Volumes and the Impact of Infection Prevention During the COVID-19 Pandemic—A National Study. *J. Clin. Med.* **2024**, *13*, 7190. https://doi.org/10.3390/jcm13237190.
4. Anastasiadou, S.; Bountzis, P.; Gkogkos, D.-E.; Karkos, P.; Constantinidis, J.; Triaridis, S.; Psillas, G. Chronic Nasal Disease and Eustachian Tube Function: What Is the Role of Tubomanometry? *J. Clin. Med.* **2024**, *13*, 6731. https://doi.org/10.3390/jcm13226731.
5. Zasadzińska-Stempniak, K.; Zajączkiewicz, H.; Kukwa, A. Correlation between Subjective Nasal Patency and Nasal Capacity in Young Adults: A Pilot Study with a Prototype Device—A Nasoorospirometer. *J. Clin. Med.* **2024**, *13*, 2506. https://doi.org/10.3390/jcm13092506.
6. Johnson, F.; Burian, N.-M.; Santer, M.; Strasser, V.; Steinbichler, T.; Hofauer, B.; Stenzl, A.; Klarer, J.; Lochbaum, R.; Lei, H.; et al. A Six-Year Examination of the Influence of Surgical Technique and Intraoperative Intraglandular Clostridium Botulinum Toxin Application in Salivary Gland Tumor Operations. *J. Clin. Med.* **2024**, *13*, 6902. https://doi.org/10.3390/jcm13226902.
7. Vater, J.; Gröschel, M.; Szczepek, A.J.; Olze, H. Electrical Ear Canal Stimulation as a Therapeutic Approach for Tinnitus—A Proof of Concept Study. *J. Clin. Med.* **2024**, *13*, 2663. https://doi.org/10.3390/jcm13092663.
8. Zwierz, A.; Komisarek, O.; Burduk, P. Parachute Technique: A New Endoscopic Method for Closing Recurrent Oronasal Fistulas in Cleft Palate Patients. *J. Clin. Med.* **2025**, *14*, 4299. https://doi.org/10.3390/jcm14124299.
9. Paperlein, F.; Klinger-König, J.; Busch, C.-J.; Scharf, C.; Beule, A.G. Maxillary Sinus Puncture: A Traditional Procedure in Decline—Insights from SHIP. *J. Clin. Med.* **2025**, *14*, 5578. https://doi.org/10.3390/jcm14155578.
10. Maiou, C.; Lachanas, V.A.; Doumas, S.N.; Kalogritsas, N.; Mpouronikou, A.; Hajiioannou, J.; Petinaki, E.; Skoulakis, C.E. Pharyngeal Mucosal Space Abscess: A Special Entity That Merits Special Management—Our Experience in 106 Cases. *J. Clin. Med.* **2025**, *14*, 1515. https://doi.org/10.3390/jcm14051515.
11. Ueha, R.; Koyama, M.; Seto, A.; Sato, T.; Goto, T.; Orimo, K.; Mitsui, J.; Yamasoba, T. Esophageal Dysmotility in Multiple System Atrophy: A Retrospective Cross-Sectional Study. *J. Clin. Med.* **2024**, *13*, 5026. https://doi.org/10.3390/jcm13175026.
12. Tarazis, K.; Garefis, K.; Chatziavramidis, A.; Konstantinidis, I. Recurrent Sialolithiasis following Intraoral Deep Hilar/Intraparenchymal Stone Removal from Wharton's Duct. *J. Clin. Med.* **2024**, *13*, 909. https://doi.org/10.3390/jcm13030909
13. Mughal, Z.; Martinez-Devesa, P.; Boukas, A.; Jeyaretna, S.; Qureishi, A. Contemporary Management of Cerebrospinal Fluid Rhinorrhoea: A Review of the Literature. *J. Clin. Med.* **2025**, *14*, 995. https://doi.org/10.3390/jcm14030995.
14. Wollny, M.; Heiser, C.; Sommer, U.; Schöbel, C.; Braun, M. Adverse Events with Hypoglossal Nerve Stimulation in the Treatment of Obstructive Sleep Apnea—A Systematic Review of Clinical Trials and Real-World Data. *J. Clin. Med.* **2024**, *13*, 4282. https://doi.org/10.3390/jcm13154282.
15. Romanowicz, A.; Komisarek, O.; Klimaszewska-Wiśniewska, A.; Antosik, P.; Naglik, K.; Czech, J.; Wrzesiński, W.; Kodzik, M.; Bodnar, M.; Grzanka, D.; et al. Evaluation of GDF15 Significance as a Biomarker in Laryngeal Squamous Cell Carcinoma. *J. Clin. Med.* **2025**, *14*, 4870. https://doi.org/10.3390/jcm14144870.

16. Fulla, M.; Quiros, B.; Clavero, O.; Gomà, M.; de Andrés-Pablo, Á.; Pavon, M.À.; Penella, A.; Alemany, L.; González-Compta, X.; Mena, M. Clinical, Histological, and HPV-Related Factors Associated to Diffuse Presentation of Exophytic Nasal Papillomas. *J. Clin. Med.* **2024**, *13*, 6638. https://doi.org/10.3390/jcm13226638.
17. Jangan, A.; Minhas, S.; Diakos, E.; Simmons, M.; Mughal, Z. Evolving Trends and Future Demands in ENT Procedures: A Nationwide 10-Year Analysis. *J. Clin. Med.* **2024**, *13*, 7850. https://doi.org/10.3390/jcm13247850.

References

1. Brimioulle, M.; Arih, I.; Pervaiz, A.; Patel, W.; Davies, A.; Sekyi-Djan, M.; Qureishi, A.; Chaidas, K. The Role of Telephone Clinics in ENT. *J. Laryngol. Otol.* **2023**, *137*, 914–920. [CrossRef] [PubMed]
2. Song, D.; Kim, T.; Lee, Y.; Kim, J. Image-Based Artificial Intelligence Technology for Diagnosing Middle Ear Diseases: A Systematic Review. *J. Clin. Med.* **2023**, *12*, 5831. [CrossRef] [PubMed]
3. Emre, E.; Cetintas, D.; Yildirim, M.; Emre, S. Vocal Fold Disorders Classification and Optimization of a Custom Video Laryngoscopy Dataset through Structural Similarity Index and a Deep Learning-Based Approach. *J. Clin. Med.* **2025**, *14*, 6899. [CrossRef] [PubMed]
4. Navarathna, N.; Kanhere, A.; Gomez, C.; Isaiah, A. Artificial Intelligence in Pediatric Otolaryngology: A State-of-the-Art Review of Opportunities and Pitfalls. *Int. J. Pediatr. Otorhinolaryngol.* **2025**, *194*, 112369. [CrossRef]
5. Chatzisouleiman, I.; Kolovou, V.; Tolley, N.; Mochloulis, G.; Katotomichelakis, M.; Chaidas, K. Radiofrequency and Microwave Ablation as Promising Minimally Invasive Treatment Options for Papillary Thyroid Microcarcinoma: A Systematic Review. *Ann. R. Coll. Surg. Engl.* 2025; *ahead of print*. [CrossRef]
6. Mouratidou, S.; Chaidas, K. Transoral Robotic Surgery for Patients with Obstructive Sleep Apnoea: A Systematic Literature Review of Current Practices. *Life* **2024**, *14*, 1700. [CrossRef]
7. Song, S.S.; Lee, Z.-H.; Yu, J.Z. Transoral Robotic Surgery (TORS) in Head and Neck Reconstruction. *J. Clin. Med.* **2025**, *14*, 5775. [CrossRef] [PubMed]

Journal of
Clinical Medicine

MDPI

Article

Recurrent Sialolithiasis following Intraoral Deep Hilar/Intraparenchymal Stone Removal from Wharton's Duct

Konstantinos Tarazis †, Konstantinos Garefis †, Angelos Chatziavramidis and Iordanis Konstantinidis *

2nd Academic ORL, Head and Neck Surgery Department Aristotle University of Thessaloniki, Papageorgiou Hospital, 56403 Thessaloniki, Greece; paulhawking29@gmail.com (K.T.); kgarefis@hotmail.com (K.G.); angchatziavram@hotmail.com (A.C.)

* Correspondence: jordan_orl@hotmail.com

† These authors contributed equally to this paper.

Abstract: (1) Background: Submandibular gland (SMG) sialolithiasis treatment has shifted significantly, favouring minimal invasiveness. Nonetheless, transoral stone removal remains viable for distal, deep hilar, and intraparenchymal stones. However, data are limited regarding recurrence and revision surgery; (2) Patients/Methods: This retrospective study included 226 patients with SMG stones treated using Wharton's duct slitting and marsupialisation over nine years; 138 had deep hilar or intraparenchymal stones, while 88 had distal stones. Of the former group, 18 experienced symptom recurrence post-surgery, 12 with stones and 6 with duct stenosis; (3) Results: Of the 126 patients without recurrent stones, 71% were male and 29% were female. Their mean age was 51.02 ± 9.36 years. The stones of the 126 patients without recurrence had a diameter of 8.3 mm ± SD: 4 mm, which was significantly smaller than those of the patients who experienced recurrence (13.8 mm ± SD: 2.4 mm; $p < 0.05$). The mean estimated stone growth recurrence rate was 8.4 ± SD: 1.8 mm per year. A secondary operation was performed 34 ± SD: 14.7 months after the first. Of the patients with recurrence, 91.7% were treated under general anaesthesia. The preferred treatment for 58.4% of patients was intraoral revision operation; the remainder underwent total gland resection. The mean follow-up period was 43 ± SD: 18 months; (4) Conclusions: The rate of revision surgery was relatively low. In recurrent SMG sialolithiasis, new stones may grow faster than the primary stones, which are already larger than those in patients without recurrence. The slitting and marsupialisation of Wharton's duct can treat recurrent cases.

Keywords: sialolithiasis; recurrence; stone; Wharton's duct; intraoral

1. Introduction

In recent decades, the management of submandibular gland (SMG) sialolithiasis has shifted notably, favouring minimally invasive procedures. The development of semirigid endoscopes has facilitated stone removal while preserving the gland. Compared to traditional open approaches, these methods present several advantages, including reduced morbidity and complication rates, along with significantly lower costs for the healthcare system [1]. However, the feasibility of endoscopic SMG stone removal may be limited by factors such as equipment availability, insufficient training, or a lack of reimbursement by the Greek National Health Service.

An alternative, commonly employed technique is the transoral approach. The transoral removal of SMG stones is indicated not only for distal stones but also for deep hilar and intraparenchymal stones. This procedure can be performed under local anaesthesia, primarily for distal stones; typically, it is performed under general anaesthesia for deep hilar stones [1]. The method involves incising Wharton's duct from the ostium to the stone's location, including the hilum, and marsupialising the submandibular duct [2].

In the current literature, SMG stone recurrence following the initial transoral removal has been reported to range from 0.5% to 19% [3–11]. The estimated growth rate for primary stones has been documented to be between 1 and 3 mm per year [12]. However, information on this growth rate in recurrence cases is lacking. Limited data are available; only three studies have exclusively addressed the recurrence rate after a primary duct-slitting and marsupialization procedure [2,3,6]. Finally, a specific protocol for managing recurrent SMG sialolithiasis after a primary intraoral procedure is also lacking.

The purpose of the current case series report is, firstly, to present our results concerning the management of recurrent SMG lithiasis treated primarily with an intraoral operation. Secondly, we sought to report the results of our long-term follow-up, focusing on the recurrent stone growth rate and the possibility of recurrence.

2. Materials and Methods

2.1. Patients

Our retrospective study was based on the medical records of 226 patients with SMG sialolithiasis who underwent slitting and marsupialisation of their Wharton's duct over nine years. Out of these 226 patients, 138 were diagnosed with deep hilar or intraparenchymal stones and underwent surgery, while 88 had distal stones. Eighteen of the 138 patients who underwent surgery experienced symptom recurrence after their initial procedures. Of these 18 patients, 12 had recurrent stones—recurrent stones group (RSG)—and 6 had duct stenosis (see Figure 1). The demographic data of the 126 patients with primary lithiasis with no recurrent stones (n-RSG), including their age, sex, and stone size, were recorded. For RSG, demographic data including age, sex, and disease history were recorded. Information regarding treatment type for the primary and recurrent diseases was collected. This information included the time elapsed between appearance of the first symptoms and the primary procedure, the time elapsed between the primary and secondary interventions, the stone size of the primary and recurrent diseases, the recurrent stone growth rate, postoperative complications, and the follow-up period (see Table 1). The size of the stone was determined in mm by its largest diameter, and measurements were taken after its removal.

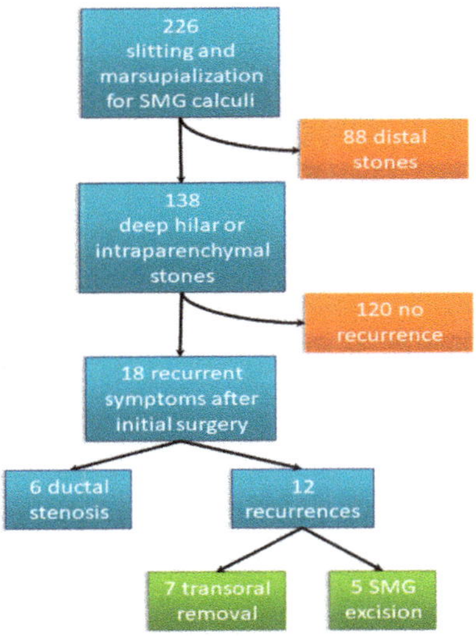

Figure 1. Patient flowchart.

Table 1. Characteristics of the 12 patients with recurrence.

	Percent (%)
Sex	71% male, 29% female
Side	42% right, 58% left
Recurrent stone location	66.7% hilo-parenchymal, 8.3% hilum 25% parenchymal
Secondary intervention	58.4% intraoral, 41.6% external
	Mean (±SD)
Age (years)	53.75 (±11.32)
Primary stone size (mm)	13.8 (±4)
Recurrent stone size (mm)	10.4 (±4.5)
Time of recurrency diagnosis (months)	30.3 (±15.4)
Time between two operations (months)	34 (±14.7)
Growth rate (mm per year)	8.4 (±1.8)
Follow-up (months)	43 (±18)

2.2. Interventions

2.2.1. Primary Surgical Procedure: Marsupialisation of Wharton's Duct

Currently, the Greek National Health Service does not reimburse sialendoscopy costs. Therefore, patients who were unable to cover this cost for their stone removal could choose a marsupialisation procedure (see Figure 2), as previously described, when necessary [2].

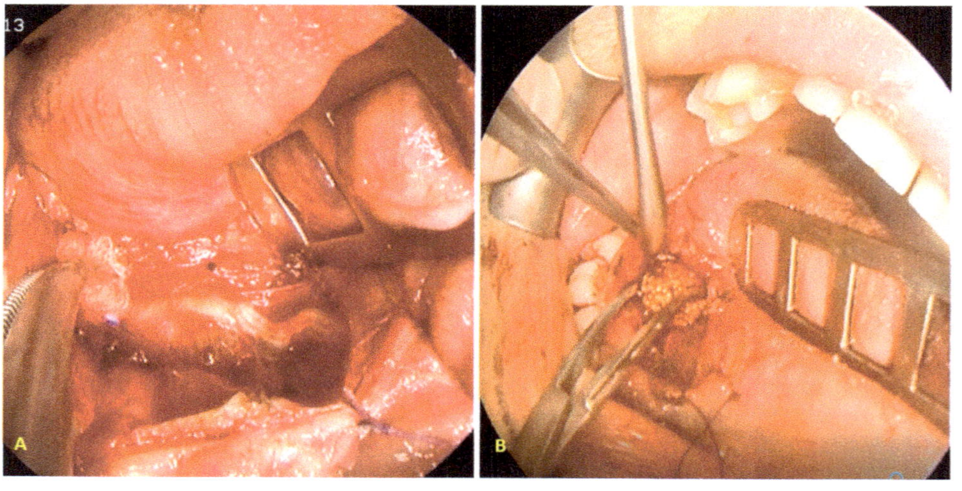

Figure 2. (**A**) The floor of the oral cavity was incised, and the lingual nerve was recognised and preserved. (**B**) The submandibular duct was slit, and the stone was removed using haemostatic forceps.

2.2.2. Revision Surgery

Patients who had experienced recurrent stones (see Figure 3) after their initial intraoral procedure were rescheduled for a secondary treatment. This treatment could involve either a secondary intraoral procedure or an open submandibulectomy.

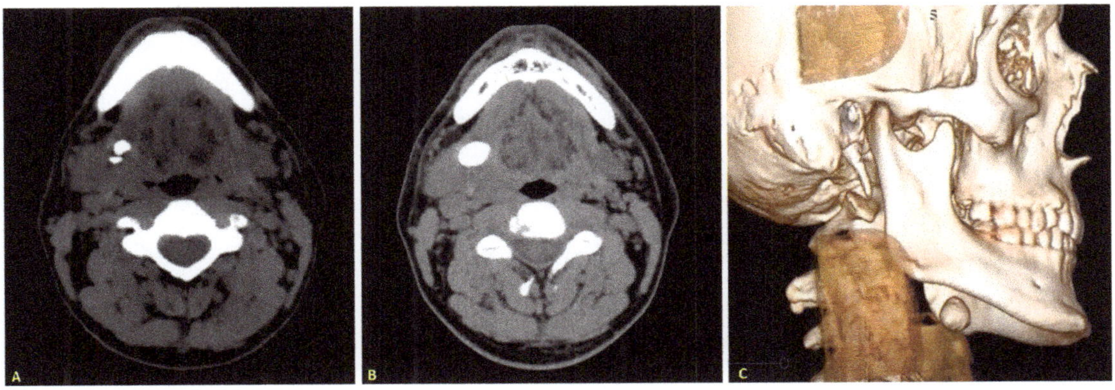

Figure 3. (**A**) CT scan shows the primary stone in the hilar region and a second, smaller stone located behind it. (**B**) CT showing the recurrent stone in the same patient after treatment using the slitting and marsupialisation approach. (**C**) Three-dimensional high-resolution computed tomography reconstruction showing the recurrent stone.

2.2.3. Secondary Intraoral Procedure

In the secondary intraoral procedure, the mucosa was carefully dissected directly at the hilar region of the affected SMG. The neo-ostium created during the previous procedure was used as a landmark. Following stone removal, the neo-ostium was enlarged as much as feasible, and the mucosa was secured with stitches to the floor of the mouth.

In all intraoral procedures, Wharton's duct was thoroughly washed with saline after removal of the stone.

2.3. *Follow-Up*

After the initial treatments, follow-up data were collected every six months, for at least two years postoperatively, primarily through physical examinations and histories of recurrent sialadenitis. Physical examinations included palpation of the gland and its duct, as well as an assessment of the gland's consistency, determining whether it was soft or hard. Evaluation of the quality of the saliva (clear, watery, viscus, purulent) was also performed. The history-taking process included questions about previous swelling or pain of the gland, observation of purulent saliva, or saliva with a sour/salty taste indicating sialadenitis, and the presence of spontaneous fragments of stones. For patients with suggestive histories of recurrent episodes, ultrasounds of the neck were performed. A computed tomography scan was performed in all cases of recurrent lithiasis and non-conclusive ultrasound examinations.

2.4. *Statistical Analyses*

Data analysis was performed using SPSS software (Version 28.0; IBM Corp., Armonk, NY, USA). Statistics were presented as the mean $\pm$ standard deviation or median with the range. T-tests and paired t-tests were employed to compare patient age and stone size, respectively, with a p-value < 0.05 considered as significant. To determine the mean growth rate of recurrent stones, we calculated the growth rate for each stone per year and then computed the mean of these rates.

3. Results

3.1. *Primary Results*

Of the 126 patients of n-RSG, 89 were male (71%), and 37 were female (29%). The mean patient age was 51.02 $\pm$ 9.36 years. Eighteen (13%) of these 138 patients experienced recurrent symptoms after their initial surgeries. Among them, 12 (8.6%) had recurrent stones (RSG) and 6 (4.4%) had duct stenosis. Of the patients of RSG, nine were male (75%), and three were female (25%). The mean patient age was 53.75 ± SD: 11.32 years.

No differences in age or gender were observed between the patients of RSG and the 126 patients of n-RSG ($p < 0.05$). A diagnosis of recurrent sialolithiasis was made 30.3 ± SD: 15.4 months after the primary operation, while the secondary operation was performed 4 months (range: 1–13 months) after the diagnosis and 34 ± SD: 14.7 months after the first operation, respectively. The new stones were located on the right SMG for five patients (42%) and on the left SMG for seven patients (58%), while the primary stones were found in 63 patients (46%) on the right side and 75 patients (54%) on the left side.

The mean recurrent stone diameter was 10.4 ± SD: 4.5 mm. In comparison, the mean primary stone diameter in the same patient group was 13.8 ± SD: 4 mm. However, the primary stone diameter for the remaining 126 patients with deep hilar or intraparenchymal SMG stones was 8.3 ± SD: 2.4 mm. A comparison between the primary stone size of the patients with recurrence and the recurrent stone size revealed a significant difference ($p < 0.05$): the primary stones were larger. More importantly, the primary stones of n-RSG were smaller in diameter than those of RSG ($p < 0.05$). For four patients (33%), the recurrent stone was larger than the primary stone upon diagnosis. Of the 12 patients with recurrence, 10 (83.3%) had primary stones larger than 10 mm in diameter. Of the same 12 patients, two had a secondary stone with a smaller diameter, lacking clinical significance, behind the primary stone, while the recurrent stone in one of them was larger in diameter than the primary stone. In the primary group of 138 patients, multiple stones (2–3) were identified in 21 patients in total. The mean estimated stone growth rate during recurrence was 8.4 ± SD: 1.8 mm per year. All patients who presented with recurrence—except for one such patient—were treated under general anaesthesia (11 of 12 or 91.7%). The preferred treatment method for seven patients (58.4%) was intraoral revision operation. The remaining patients (5 of 12 or 41.6%) were treated via total gland resection. The mean follow-up period was 43 ± SD: 18 months.

The data of the patients who were diagnosed with recurrence are presented in Table 1.

3.2. *Complications after Revision Treatment*

Only two complications occurred after the revision surgery. The first was stenosis of the neo-ostium in two patients (16.6%). This condition was treated with a dilation procedure under sialendoscopy. Secondly, one patient (8.3%) presented with temporary lingual nerve hypoesthesia that lasted for two weeks after the procedure. Appointments for re-evaluation after the revision surgery were scheduled, and during the follow-ups, no major complications occurred.

Of the seven patients who had undergone secondary transoral surgeries, only one (14.3%) had experienced a recurrence 42 months later. The third stone had a diameter of 3.5 mm. It was observed to be impacted at the stenosed neo-ostium, and it was removed under local anaesthesia. In cases where total gland resection was needed, we documented temporary paralysis of the marginal branch of the facial nerve in one patient (8.3%). Also, one patient (8.3%) experienced postoperative oedema in the submandibular region. It subsided after 48 h with the use of corticosteroids.

4. Discussion

The intraoral procedure to treat SMG sialolithiasis is well known and has been previously described [13–18]. It includes duct slitting and marsupialisation procedures [2–11,13–25]. However, the literature does not clarify whether a secondary intraoral procedure can be performed. To our knowledge, limited data are available on recurrent SMG sialolithiasis and its treatment.

The main findings of our study are as follows:

1. The rate of revision surgery in our patient cohort was 8.6%. This rate was relatively low, and it aligned with that reported in similar case series [2–11].

2. The mean primary stone size in patients without recurrence (8.3 mm in diameter) was significantly smaller than that in patients with recurrence (13.8 mm).
3. Secondary intraoral stone removal intervention could be an option even in revision cases (58.4%) as part of the gland preservation strategy.
4. The mean time (34 months) between the primary procedure and the secondary intervention as well as the stone growth rate (8.4 mm in diameter per year) during recurrence indicated a significant acceleration in stone formation. We have reported these findings for the first time in the literature.

First, in comparing the recurrence rate in our case series with that in the current literature, we found that approximately 8.6% of our patients had been diagnosed with a second stone during the follow-up period. In two previous studies, patients with SMG sialolithiasis were treated with the same intraoral slitting procedure, and recurrence rates between 1% and 4.6% were reported [2,3,6]. Throughout the remaining previous studies in which patients were treated with a similar transoral operation, recurrence rates of 0.5–19% were reported [3–11]. One review compared intraoral ductotomy with or without ductoplasty and slitting and marsupialisation techniques. Its authors concluded that the latter were associated with lower rates of distal duct stenosis postoperatively and were preferred in cases where multiple stones were present [24]. Furthermore, three studies suggested that a major contributing factor in stone recurrence is the presence of microcalculi and debris within the gland and/or the lumen of the duct after the initial approach [4,10,11]. First described in a case series by Cappacio et al. [4], the fragments of the stone and small stones left inside the duct were proposed as a probable cause of recurrence. Another study supported this notion, attributing the low recurrence rate to the postoperative use of endoscopy and dilation, which prevent symptomatic impacted stones [11]. Additionally, Galli et al. demonstrated that stone size and gland topography diameter (GTD) classification did not correlate with recurrence; instead, early recurrences were attributed to the remaining debris [10]. In both of these series, the duct was thoroughly washed after stone removal to prevent symptom reappearance, as it had been for our patients [10,26]. On the contrary, our results show that larger stones are associated with an increased recurrence rate. We hypothesise that the substantial size of recurrent stones gradually destroys the ductal system's architecture, creating a larger and less functional ductal system. This mechanism seemed more probable in our series, as we removed the stones intraorally without leaving fragments.

Second, in individuals without recurrence, the mean size of the initial stones was 8.3 mm in diameter—significantly less than in patients who experienced recurrence (13.8 mm). Conversely, the mean primary stone size in cases with recurrence was 13.8 mm, which was significantly larger than the recurrent stones (10.4 mm). However, in 33% of patients, the recurrent stone was larger than the primary stone. Moreover, 83.3% of the patients who experienced recurrence had primary stones measuring more than 10 mm in diameter. In a retrospective cohort study by Zhang et al., 118 patients with proximal submandibular stones over 10 mm in diameter were treated similarly to our study. During the follow-up period, 14.4% experienced recurrent symptoms, with 3.4% developing newly formed stones [5]. In our series, 13% of patients had recurrent symptoms, and 8.6% developed newly formed stones. Zhang et al. suggested that stone size does not contribute to chronic obstructive symptoms or inflammation [5]. Another study demonstrated that symptoms recurred more frequently in patients with stones located in the proximal and hilar portions of the duct, which was not related to the size of the primary stone, in contrast with our data [9]. A retrospective study involving 378 patients concluded that the average stone size and stone location in the duct did not correlate with more complications, though a specific stone recurrence rate was not specified [7].

Third, our results show that a secondary transoral procedure could be an option in recurrence cases. The percentage of gland excision was low, as this procedure was employed for 3.62% of all patients. Although no specific algorithm dictating the actions to be taken in recurrence cases after intraoral procedures is available, we agree with the authors of the most current literature regarding the use of a secondary transoral approach as the preferred method in recurrent lithiasis [1,9,27]. We also propose the use of the transoral procedure in recurrence cases, especially those with easily palpable stones, to cut precisely above the stone with recognition and protection of lingual nerve, if possible. However, the transoral procedure should be avoided in excessive fibrosis cases, developed from the primary surgery, to avoid injury of the nerve and duct's restenosis.

Finally, during our follow-up period, we observed the stones formed in patients experiencing recurrence had a remarkably accelerated growth rate of 8.4 mm in diameter per year, compared to the growth rate of 1–3 mm per year described in the literature for primary stones [12]. However, we could not directly compare the growth rate of recurrent stones with that of primary ones in our patients since we could only rely on their histories of primary symptoms, and stones may be symptomless. Recurrence was found to have occurred, on average, 30.3 months after the initial transoral removal, and a secondary operation was conducted about four months after the diagnosis and 34 months after the initial surgery.

Our study's main limitations include its small number of recurrent sialolithiasis cases, though the main patient group was sufficient in size. Additionally, our study was retrospective, so we could not determine the growth rates of patients' primary stones. Lastly, salivary stones have three-dimensional irregular sizes and their growth in different directions may vary; therefore, the growth rates may differ.

5. Conclusions

The intraoral procedure involving slitting and marsupialisation of Wharton's duct can be used to treat recurrent SMG sialolithiasis. Its low complication and recurrence rates confirm its efficacy and safety—even in revision cases—minimising the possibility of total gland excision. The hilar location may be associated with higher relapse rates. Finally, newly formed stones might exhibit higher growth rates than primary stones in patients with recurrent disease.

Author Contributions: Conceptualization, I.K. and K.T.; methodology, K.G.; software, A.C.; validation, I.K., K.G. and K.T.; formal analysis, K.G.; investigation, K.T.; resources, K.G.; data curation, K.T.; writing—original draft preparation, K.T.; writing—review and editing, I.K., A.C. and K.G.; visualization, I.K.; supervision, I.K.; project administration, I.K. All authors have read and agreed to the published version of the manuscript.

Funding: This research received no external funding.

Institutional Review Board Statement: The study was conducted in accordance with the Declaration of Helsinki and approved by the Institutional Review Board of Papageorgiou Hospital Thessaloniki Greece (protocol code 2023-B2015-259 and date of approval 31 March 2023).

Informed Consent Statement: Informed consent was obtained from all subjects involved in the study.

Data Availability Statement: The data presented in this study are available upon request from the corresponding author.

Conflicts of Interest: The authors declare no conflicts of interest.

References

1. Koch, M.; Mantsopoulos, K.; Muller, S.; Sievert, M.; Iro, H. Treatment of sialolithiasis: What has changed? An update of the treatment algorithms and a review of the literature. *J. Clin. Med.* **2022**, *11*, 231. [CrossRef]
2. Zenk, J.; Constantinidis, J.; Al-Kadah, B.; Iro, H. Transoral removal of submandibular stones. *Arch. Otolaryngol. Head Neck Surg.* **2001**, *127*, 432–436. [CrossRef]
3. Nahlieli, O.; Shacham, R.; Zagury, A.; Bar, T.; Yoffe, B. The ductal stretching technique: An endoscopic-assisted technique for removal of submandibular stones. *Laryngoscope* **2007**, *117*, 1031–1035. [CrossRef]
4. Capaccio, P.; Clemente, I.A.; McGurk, M.; Bossi, A.; Pignataro, L. Transoral removal of hiloparenchymal submandibular calculi: A long-term clinical experience. *Eur. Arch. Oto-Rhino-Laryngol.* **2011**, *268*, 1081–1086. [CrossRef]
5. Zhang, L.; Escudier, M.; Brown, J.; Capaccio, P.; Pignataro, L.; McGurk, M. Long-term outcome after intraoral removal of large submandibular gland calculi. *Laryngoscope* **2010**, *120*, 964–966. [CrossRef]

6. Schapher, M.; Mantsopoulos, K.; Messbacher, M.E.; Iro, H.; Koch, M. Transoral submandibulotomy for deep hilar submandibular gland sialolithiasis. *Laryngoscope* **2017**, *127*, 2038–2044. [CrossRef]
7. Holden, A.M.; Man, C.B.; Samani, M.; Hills, A.J.; McGurk, M. Audit of minimally-invasive surgery for submandibular sialolithiasis. *Br. J. Oral Maxillofac. Surg.* **2019**, *57*, 582–586. [CrossRef] [PubMed]
8. Roh, J.L.; Park, C.I. Transoral removal of submandibular hilar stone and sialodochoplasty. *Otolaryngol. Head Neck Surg.* **2008**, *139*, 235–239. [CrossRef] [PubMed]
9. Kim, J.K.; Shin, S.M.; Lee, H.; Lee, S. Factors affecting long-term outcome of transoral surgery for submandibular stones: A follow-up study of 125 patients. *Clin. Otolaryngol.* **2016**, *41*, 365–370. [CrossRef] [PubMed]
10. Galli, P.; Ceva, A.; Foletti, J.M.; Iline, N.; Giorgi, R.; Chossegros, C.; Graillon, N. Salivary Gland Lithiasis Recurrence After Minimally-Invasive Surgery: Incidence, Risk Factors and Prevention. *Laryngoscope* **2020**, *131*, 794–799. [CrossRef] [PubMed]
11. Zhao, Y.N.; Zhang, Y.Q.; Zhang, L.Q.; Xie, X.Y.; Liu, D.G.; Yu, G.Y. Treatment strategy of hilar and intraglandular stones in wharton's duct: A 12-year experience. *Laryngoscope* **2020**, *130*, 2360–2365. [CrossRef]
12. Truijllo, O.; Drusin, M.A.; Rahmati, R. Rapid recurrent sialolithiasis: Altered stone composition and potential factors for recurrence. *Laryngoscope* **2016**, *127*, 1365–1368. [CrossRef]
13. Rontal, M.; Rontal, E. The use of sialodochoplasty in the treatment of benign inflammatory obstructive submandibular gland disease. *Laryngoscope* **1987**, *97*, 1417–1421. [CrossRef]
14. Sobol, S.; Spector, G.J. Sialodochotomy and sialolithectomy for acute calculous submaxillary sialadenitis. *Laryngoscope* **1979**, *89*, 1864–1866. [CrossRef]
15. van den Akker, H.P.; Busemann-Sokole, E. Submandibular gland function following transoral sialolithectomy. *Oral Surg. Oral Med. Oral Pathol.* **1983**, *56*, 351–356. [CrossRef]
16. Seward, G.R. Anatomic surgery for salivary calculi, part II: Calculi in the anterior part of the submandibular duct. *Oral Surg. Oral Med. Oral Pathol.* **1968**, *25*, 287–293. [CrossRef]
17. Seward, G.R. Anatomic surgery for salivary calculi, part III: Calculi in the posterior part of the submandibular duct. *Oral Surg. Oral Med. Oral Pathol.* **1968**, *25*, 525–531. [CrossRef]
18. Seward, G.R. Anatomic surgery for salivary calculi, part IV: Calculi in the intraglandular part of the submandibular duct. *Oral Surg. Oral Med. Oral Pathol.* **1968**, *25*, 670–678. [CrossRef] [PubMed]
19. McGurk, M.; Makdissi, J.; Brown, J.E. Intra-oral removal of stones from the hilum of the submandibular gland: Report of technique and morbidity. *Int. J. Oral Maxillofac. Surg.* **2004**, *33*, 683–686. [CrossRef] [PubMed]
20. Mulcahy, C.F.; Fassas, S.; Lloyd, A.; Strum, D.; Badger, C.; Joshi, A. Modified Marionette Technique for Unassisted In-Office Access to the Submandibular Duct. *Laryngoscope* **2021**, *131*, 1016–1018. [CrossRef] [PubMed]
21. Combes, J.; Karavidas, K.; McGurk, M. Intraoral removal of proximal submandibular stones—An alternative to sialadenectomy? *Int. J. Oral Maxillofac. Surg.* **2009**, *38*, 813–816. [CrossRef]
22. Matsunobu, T.; Kurioka, T.; Miyagawa, Y.; Araki, K.; Tamura, A.; Niwa, K.; Tomifuji, M.; Yamashita, T.; Shiotani, A. Minimally invasive surgery of sialolithiasis using sialendoscopy. *Auris Nasus Larynx* **2014**, *41*, 528–531. [CrossRef] [PubMed]
23. Schwartz, N.; Hazkani, I.; Goshen, S. Combined approach sialendoscopy for management of submandibular gland sialolithiasis. *Am. J. Otolaryngol.* **2015**, *36*, 632–635. [CrossRef] [PubMed]
24. Saga-Gutierrez, C.; Chiesa-Estomba, C.M.; Larruscain, E.; González-García, J.Á.; Sistiaga, J.A.; Altuna, X. Transoral sialolitectomy combined with sialoendoscopy versus open submaxilectomy for the management of hilar lithiasis of the submandibular gland. *Acta Otorrinolaringol. Esp.* **2019**, *70*, 342–347. [CrossRef] [PubMed]
25. Saga-Gutierrez, C.; Chiesa-Estomba, C.M.; Larruscain, E.; González-García, J.Á.; Sistiaga, J.A.; Altuna, X. Transoral Sialolitectomy as an Alternative to Submaxilectomy in the Treatment of Submaxillary Sialolithiasis. *Ear Nose Throat J.* **2019**, *98*, 287–290. [CrossRef] [PubMed]
26. Foletti, J.M.; Graillon, N.; Avignon, S.; Guyot, L.; Chossegros, C. Salivary Calculi Removal by Minimally Invasive Techniques: A Decision Tree Based on the Diameter of the Calculi and Their Position in the Excretory Duct. *J. Oral Maxillofac. Surg.* **2018**, *76*, 112–118. [CrossRef]
27. Iro, H.; Zenk, J.; Escudier, M.P.; Nahlieli, O.; Capaccio, P.; Katz, P.; Brown, J.; McGurk, M. Outcome of minimally invasive management of salivary calculi in 4,691 patients. *Laryngoscope* **2009**, *119*, 263–268. [CrossRef]

Journal of
Clinical Medicine

MDPI

Article

The COVID-19 Tracheostomy Experience at a Large Academic Medical Center in New York during the First Year

Dhruv Patel [1,2,3], Anthony Devivo [1,4], Evan Leibner [1,4,*], Atinuke Shittu [1], Usha Govindarajulu [5], Pranai Tandon [6], David Lee [2], Randall Owen [2], Gustavo Fernandez-Ranvier [2], Robert Hiensch [6], Michael Marin [2], Roopa Kohli-Seth [1,2] and Adel Bassily-Marcus [1,2]

1 Institute for Critical Care Medicine, Icahn School of Medicine at Mount Sinai, New York, NY 10029, USA; dhruv.patel@mountsinai.org (D.P.); anthony.devivo@mountsinai.org (A.D.); adel.bassily-marcus@mountsinai.org (A.B.-M.)
2 Department of Surgery, Icahn School of Medicine at Mount Sinai, New York, NY 10029, USA
3 Department of Medicine, Icahn School of Medicine at Mount Sinai, New York, NY 10029, USA
4 Department of Emergency Medicine, Icahn School of Medicine at Mount Sinai, New York, NY 10029, USA
5 Center for Biostatistics, Department of Population Health Science and Policy, Icahn School of Medicine at Mount Sinai, New York, NY 10029, USA
6 Department of Medicine, Division of Pulmonary, Critical Care, and Sleep Medicine, Icahn School of Medicine at Mount Sinai, New York, NY 10029, USA
* Correspondence: evan.leibner@mountsinai.org; Tel.: +1-212-241-8867; Fax: +1-212-860-3669

Abstract: Background: New York City was the epicenter of the initial surge of the COVID-19 pandemic in the United States. Tracheostomy is a critical procedure in the care of patients with COVID-19. We hypothesized that early tracheostomy would decrease the length of time on sedation, time on mechanical ventilation, intensive care unit length of stay, and mortality. **Methods:** A retrospective analysis of outcomes for all patients with COVID-19 who underwent tracheostomy during the first year of the COVID-19 pandemic at the Mount Sinai Hospital in New York City, New York. All adult intensive care units at the Mount Sinai Hospital, New York. Patients/subjects: 888 patients admitted to intensive care with COVID-19. Results: All patients admitted to the intensive care unit with COVID-19 (888) from 1 March 2020 to 1 March 2021 were analyzed and separated further into those intubated (544) and those requiring tracheostomy (177). Of those receiving tracheostomy, outcomes were analyzed for early (≤12 days) or late (>12 days) tracheostomy. Demographics, medical history, laboratory values, type of oxygen and ventilatory support, and clinical outcomes were recorded and analyzed. **Conclusions:** Early tracheostomy resulted in reduced duration of mechanical ventilation, reduced hospital length of stay, and reduced intensive care unit length of stay in patients admitted to the intensive care unit with COVID-19. There was no effect on overall mortality.

Keywords: COVID-19; tracheostomy; ICU length of stay; ARDS

1. Introduction

The initiation and use of a tracheostomy in the intensive care unit (ICU) has become an increasingly common procedure in patients who require prolonged critical care, have difficulty weaning from the ventilator, and/or have failed trials of extubation. Over one-third of patients who require greater than two days of mechanical ventilation in the ICU require tracheostomy [1]. Over the past several decades, extensive literature has been published evaluating the potential advantages of tracheostomy over prolonged endotracheal intubation, as well as the timing for when this procedure should be performed. Tracheostomy has repeatedly been shown to significantly decrease ventilator-associated pneumonia and the duration of time requiring mechanical ventilation, shorten duration of continuous sedation, and decrease the length of stay in the ICU when performed within the first seven to ten days of endotracheal intubation [2–5]. While it is a continued point of contention within the field of critical care, there is some evidence supporting an overall improvement in long-term mortality in patients who undergo early tracheostomy [5,6].

In light of the worldwide increase in patients developing acute respiratory distress syndrome (ARDS) after contracting the SARS-CoV-2 virus leading to the development of COVID-19 pneumonia, the critical care community has seen a subsequent increase in patients requiring prolonged mechanical ventilation, high-dose sedation, and lengthened ICU stays, often inevitably requiring tracheostomy. Previous data suggest that up to 15% of hospitalized patients with COVID-19 pneumonia require intubation and mechanical ventilatory support [7]. Furthermore, data from a large institution in the southern United States from 2020 found that over 80% of patients who met the criteria for ICU admission required mechanical ventilatory support [8]. While the majority of patients admitted to ICUs in the setting of COVID-19 pneumonia, particularly during the initial outbreak of the SARS-CoV-2 pandemic, required mechanical ventilation, upwards of 60% needed long-term mechanical ventilatory support necessitating tracheostomy [9]. The vast number of patients requiring tracheostomy and long-term mechanical ventilatory support has raised numerous questions regarding procedure safety, appropriate timing, and long-term outcome benefits in COVID-19.

While there is substantial evidence supporting the advantages and benefits of early tracheostomy in the setting of acute hypoxic respiratory failure, COVID-19 presented a plethora of unique circumstances that caused initial delays in the performance of tracheostomies. Early on in the COVID-19 pandemic, delays in tracheostomy occurred in the setting of safety concerns for the team performing the procedure, which is considered aerosol-generating [10]. Given these concerns, initial guidelines suggested delaying tracheostomy until at least day ten and then only if the patient was showing signs of clinical improvement [11]. These concerns have since been mitigated with evidence reassuring that tracheostomy can be performed safely and with low rates of COVID-19 transmission when appropriate enhanced personal protective equipment (PPE) is utilized [7,12–14]. A retrospective study from the United Kingdom assessed viral transmission in their tracheostomy team after the performance of one hundred tracheostomies over the course of six weeks and found no healthcare provider transmission attributable to the procedure [9]. A meta-analysis of current literature assessing outcomes of tracheostomies in the setting of COVID-19 pneumonia found that 94.8% of studies reported no SARS-CoV-2 transmission amongst healthcare provider teams who performed the tracheostomies [7].

Aside from safety concerns related to potential viral transmission, the performance of early tracheostomies for patients with COVID-19 pneumonia has been hindered by the prolonged critical acuity, high ventilator requirements, and profoundly high mortality initially found to be associated with COVID-19 patients requiring mechanical ventilatory support [15,16]. Prior to the COVID-19 pandemic, high ventilator demand was often defined as a Positive End Expiratory Pressure of greater than or equal to 10–12 cm H20 or an FIO2 > 50–70% [17,18]. As subsequent data have become available throughout the pandemic, it has been found that tracheostomies can be performed safely on patients who are critically ill, with reasonably high ventilator requirements, and without increased complications related to oxygenation [19]. In addition, despite initial mortality reports of patients with ARDS in the setting of COVID-19 pneumonia being nearly 80%, current data suggest that improved treatment modalities, resources, and overall management have decreased ICU mortality despite mechanical ventilator requirements to between 26.5 and 44% [8,9,20].

While the international academic community has accrued a substantial amount of data on the benefits of early tracheostomy in regard to ICU length of stay, as well as ventilator-free days, questions remain regarding the optimal time to perform an early tracheostomy in order to obtain the best possible outcomes. This is particularly important when taking into consideration the immense quantities of sedation and long-term paralysis many COVID-19 patients have been noted to require in order to maintain adequate gas exchange in the setting of ventilator dyssynchrony [21,22]. Prior to the COVID-19 pandemic, evidence with regard to the timing of tracheostomy in patients who require prolonged mechanical ventilation suggested a significant decrease in continuous intravenous sedation when performed early [23–25]. Given the profoundly high dosages of continuous intravenous sedatives that have been noted to be required to achieve adequate sedation and ventilator synchrony in the setting ARDS from COVID-19 pneumonia, ascertaining adequate data to answer the question of whether not early tracheostomy can assist in decreasing sedative requirements particularly prudent [22,26]. In the retrospective data we have collected and analyzed below, we present some evidence to support the notion that early tracheostomy, when compared to delayed, can facilitate decreasing days of continuous intravenous sedation, as well as ICU length of stay.

2. Methods

We searched our medical records for all patients admitted with a positive SARS-CoV-2 PCR test between 1 March 2020 and 1 March 2021. For all relevant baseline covariates, we computed means, standard deviation, and range (min and max) for all continuous ones and frequency and percent for categorical ones. In addition, we compared each covariate between groups, which were defined by dichotomizing tracheostomy at day 12, by either using a two-sided two-sample *t*-test for a continuous covariate or a Pearson chi-square test of association for a categorical covariate. We then compared each of the following outcomes between groups: continuous sedation, hospital LOS or ICU LOS, days on ventilator from initial intubation to date weaned, and days of continuous paralytics. We also created a histogram of tracheostomies by day. Finally, we created a Kaplan–Meier survival probability plot for the time to death with right censoring. All analyses were conducted at the 0.05 level of significance and were analyzed in SAS Version 9.4 and also R version 4.0.3. The study was reviewed by the Mount Sinai Hospital IRB # 20-00584.

3. Results

During the first year of the COVID-19 pandemic in New York City, between 1 March 2020 and 1 March 2021, the Mount Sinai Hospital admitted 3672 patients with COVID-19 pneumonia, of which 888 (24.8%) patients required an ICU stay, among which 544 (14.81%) required mechanical ventilation. Among the 544 patients who required mechanical ventilation, 177 (32.53%) underwent tracheostomy. The demographics of these patients are shown in Table 1. Among the patients who were on mechanical ventilation, a total of 177 (32.53%) underwent tracheostomy. Most of them were bedside percutaneous tracheostomy and were performed by Intensivists, General Surgery, Cardiothoracic Surgery, and Otolaryngology. Table 2 shows the demographics of the patients in each group along with the degree of elevation in inflammatory markers as well the extent of impact the disease process had on gas exchange, including the highest PCO2 as well as lowest PaO2 and PaO2:FiO2 ratios. Of the total tracheostomies performed in the setting of severe COVID-19 pneumonia during this timeframe, 74 (41.81%) were carried out on or before day 12 of mechanical ventilation, while 103 (58.19%) were carried out after day 12; further details can be seen in Table 3.

Table 1. Demographics of patients admitted with COVID-19 to MSH.

Demographics of Patients Admitted with COVID-19 to MSH, Requiring ICU Stay, and Mechanical Ventilation			
Patients Admitted from 1 March 2020 to 1 March 2021			
Characteristic	**All Patients**	**ICU Patients**	**Intubated Patients**
	N = 3672 [1]	**N = 888** [1]	**N = 544** [1]
Age	61(18)	62(16)	63(14)
Gender			
F	1649 (45%)	333 (38%)	200 (37%)
M	2022 (55%)	555 (62%)	344 (63%)
U	1 (<0.1%)	0 (0%)	0 (0%)
BMI	29(8)	30(8)	31(8)

Table 1. *Cont.*

Demographics of Patients Admitted with COVID-19 to MSH, Requiring ICU Stay, and Mechanical Ventilation			
Patients Admitted from 1 March 2020 to 1 March 2021			
Characteristic	**All Patients** N = 3672 [1]	**ICU Patients** N = 888 [1]	**Intubated Patients** N = 544 [1]
Race			
White	1114 (30%)	239 (27%)	139 (26%)
Black	737 (20%)	156 (18%)	84 (15%)
Hispanic	849 (23%)	211 (24%)	140 (26%)
Asian	174 (4.7%)	47 (5.3%)	31 (5.7%)
Native American or Pacific Islander	21 (0.6%)	3 (0.3%)	3 (0.6%)
Other	777 (21%)	232 (26%)	147 (27%)
History of Diabetes	1434 (39%)	417 (47%)	274 (50%)
History of Hypertension	2228 (61%)	585 (66%)	365 (67%)
History of Chronic Lung Disease	678 (19%)	187 (21%)	106 (19%)
History of Chronic Liver Disease	320 (8.7%)	116 (13%)	77 (14%)
History of Renal Failure	746 (20%)	224 (25%)	137 (25%)
History of Heart Failure	602 (16%)	196 (22%)	122 (22%)
HIV/AIDS	77 (2.1%)	19 (2.1%)	14 (2.6%)
History of Alcohol or Substance Use Disorder	156 (4.3%)	49 (5.5%)	29 (5.3%)
BMI ≥ 30.0	1257 (39%)	367 (44%)	229 (44%)
Hospital Length of Stay in Days	7 (4, 14)	16 (9, 28)	20 (12, 34)
Died	618 (17%)	370 (42%)	313 (58%)
Discharged out of Hospital	3053 (83%)	518 (58%)	231 (42%)
Routine Discharge to Home	2496 (68%)	330 (37%)	97 (18%)
Not Routine Discharge to Home	557 (15%)	188 (21%)	134 (25%)

[1] Mean (SD); n (%); median (IQR).

Table 2. Demographics of patients who underwent tracheostomy during the study period.

Demographics of Patients Who Underwent Tracheostomy during the Study Period			
Characteristic	**Trach after Day 12, N = 103** [1]	**Trach on or before Day 12, N = 74** [1]	***p*-Value** [2]
Age	61 (14)	63 (15)	0.12
Gender			0.5
Female	36 (35%)	22 (30%)	
Male	67 (65%)	52 (70%)	
Race			0.12
African American	14 (14%)	10 (14%)	
Asian Indian	4 (3.9%)	1 (1.4%)	
Bangladeshi	1 (1.0%)	1 (1.4%)	
Filipino	3 (2.9%)	0 (0%)	
Haitian	2 (1.9%)	0 (0%)	
Pakistani	1 (1.0%)	1 (1.4%)	
Trinidadian	0 (0%)	2 (2.7%)	
White	23 (22%)	24 (32%)	
Geography			0.6
Bolivian	1 (1.0%)	0 (0%)	
Dominican	4 (3.9%)	2 (2.7%)	
Ecuadorian	8 (7.8%)	2 (2.7%)	
Latin American	7 (6.8%)	4 (5.4%)	
Latina American	1 (1.0%)	1 (1.4%)	
Mexican	7 (6.8%)	2 (2.7%)	
Peruvian	0 (0%)	1 (1.4%)	
Puerto Rican	3 (2.9%)	4 (5.4%)	
South American Indian	1 (1.0%)	0 (0%)	
Spaniard	0 (0%)	1 (1.4%)	
Unknown/Other	74 (72%)	53 (72%)	
max_PaCO2	74 (20)	64 (17)	<0.001
max_D_DIMER	15.2 (15.4)	11.3 (8.0)	0.040
max_CREATININE	4.2 (4.0)	3.9 (3.2)	0.8
max_CRP	297 (108)	269 (107)	0.039
max_FERRITIN	3826 (4666)	3452 (3639)	0.8
min_PaO2	55 (17)	57 (11)	0.3
min_PFRatio_Streaming	79 (52)	82 (36)	0.2

[1] Mean (SD); n (%). [2] Wilcoxon rank sum test; Pearson's Chi-squared test; Fisher's exact test.

Table 3. Outcomes for early vs. late tracheostomy.

	Early Tracheostomy (≤12 Days) n = 74	Late Tracheostomy (>12 Days) n = 103
Sedation pre-tracheostomy	9.64	8.13
Sedation post-tracheostomy	10.21	15.64
Total days on sedation	19.86	23.85
ICU LOS	23.66	67.91
Hospital LOS	33.2	88.8
	n = 48	n = 75
Days on paralytics	5.79	9.66
	n = 25	n = 43
Days on mechanical ventilator, intubation to date weaned	22.96	34.72
	n = 21	n = 36
Days on mechanical ventilator, adjusted for mortality	23.04	34.44

We noted that patients who had tracheostomy performed on or before 12 days of mechanical ventilation spent significantly less time on sedation (10.21 vs. 15.64, 95% CI of difference: −6.85, −4.00) before tracheostomy. Post-tracheostomy patients with early tracheostomy spent 9.64 days on sedation compared to 8.13 days for patients who underwent tracheostomy after 12 days (95% CI of difference: −1.70, 4.72). However, when looking at total days requiring continuous sedation while on mechanical ventilator, the early tracheostomy group spent significantly fewer days (19.89 days, 95% CI: 16.72, 23.00) compared to the later tracheostomy group (23.81 days, 95% CI: 21.71, 25.92). Similarly, the early tracheostomy group required paralytics for a mean of 5.79 days as compared to the late tracheostomy group, which required paralytics for 9.66 days (95% CI: −6.11, −1.64). This difference was also reflected in the Intensive care unit length of stay (LOS) which was 23.66 days (95% CI: 14.31, 33.01) in the early tracheostomy group compared to 67.91 days (95% CI: 0, 139.8) in the late tracheostomy group; and also in the hospital length of stay (LOS) which was 33.2 days (95% CI: 19.25, 47.16) in the early tracheostomy group, compared to 88.8 days (95% CI: 18.48, 159.1) in the late tracheostomy group. A total of 25 patients in the early tracheostomy group and 43 patients in the late ventilator group were off the mechanical ventilator at the end of the follow-up period. The early tracheostomy group spent an average of 22.9 days (95% CI: 18.65, 27.27) on the mechanical ventilator, which was significantly shorter than the late tracheostomy group, which was 34.72 days (95% CI: 30.43, 39.00). There were four deaths in the early tracheostomy group and seven in the late tracheostomy group. After adjusting for people who died, patients in the early group spent 23.04 days (95% CI: 17.95, 28.14) vs. 34.44 days (95% CI: 29.84, 39.04) in the late tracheostomy group from intubation to being weaned off mechanical ventilation, as can be seen in Table 3. Additionally, the dispositions of the patients based on early vs. late tracheostomy can be seen in Table 4.

Table 4. Discharge disposition.

Group	Disposition							
	Acute Rehabn (%)	Deceased n (%)	Home n (%)	LTACH n (%)	SAR n (%)	SNF n (%)	Transfer to Another Hospital n (%)	Total
Early Trach	11 (6.21%)	38 (21.47%)	9 (5.08%)	12 (6.78%)	2 (1.13%)	1 (0.56%)	1 (0.56%)	74 (41.81%)
Late Trach	18 (10.17%)	40 (22.60%)	7 (3.95%)	24 (13.56%)	7 (3.95%)	3 (1.69%)	4 (2.26%)	103 (58.19%)
Total	29 (16.38%)	78 (44.07%)	16 (9.04%)	36 (20.34%)	9 (5.08%)	4 (2.26%)	5 (2.82%)	177 (100.00%)

4. Discussion

There remains a lack of evidence to guide whether patients with ARDS in the setting of COVID-19 pneumonia would incur the same benefits that have previously been found to be associated with early tracheostomy in patients requiring prolonged mechanical ventilation. As the pandemic has progressed and knowledge of the COVID-19 pneumonia disease process has continued to advance, the safety and advantages of early tracheostomy have become more evident. The largest pooled data study to date, a systematic review and meta-analysis of 69 non-randomized studies including 4669 patients, assessed the benefits and timing of tracheostomy. This study showed a significant overall decrease in mortality in those patients who underwent tracheostomy in comparison to those who continued to be managed on mechanical ventilation via endotracheal tube. In addition, early tracheostomy and late tracheostomy (defined as before or after day fourteen of endotracheal intubation) were assessed.

It was determined that patients who underwent early tracheostomy had a shorter ICU length of stay but no significant difference in timing of weaning from mechanical ventilatory support or tracheostomy decannulation [7]. With regard to additional endpoints after tracheostomy, a systematic review and meta-analysis by Benito et al. assessed the success of and time to tracheostomy decannulation in a pooled group of 3234 patients from eighteen studies and found that, while the overall post-tracheostomy mortality was 13.1%, nearly 35% of patients were successfully decannulated, with a mean decannulation time of 18.6 days [27].

More recent literature has shown that patients with COVID-19 once intubated have high rates of extubation failure with low use of prophylactic noninvasive ventilation (NIV). [28] Additional studies have shown that extubation to NIV can decrease the rates of reintubation but without increasing length of stay or mortality. [29]

Our study looked at tracheostomies' outcomes for all COVID-19 patients at Mount Sinai Hospital based on the timing of the tracheostomy over a period of 1 year. This included the initial pandemic wave and then the second wave of SARS-CoV-2 in a major New York City hospital. During this time, our understanding of the disease evolved, as did the management. Our institution decided to follow our standard of care, with a goal of tracheostomy prior to day 12 for all our patients with prolonged mechanical ventilation [30]. This was carried out to both continue with the current practice at our institution as well as out of necessity. With the initial surge of patients, even while greatly expanding our ICU capacity, we would have very quickly run out of ICU beds without the ability to decompress the ICU [31]. The actual time to tracheotomy was influenced by several factors, including but not limited to high fio2 requirement on the vent and inability to tolerate the procedure, religious beliefs, and patient/family choice, etc. While we did our best to account for cofactors, it was not possible to account for the rapidly changing and evolving therapies and their influence on the overall outcome, as this is a retrospective analysis.

5. Conclusions

COVID-19 has been a worldwide pandemic, resulting in the loss of millions of people across the world. In March 2020, New York City became ground zero across the world in COVID-19 cases and deaths. At hospitals across New York City, the number of patients with severe ARDS and respiratory failure quickly overwhelmed the health system. At Mount Sinai Hospital, we surged from 104 ICU beds to 235 ICU beds [31]. With this being a new and unknown respiratory illness, there was a concern for the risk of performing tracheostomies prior to day 21 for the risk of infection to the physician team [30,32–34]. It was in this context that we, as an institute, decided to continue performing early tracheostomies when possible. We found that early tracheostomy, even in the patients with SARS-CoV-2 severe pneumonia, was safe, with no cases of known transmission to the operator. We also observed a reduction in the use of sedation, paralytics, and ICU days for these patients. As more effective therapies have been developed and a large amount of the population has been vaccinated, early tracheostomy has become a standard.

Author Contributions: Conceptualization, E.L., A.B.-M. and A.D.; methodology, P.T. and U.G.; formal analysis, P.T. and U.G.; investigation, E.L., D.L., A.B.-M., D.P., R.H. and A.D.; data curation, A.D. and P.T.; writing—original draft preparation, A.D., D.P. and P.T.; writing—review and editing, E.L., A.B.-M., R.O. and G.F.-R.; supervision, M.M. and R.K.-S.; project administration, A.S.; funding acquisition, E.L. and R.K.-S. All authors have read and agreed to the published version of the manuscript.

Funding: This research received no external funding.

Institutional Review Board Statement: The study was conducted in accordance with the Declaration of Helsinki, and approved by the Institutional Review Board of Mount Sinai Hospital protocol code 20-00584 and 4/30/2020).

Informed Consent Statement: Patient consent was waived due to being a retrospective database review.

Data Availability Statement: Dataset available on request from the authors.

Conflicts of Interest: The authors declare no conflicts of interest.

References

1. Quality of Life After Mechanized Ventilation in the Elderly Study Investigators. 2-month mortality and functional status of critically ill adult patients receiving prolonged mechanical ventilation. *Chest* **2002**, *121*, 549–558. [CrossRef] [PubMed]
2. Chorath, K.; Hoang, A.; Rajasekaran, K.; Moreira, A. Association of Early vs Late Tracheostomy Placement with Pneumonia and Ventilator Days in Critically Ill Patients: A Meta-analysis. *JAMA Otolaryngol. Head Neck Surg.* **2021**, *147*, 450–459. [CrossRef] [PubMed]
3. Zheng, Y.; Sui, F.; Chen, X.K.; Zhang, G.C.; Wang, X.W.; Zhao, S.; Song, Y.; Liu, W.; Xin, X.; Li, W.X. Early versus late percutaneous dilational tracheostomy in critically ill patients anticipated requiring prolonged mechanical ventilation. *Chin. Med. J.* **2012**, *125*, 1925–1930. [PubMed]
4. Herritt, B.; Chaudhuri, D.; Thavorn, K.; Kubelik, D.; Kyeremanteng, K. Early vs. late tracheostomy in intensive care settings: Impact on ICU and hospital costs. *J. Crit. Care* **2018**, *44*, 285–288. [CrossRef] [PubMed]
5. Hosokawa, K.; Nishimura, M.; Egi, M.; Vincent, J.L. Timing of tracheotomy in ICU patients: A systematic review of randomized controlled trials. *Crit. Care* **2015**, *19*, 424. [CrossRef] [PubMed]
6. Andriolo, B.N.; Andriolo, R.B.; Saconato, H.; Atallah, A.N.; Valente, O. Early versus late tracheostomy for critically ill patients. *Cochrane Database Syst. Rev.* **2015**, *1*, CD007271. [CrossRef] [PubMed]
7. Staibano, P.; Levin, M.; McHugh, T.; Gupta, M.; Sommer, D.D. Association of Tracheostomy with Outcomes in Patients with COVID-19 and SARS-CoV-2 Transmission Among Health Care Professionals: A Systematic Review and Meta-analysis. *JAMA Otolaryngol. Head Neck Surg.* **2021**, *147*, 646–655. [CrossRef] [PubMed]
8. Oliveira, E.; Parikh, A.; Lopez-Ruiz, A.; Carrilo, M.; Goldberg, J.; Cearras, M.; Fernainy, K.; Andersen, S.; Mercado, L.; Guan, J.; et al. ICU outcomes and survival in patients with severe COVID-19 in the largest health care system in central Florida. *PLoS ONE* **2021**, *16*, e0249038. [CrossRef]
9. Queen Elizabeth Hospital Birmingham C-at. Safety and 30-day outcomes of tracheostomy for COVID-19: A prospective observational cohort study. *Br. J. Anaesth.* **2020**, *125*, 872–879. [CrossRef]
10. Ferri, E.; Boscolo Nata, F.; Pedruzzi, B.; Campolieti, G.; Scotto di Clemente, F.; Baratto, F.; Cristalli, G. Indications and timing for tracheostomy in patients with SARS CoV2-related. *Eur. Arch. Otorhinolaryngol.* **2020**, *277*, 2403–2404. [CrossRef]
11. McGrath, B.A.; Brenner, M.J.; Warrillow, S.J. Tracheostomy for COVID-19: Business as usual? *Br. J. Anaesth.* **2020**, *125*, 867–871. [CrossRef] [PubMed]
12. Smith, D.; Montagne, J.; Raices, M.; Dietrich, A.; Bisso, I.C.; Las Heras, M.; San Roman, J.E.; Garcia Fornari, G.; Figari, M. Tracheostomy in the intensive care unit: Guidelines during COVID-19 worldwide pandemic. *Am. J. Otolaryngol.* **2020**, *41*, 102578. [CrossRef] [PubMed]
13. Takhar, A.; Walker, A.; Tricklebank, S.; Wyncoll, D.; Hart, N.; Jacob, T.; Arora, A.; Skilbeck, C.; Simo, R.; Surda, P. Recommendation of a practical guideline for safe tracheostomy during the COVID-19 pandemic. *Eur. Arch. Otorhinolaryngol.* **2020**, *277*, 2173–2184. [CrossRef] [PubMed]
14. Bassily-Marcus, A.; Leibner, E.S.; Kohli-Seth, R. Tracheostomy for Coronavirus Disease 2019 Patients: Maintaining the Standard of Care. *Crit. Care Explor.* **2020**, *2*, e0190. [CrossRef]
15. Wu, C.; Chen, X.; Cai, Y.; Xia, J.; Zhou, X.; Xu, S.; Huang, H.; Zhang, L.; Zhou, X.; Du, C.; et al. Risk Factors Associated with Acute Respiratory Distress Syndrome and Death in Patients with Coronavirus Disease 2019 Pneumonia in Wuhan, China. *JAMA Intern. Med.* **2020**, *180*, 934–943. [CrossRef] [PubMed]
16. Yang, X.; Yu, Y.; Xu, J.; Shu, H.; Xia, J.; Liu, H.; Wu, Y.; Zhang, L.; Yu, Z.; Fang, M.; et al. Clinical course and outcomes of critically ill patients with SARS-CoV-2 pneumonia in Wuhan, China: A single-centered, retrospective, observational study. *Lancet Respir. Med.* **2020**, *8*, 475–481. [CrossRef]
17. Beiderlinden, M.; Groeben, H.; Peters, J. Safety of percutaneous dilational tracheostomy in patients ventilated with high positive end-expiratory pressure (PEEP). *Intensive Care Med.* **2003**, *29*, 944–948. [CrossRef] [PubMed]

18. Rashid, A.O.; Islam, S. Percutaneous tracheostomy: A comprehensive review. *J. Thorac. Dis.* **2017**, *9* (Suppl. 10), S1128–S1138. [CrossRef]
19. Murphy, P.; Holler, E.; Lindroth, H.; Laughlin, M.; Simons, C.J.; Streib, E.W.; Boustani, M.; Ortiz, D. Short-term Outcomes for Patients and Providers After Elective Tracheostomy in COVID-19-Positive Patients. *J. Surg. Res.* **2021**, *260*, 38–45. [CrossRef]
20. Roedl, K.; Jarczak, D.; Thasler, L.; Bachmann, M.; Schulte, F.; Bein, B.; Weber, C.F.; Schafer, U.; Veit, C.; Hauber, H.P.; et al. Mechanical ventilation and mortality among 223 critically ill patients with coronavirus disease 2019: A multicentric study in Germany. *Aust. Crit. Care* **2021**, *34*, 167–175. [CrossRef]
21. Adams, C.D.; Altshuler, J.; Barlow, B.L.; Dixit, D.; Droege, C.A.; Effendi, M.K.; Heavner, M.S.; Johnston, J.P.; Kiskaddon, A.L.; Lemieux, D.G.; et al. Analgesia and Sedation Strategies in Mechanically Ventilated Adults with COVID-19. *Pharmacotherapy* **2020**, *40*, 1180–1191. [CrossRef] [PubMed]
22. Flinspach, A.N.; Booke, H.; Zacharowski, K.; Balaban, U.; Herrmann, E.; Adam, E.H. High sedation needs of critically ill COVID-19 ARDS patients-A monocentric observational study. *PLoS ONE* **2021**, *16*, e0253778. [CrossRef] [PubMed]
23. Young, D.; Harrison, D.A.; Cuthbertson, B.H.; Rowan, K.; TracMan, C. Effect of early vs late tracheostomy placement on survival in patients receiving mechanical ventilation: The TracMan randomized trial. *JAMA* **2013**, *309*, 2121–2129. [CrossRef] [PubMed]
24. Rumbak, M.J.; Newton, M.; Truncale, T.; Schwartz, S.W.; Adams, J.W.; Hazard, P.B. A prospective, randomized, study comparing early percutaneous dilational tracheotomy to prolonged translaryngeal intubation (delayed tracheotomy) in critically ill medical patients. *Crit. Care Med.* **2004**, *32*, 1689–1694. [CrossRef] [PubMed]
25. Meng, L.; Wang, C.; Li, J.; Zhang, J. Early vs late tracheostomy in critically ill patients: A systematic review and meta-analysis. *Clin. Respir. J.* **2016**, *10*, 684–692. [CrossRef] [PubMed]
26. Hanidziar, D.; Bittner, E.A. Sedation of Mechanically Ventilated COVID-19 Patients: Challenges and Special Considerations. *Anesth. Analg.* **2020**, *131*, e40–e41. [CrossRef] [PubMed]
27. Benito, D.A.; Bestourous, D.E.; Tong, J.Y.; Pasick, L.J.; Sataloff, R.T. Tracheotomy in COVID-19 Patients: A Systematic Review and Meta-analysis of Weaning, Decannulation, and Survival. *Otolaryngol. Head Neck Surg.* **2021**, *165*. 398–405. [CrossRef] [PubMed]
28. Boniatti, V.M.C.; Pereira, C.R.; Costa, G.M.; Teixeira, M.C.; Werlang, A.P.; Martins, F.T.M.; Marques, L.D.S.; Nedel, W.L.; Boniatti, M.M. Extubation failure and the use of noninvasive ventilation during the weaning process in critically ill COVID-19 patients. *Crit. Care Sci.* **2023**, *35*, 163–167. [CrossRef]
29. Cammarota, G.; Vaschetto, R.; Azzolina, D.; De Vita, N.; Olivieri, C.; Ronco, C.; Longhini, F.; Bruni, A.; Colombo, D.; Pissaia, C.; et al. Early extubation with immediate non-invasive ventilation versus standard weaning in intubated patients for coronavirus disease 2019: A retrospective multicenter study. *Sci. Rep.* **2021**, *11*, 13418. [CrossRef]
30. Noah, P.; Parker, M.; Bradley, A.; Schiff, M.D.; Mark, A.; Fritz, M.D.; Sarah, K.; Rapoport, M.D.; Sam Schild, M.D.; Kenneth, W.; et al. *Tracheotomy Recommendations during the COVID-19 Pandemic*; American Academy of Otolaryngology-Head and Neck Surgery: Alexandria, VA, USA, 2020.
31. Wang, J.; Leibner, E.; Hyman, J.B.; Ahmed, S.; Hamburger, J.; Hsieh, J.; Dangayach, N.; Tandon, P.; Gidwani, U.; Leibowitz, A.; et al. The Mount Sinai Hospital Institute for critical care medicine response to the COVID-19 pandemic. *Acute Crit. Care* **2021**, *36*, 201–207. [CrossRef]
32. Michetti, C.P.; Burlew, C.C.; Bulger, E.M.; Davis, K.A.; Spain, D.A.; the Critical Care and Acute Care Surgery Committees of the American Association for the Surgery of Trauma. Performing tracheostomy during the COVID-19 pandemic: Guidance and recommendations from the Critical Care and Acute Care Surgery Committees of the American Association for the Surgery of Trauma. *Trauma Surg. Acute Care Open* **2020**, *5*, e000482. [CrossRef] [PubMed]
33. Sommer, D.D.; Engels, P.T.; Weitzel, E.K.; Khalili, S.; Corsten, M.; Tewfik, M.A.; Fung, K.; Cote, D.; Gupta, M.; Sne, N.; et al. Recommendations from the CSO-HNS taskforce on performance of tracheotomy during the COVID-19 pandemic. *J. Otolaryngol. Head Neck Surg.* **2020**, *49*, 23. [CrossRef] [PubMed]
34. Chao, T.N.; Braslow, B.M.; Martin, N.D.; Chalian, A.A.; Atkins, J.; Haas, A.R.; Rassekh, C.H. Tracheotomy in Ventilated Patients with COVID-19. *Ann. Surg.* **2020**, *272*, e30–e32. [CrossRef] [PubMed]

Journal of
Clinical Medicine

MDPI

Article

Correlation between Subjective Nasal Patency and Nasal Capacity in Young Adults: A Pilot Study with a Prototype Device—A Nasoorospirometer

Katarzyna Zasadzińska-Stempniak *, Hanna Zajączkiewicz and Andrzej Kukwa

Department of Otorhinolaryngology, Head and Neck Diseases, School of Medicine, University of Warmia and Mazury in Olsztyn, al. Warszawska 30, 10-082 Olsztyn, Poland
* Correspondence: katarzyna.zasadzinska@uwm.edu.pl; Tel.: +48-89-524-5631

Abstract: Background: Nasal airway obstruction (NAO) is characterised by high resistance in the nasal cavity with a collapsible and narrowed upper airway and is an integral part of OSA pathophysiology. The literature demonstrates that the identification of high-risk OSA in the young adult population leads to the prevention of later health consequences. A nasoorospirometer is a prototype device that measures nasal capacity during inspiration. The basis for measurement is a Wheatstone bridge and a thermal anemometer. The parameters are recorded via hot wire anemometry (HTA) with velocity measurements in the airflow field. Therefore, this pilot study aimed to test the feasibility of the device by examining a young adult sample. The secondary aim was to determine whether subjective NAO correlates with nasal capacity and whether NAO corresponds with anthropometric parameters and individual risk of OSA. **Methods**: A group of 31 participants (mean age 24.9 years) underwent a thorough laryngological examination. The nasoorospirometer was used to measure objective NAO (nasal capacity), the NOSE scale was used to gain subjective NAO evaluation, and the Berlin Questionnaire for the risk of OSA. **Results**: A correlation analysis confirmed no significant associations between the subjective and objective measures ($p > 0.05$). Higher BMI and neck circumference are associated with lower NAO and higher nasal patency in the population of young adults (r: 0.32–0.45; $p < 0.05$). The risk of OSA showed no statistically significant association ($p > 0.05$). **Conclusions**: We presented three methods of NAO assessment: subjective participant evaluation, objective nasoosopirometry, and objective laryngological assessment. However, the use of a nasoorospirometer with anthropometric measures in young adults needs to be verified in future studies.

Keywords: sleep apnea syndrome; sleep health; obstructive sleep apnea; screening; sleep study; young adults; disease severity

1. Introduction

Obstructive sleep apnea (OSA) is a condition primarily associated with the narrowing of the upper airways, which is characterized by repeated episodes of total or partial pharyngeal occlusion during sleep. Moreover, high resistance in the nasal cavity with a collapsible and narrowed upper airway is the typical feature of nasal airway obstruction (NAO) [1,2]. Various degrees of NAO and increased nasal resistance often accompany OSA and increase the risk of snoring [3–7]. Further, isolated nasal surgery can possibly improve OSA subjectively, especially in patients with NAO, or improve treatment effectiveness with continuous positive airway pressure (CPAP) [8–10]. Other factors that increase the risk of OSA are high body-mass index (BMI) and increased neck circumference (NC). Unfortunately, data on the association of NAO with BMI and NC are scarce. Only a few studies have compared the occurrence of NAO in different body weight status groups and explored the association between anthropometric measures and NAO occurrence [11–13]. The literature demonstrates that the identification of a high risk of OSA in the young adult population leads to the prevention of later health consequences [14,15]. This age group may have an unconscious nasal patency disorder that increases the risk of OSA. In the case of early OSA risk detection, it is possible to prevent the consequences to which developed OSA leads, e.g., stroke, pulmonary hypertension, and atrial fibrillation [16–18].

Due to the low availability of full polysomnography (PSG) studies, simplified strategies to diagnose or suspect OSA are being proposed, among them non-contact biomotion sensors, and sleep switch devices [19]. Since NAO is a frequent condition in OSA, its assessment can indicate a possible sleep disorder. By examining NAO parameters, e.g., nasal capacity, we could determine a predisposition to OSA. The addition of an NAO assessment to anthropometric measures can provide relevant information for OSA prediction and may perhaps become a screening test for the risk of OSA.

This study aimed to test the feasibility of the prototype device, the nasoorospirometer, to refine the technique and identify flaws. The secondary aims were to analyse nasal capacity in young adults and investigate whether subjective NAO correlates with nasal capacity. Moreover, we aimed to evaluate whether NAO correlates with anthropometric parameters and the risk of OSA. We hypothesized that subjective and objective nasal obstruction do not correlate with each other.

2. Materials and Methods

2.1. Study Design

We conducted a pilot cross-sectional study. Our study recruitment comprised 31 students and employees recruited from the University of Warmia and Mazury in Olsztyn, Poland, in 2022.

Subjects were included if they filled the following criteria:

(1) aged between 18–30 years;
(2) gave their written informed consent for the examination with a nasoorospirometer prototype device.

The exclusion criteria were:

(1) the active upper respiratory tract infection;
(2) history of neoplastic or autoimmune processes;
(3) uncontrolled chronic disease;
(4) current pregnancy.

Ethical approval was obtained from the ethics committee of the University of Warmia and Mazury (reference number 23/2020). All participants gave written informed consent.

Baseline characteristics of the participants (age, gender, weight, height, and neck circumference) and prior medical history were collected from the participants using a standard questionnaire.

Participants filled out the Nasal Obstruction Symptom Evaluation (NOSE) score to collect information on their subjective symptoms. This is a five-item scale in which an individual participant reports over the past month if he or she reports the symptoms of nasal congestion, nasal obstruction, difficulty breathing through the nose, difficulty sleeping, and sensation of air hunger using a scale from 0 (no problem) to 4 (severe problem). The numbers are summed up and multiplied by 5 to get a score ranging from 0 (no) symptoms to 100 (severe) symptoms [15].

A laryngological examination with otoscopy, nasal endoscopy, and laryngoscopy was conducted according to an established scheme before the examination with a nasoorospirometer. The examination was carried out in all subjects by the same otorhinolaryngologist with 10 years of clinical experience. The presence of anatomic nasal airway obstruction (deviated septum, medically resistant turbinate hypertrophy, or nasal valve dysfunction) was determined. Data were obtained at the same time to decrease the influence of the nasal cycle. The study was conducted in a controlled constant-temperature room to minimize the effect of the surroundings on the nasal mucosa.

The neck circumference was measured at the mid-neck, between the midline of the cervical spine and the midline of the neck, with the participant standing upright and facing forward, with arms relaxed. The circumference was measured just below the protrusion in men with a laryngeal protrusion [19].

The Berlin questionnaire (BQ) was administered to determine risk factors for obstructive sleep apnea (OSA). This questionnaire contains 10 questions on the following three categories: snoring (category 1, items 1–5), daytime somnolence (category 2, items 6–9), and presence of obesity or hypertension (category 3, item 10). High risk in at least two categories is considered high risk for OSA [14].

2.2. Nasoorospirometer

The nasoorospirometer provides the following objective measurements of NAO: unilateral and total inhale number, mean capacity, duration of the inhalation, and maximum and minimum capacity. We analysed the aforementioned parameters during inspiration. The same technician examined each subject for 2 min and read the data.

Both nostrils were tested simultaneously. A single measurement takes about a few seconds, and the entire testing process is completed in two minutes. After powering on the device and starting the computer program, calibration is carried out simply by complying with the on-screen instructions. The calibration should be performed each time the device is opened. The participant should be seated and not change position during the test. Swallowing should be avoided during measurements. The participant was instructed to breathe casually. To obtain a natural breathing pattern, participants were asked to scroll the Internet.

Figure 1 presents the placement of the mask with the sensors on the participant's face. The device is composed of a face mask, a central processing unit, and a computer. The oronasal mask is divided into sealed nasal and oral compartments with sensors: two nasal and one oral. The basis of data acquisition is three sensors that detect the nasal airflow and alterations in the turbulence kinetic energy transfer. Our group described our prototype device's principles of operation and configuration [20]. An example of the result from the measurements is shown in Figure 2.

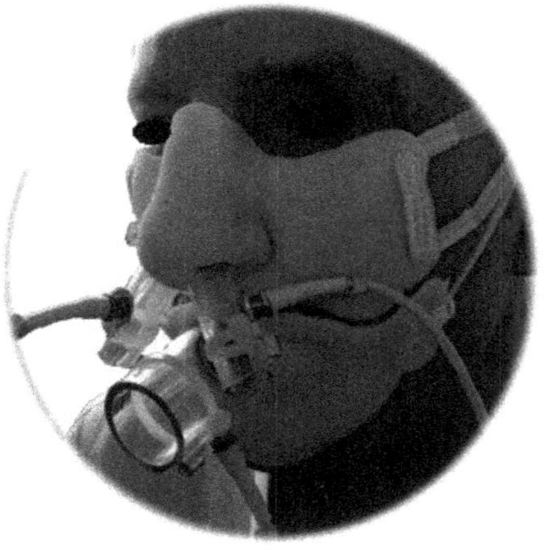

Figure 1. Placement of the printed mask with sensors on the patient's face.

Each orifice has a sensor that detects parameters: inhale/exhale number, capacity, and breath length. Two independent sensors connected to a differential pressure transducer and an amplifier were attached to the nasal and oral compartments. The basis for measurement is a Wheatstone bridge and thermal anemometer. The parameters are recorded via hot wire anemometry (HTA) with velocity measurements in the flow field. Applying HTA allows for the calculation of instantaneous flow velocity based on electrical voltage measurements. The nasal airflow alters turbulent kinetic energy, which is the basis of data acquisition. Airflow data from the nasoorospirometer were acquired using LabVIEW (National Instruments, Texas, UT, USA) and synchronized with the system.

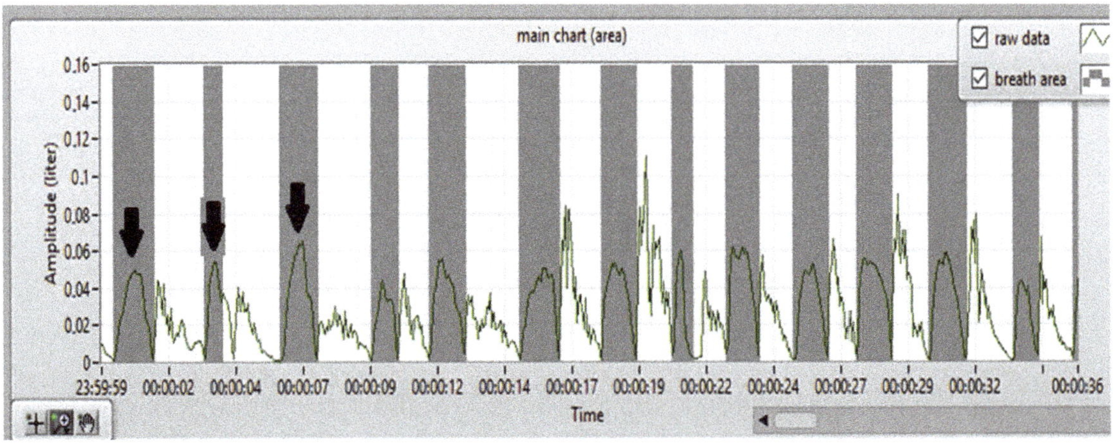

Figure 2. An example cutout of the result obtained from the device. The figure shows a measurement of nasal capacity from one nostril as a function of time. Vertical arrows indicate inspiration.

2.3. Statistical Analysis

The study characteristics were summarized using mean and standard deviation for continuous traits and number and percentage for categorical traits. The correlation between objective, subjective, and anthropometric measures was assessed using Spearman's correlation coefficients. Differences in objective nasal patency between groups with a low and a high risk of OSA were assessed using the Mann–Whitney U test. A two-sided $p < 0.05$ was considered statistically significant. All analyses were conducted in R (version 4.1.0, R Foundation for Statistical Computing, Vienna, Austria).

3. Results

The baseline characteristics of study participants are summarised in Table 1. Among the 31 participants included in this study, 13 were female, and 18 were male. The mean age of the participants was 24.9 (SD: 2.6) years. The mean BMI of the participants was 23.7 (SD: 4.5) kg/m^2. The mean NC was 35.3 (SD: 3.9) cm. Five participants had a high risk of OSA in BQ; the rest had a low risk. Six participants had severe symptoms according to the NOSE score, nine moderate, and 14 mild. Two had no symptoms, while none of the participants had extreme symptoms. Sixteen participants had nasal obstruction according to the examining laryngologist.

Correlation coefficients between objective nasal patency measures obtained with nasoorospirometry and subjective nasal patency are presented in Table 2. Mean capacity showed a moderate-to-high correlation with mean capacity variability, mean time, minimum, maximum, and sum capacity (r: 0.51–0.88). Mean capacity variability was inversely correlated with inhale number (r: −0.59) and positively with the mean time, its variability, and maximum capacity (r: 0.54–0.73). None of the nasoorospirometry parameters showed a significant correlation with the subjective NOSE score ($p > 0.05$).

Body mass index showed a significant correlation (Table 3) only with mean time (r: 0.40). In contrast, neck circumference showed a moderate-to-high positive correlation with mean, maximum, minimum, and sum capacity (r: 0.32–0.45).

Table 1. Sample characteristics.

Characteristic	*n* (%)
N of participants	31 (100%)
Age at recruitment (years)	24.9 (±2.57)
Gender: Male Female	 18 (58%) 13 (42%)
BMI (kg/m^2)	23.72 ± 4.5
NC	35.32 (±3.94)
BQ High low	 5 (16%) 26 (84%)
NOSE SCORE Severe Moderate mild No symptoms	Mean: 28.4 6 (20%) 9 (29%) 14 (45%) 2 (6%)
Nasal obstruction	16 (52%)
Earlier septoplasty	2 (6%)

BMI—body mass index; NC—neck circumference; BQ—Berlin questionnaire; NOSE—nasal obstruction symptom evaluation.

Table 2. Spearman's correlation coefficients between objective and subjective nasal patency.

	Mean Capacity (R + L) [l]	Mean Capacity (R + L) std [l]	Inhale Number (R + L)/min	Mean Time (R + L) [std(s)]	Mean Time (R + L) [s]	Max Capacity (R + L)	Min Capacity (R + L)	Sum Capacity (R + L)
Mean Capacity (R + L) std [l]	**0.51** **$p = 0.003$**							
Inhale number (R + L)/min	−0.35 $p = 0.054$	**−0.59** **$p < 0.001$**						
Mean time (R + L) [std(s)]	0.20 $p = 0.27$	**0.71** **$p < 0.001$**	**−0.40** **$p < 0.026$**					
Mean time (R + L) [s]	**0.64** **$p < 0.001$**	**0.54** **$p < 0.001$**	**−0.67** **$p < 0.001$**	**0.45** **$p < 0.011$**				
Max capacity (R + L)	**0.88** **$p < 0.001$**	**0.73** **$p < 0.001$**	**−0.39** **$p < 0.028$**	**0.40** **$p < 0.024$**	**0.65** **$p < 0.001$**			
Min capacity (R + L)	**0.55** **$p < 0.001$**	−0.10 $p < 0.59$	−0.20 $p < 0.28$	−0.07 $p < 0.69$	**0.38** **$p < 0.034$**	**0.42** **$p < 0.019$**		
Sum capacity (R + L)	**0.63** **$p < 0.001$**	0.07 $p < 0.72$	0.27 $p < 0.14$	−0.13 $p < 0.5$	0.16 $p < 0.4$	**0.52** **$p < 0.003$**	**0.39** **$p < 0.03$**	
NOSE score	0.18 $p < 0.33$	0.03 $p < 0.86$	−0.02 $p < 0.93$	−0.14 $p < 0.45$	0.19 $p < 0.31$	0.11 $p < 0.56$	−0.02 $p < 0.9$	−0.14 $p < 0.46$

Bolded are correlation coefficients that are statistically significant ($p < 0.05$). Max—maximum; Min—minimum; R—right; L—left; Sum—summed; std—standard deviation; min—minute.

Table 3. Correlation between nasoorospirometry parameters and anthropometric measures.

Measure	Body Mass Index	Neck Circumference
Mean Capacity (R + L) [l]	0.27 $p = 0.14$	**0.45** **$p = 0.01$**
Mean Capacity (R + L) std [l]	0.21 $p = 0.27$	0.21 $p = 0.27$

Table 3. *Cont.*

Measure	Body Mass Index	Neck Circumference
Inhale number (R + L)/min	−0.22 $p = 0.22$	−0 04 $p = 0.83$
Mean time (R + L) [std(s)]	0.07 $p = 0.7$	0.09 $p = 0.61$
Mean Time (R + L) [s]	**0.40** **$p = 0.03$**	0.34 $p = 0.06$
Max capacity (R + L)	0.23 $p = 0.2$	**0.44** **$p = 0.014$**
Min capacity (R + L)	0.19 $p = 0.32$	**0.32** **$p = 0.04$**
Sum capacity (R + L)	0.00 $p = 1$	**0.38** **$p = 0.03$**

Bolded are correlation coefficients that are statistically significant ($p < 0.05$). Max—maximum; Min—minimum; R—right; L—left; Sum—summed; std—standard deviation; min—minute.

Table 4 presents a comparison of nasoorospirometry parameters between groups with a low and high risk of OSA. None of the parameters showed a statistically significant difference ($p > 0.05$).

Table 4. Comparison of objective nasal patency measures according to the risk in the Berlin Q.

Measure	Low Risk, $n = 26$	High Risk, $n = 5$	p-Value
Inhale number (R + L)	24 (13, 29)	30 (24, 37)	0.3
Mean Capacity (R + L) [l]	0.47 (0.33, 0.67)	0.43 (0.31, 0.45)	0.6
Mean Capacity (R + L) std [l]	0.15 (0.10, 0.22)	0.12 (0.08, 0.20)	0.7
Inhale number (R + L)/min	12.6 (10.4, 17.6)	14.3 (11.7, 17.7)	0.8
Mean time (R + L) [std(s)]	0.35 (0.27, 0.48)	0.36 (0.22, 0.47)	0.7
Mean Time (R + L) [s]	1.66 (1.35, 2.01)	1.64 (1.55, 1.86)	>0.9
Max capacity (R + L)	0.75 (0.58, 1.01)	0.75 (0.49, 0.75)	0.7
Min capacity (R + L)	0.16 (−0.02, 0.39)	0.17 (0.12, 0.19)	>0.9
Sum capacity (R + L)	12.4 (7.0, 16.0)	10.8 (9.2, 16.0)	0.8

Values are median and interquartile range. p value was derived from the Mann–Whitney U test. Max—maximum; Min—minimum; R—right; L—left; Sum—summed; std—standard deviation; min—minute.

4. Discussion

In this study, we used an innovative method of nasal airway obstruction assessment. We investigated the association between anthropometric parameters (neck circumference and BMI) and nasal capacity. We found that there is no evidence for the correlation between subjective and objective nasal patency. In addition, we showed that higher BMI and neck circumference are associated with lower NAO and higher nasal patency in the population of young adults.

We may evaluate nasal airway obstruction with subjective and objective methods. Among the former, there are different types of questionnaires, among others, the NOSE score. A golden standard tool for objective NAO measurements would be a simple, cheap, non-invasive, and reproducible method. The most accepted and readily available are rhinomanometry, acoustic rhinometry, and peak inspiratory nasal flow [21–23]. Computational fluid dynamics [15,24] and acoustic analysis of breathing signals [25] are distinguished among the recently developed, with promising evidence of the ability to identify the actual anatomical point responsible for the patient's perceived nasal obstruction. We invented a prototype modular device, a nasoorospirometer, designed for nasal breathing analysis [20].

The objective assessment of nasal patency has long been a topic that remains evolving despite many possible modalities. This is because the obtained findings of the accurate nasal patency assessment often do not correspond to the patient's subjective patency [26–29]. In addition, examinations performed using different methods may not be comparable, and reproducibility rates may differ between clinical centres [27,28,30]. However, an accurate patency assessment may be beneficial for several reasons, including grading of patency impairment, treatment design, and evaluation of patency therapeutic outcomes.

Our result confirming that the perception of NAO does not correlate with objective measurements is in accordance with another study on the subjective perception of nasal patency [27,31]. The perception of a patent nose is the result of a number of variables, such as the cooling of the air [32,33] and nasal anatomical (e.g., septal deviation) and mucosal causes (e.g., the nasal cycle of the inferior turbinate, sinusitis, rhinorrhea) [24,34]. Our study was conducted in a controlled constant-temperature room to determine the effect of the surroundings on the nasal mucosa. Andre et al. published a systematic review, analysing 16 studies on this subject, concluding that the correlation between objective and subjective sensation remains uncertain [27]. The presence or absence of correlation was equally distributed among all the 16 analysed studies and did not depend on the study's level of evidence. However, the subjective assessment tool in all the studies that comprised this systematic review was either a Visual Analog Scale or non-validated questionnaires. Our study used a validated NOSE score, which is more valuable. Other studies confirmed poor correlation between subjective and objective measurements. There was no difference when the VAS or NOSE scores were applied [30,31]. Moreover, the studies that assessed subjective unilateral perception were more likely to have a correlation with objective measurements [24,27]. Although we assessed nostrils bilaterally, future studies might focus on a separate nostril examination.

The results of the studies analysing the association between anthropometric measures and NAO assessment are ambiguous. Our study found an association between higher BMI having higher bilateral mean capacity and lower NAO. Moreover, weight had a stronger correlation with mean capacity than height. This is contrary to previous research by Agarwal et al., where the rhinometric measures were reduced in obese patients with OSA [11]. On the other hand, Kemppainen et al. found no correlation between BMI and the results of rhinometry measurements. What is more, there were no significant changes in rhinometric values, even though a significant weight loss was achieved [12].

We found that NC correlates with nasal airway obstruction. It is comparable with the results of another study, where oronasal breathing was associated with BMI and NC [13]. Nascimento et al. performed a full night of in-laboratory polysomnography and assessed nasal breathing with pneumotachographs after that. This NAO assessment methodology may be similar to our nasoorospirometer study.

Contrary to the general consensus, we found that higher BMI and NC are associated with lower NAO. Our results may indicate that NAO may be caused not only by local causes but also by external extra-nasal causes, as also shown in other studies [1,35]. Blomster et al. showed that NAO was significantly lower in OSA patients after weight loss, which may be related to adipose tissue loss in the nasal cavity as well [36]. These findings imply that an NAO should be approached as a systemic problem, not a purely site-specific one.

In our study, we objectively characterised multiple anatomic deformities that caused NAO in each patient, although they did not correlate with subjective assessment. Contrary to the literature, specific objective measurements of NAO were correlated to subjective measures of nasal obstruction [37]. Although the group in the aforementioned study was small, it may be possible to define a nasal mean capacity pattern for each abnormality type of NAO in future studies, as was already suggested previously [24].

Some limitations of this study must be acknowledged. First, the results might be challenged due to limited measurements conducted with this device. For sure, we need more studies to test the accuracy and effectiveness of the device. However, prior research has already indicated no significant correlation between subjective and classical objective nasal obstruction assessment, which makes our results reliable. Second, we used bilateral assessment, which may negatively influence the result's reliability, so a study assessing each nostril separately should be adopted in future research. Moreover, another limitation is the lack of data necessary to calculate the minimum sample size based on previous studies. Our study sample was relatively small, but its pilot character explains this. Moreover, other studies on this subject were also on small populations [15,24,33].

In this study, the mean NOSE score of 28.4 suggests that most subjects did not experience a relevant subjective nasal obstruction. Moreover, we suspect the presence of selection bias. Despite the expectation of greater representation of OSA patients, the recruited group had a small number of such patients. Clearly, larger observational studies need to be conducted to confirm our results. Adding a PSG and not only an assessment of OSA risk through a validated questionnaire may clarify the association better in future studies.

We presented three methods of NAO assessment: subjective patient evaluation, objective nasoosopirometry, and objective laryngological assessment. When used separately, they can only show part of the clinical picture, so we suggest that they should complement each other.

5. Conclusions

NAO is an integral part of OSA pathophysiology. The nasoorospirometer is a simple, cheap, and non-invasive method. By analysing objective NAO with anthropometric measures, NC and BMI might be effective in diagnosing OSA predisposition. Higher BMI and NC were noted to be associated with lower NAO in the population of young adults. Moreover, no evidence for the correlation between subjective and objective nasal patency was observed. The results of this pilot study are encouraging; however, the usage of NAO with anthropometric measures needs to be verified in future studies.

Author Contributions: Conceptualization, K.Z.-S.; methodology, K.Z.-S.; software, K.Z.-S.; validation, K.Z.-S. and H.Z.; formal analysis, K.Z.-S.; H.Z. investigation, K.Z.-S.; resources, K.Z.-S.; data curation, K.Z.-S.; writing—original draft preparation, K.Z.-S.; writing—review and editing K.Z.-S. and H.Z.; visualization, K.Z.-S. supervision, H.Z. and A.K.; project administration, K.Z.-S.; funding acquisition, H.Z. All authors have read and agreed to the published version of the manuscript.

Funding: This research received no external funding.

Institutional Review Board Statement: The study was conducted in accordance with the Declaration of Helsinki and approved by the Institutional Review Board (or Ethics Committee) of the University of Warmia and Mazury (reference number 23/2020, 25 April 2020).

Informed Consent Statement: Informed consent was obtained from all subjects involved in the study.

Data Availability Statement: Data available on request due to restrictions, e.g., privacy or ethics. The data presented in this study are available on request from the corresponding author. The data are not publicly available due to the protection of personal data.

Acknowledgments: Special thanks to Jakub Morze.

Conflicts of Interest: The authors declare no conflicts of interest.

References

1. Lu, Y.; Li, S.; Jin, H.; Song, L.; Li, Y.; Zhong, N.; Zhang, X. High nasal resistance may be a result rather than a cause of obstructive sleep apnea. *Eur. Arch. Otorhinolaryngol.* **2014**, *271*, 2999–3003. [CrossRef] [PubMed]
2. Young, T.; Finn, L.; Kim, H.; Palta, M.; Dempsey, J.; Skatrud, J. Nasal obstruction as a risk factor for sleep-disordered breathing. The University of Wisconsin Sleep and Respiratory Research Group. *J. Allergy Clin. Immunol.* **1997**, *99*, S757–S762. [CrossRef] [PubMed]
3. Banabilh, S.M.; Suzina, A.H.; Mohamad, H.; Dinsuhaimi, S.; Samsudin, A.R.; Singh, G.D. Assessment of 3-D nasal airway morphology in Southeast Asian adults with obstructive sleep apnea using acoustic rhinometry. *Clin. Oral Investig.* **2010**, *14*, 491–498. [CrossRef] [PubMed]
4. Liu, S.A.; Su, M.C.; Jiang, R.S. Nasal patency measured by acoustic rhinometry in East Asian patients with sleep-disordered breathing. *Am. J. Rhinol.* **2006**, *20*, 274–277. [CrossRef] [PubMed]
5. Hoel, H.C.; Kvinnesland, K.; Berg, S. Impact of nasal resistance on the distribution of apneas and hypopneas in obstructive sleep apnea. *Sleep Med.* **2020**, *71*, 83–88. Available online: https://pubmed.ncbi.nlm.nih.gov/32502854/ (accessed on 31 October 2023). [CrossRef] [PubMed]

6. Zeng, B.; Ng, A.T.; Qian, J.; Petocz, P.; Darendeliler, M.A.; Cistulli, P.A. Influence of nasal resistance on oral appliance treatment outcome in obstructive sleep apnea. *Sleep* **2008**, *31*, 543–547. [CrossRef] [PubMed]
7. Zamarrón, C.; Gude, F.; Alvarez, J.M.; Rivera, M.; Gonzalez, F.J.; Rodriguez, J.R. Airway disorders and pulmonary function in snorers. A population-based study. *Respir. Med.* **2000**, *94*, 835–840. [CrossRef] [PubMed]
8. Park, D.-Y.; Cho, J.H.; Jung, Y.G.; Choi, J.H.; Kim, D.-K.; Kim, S.-W.; Kim, H.J.; Kim, H.Y.; Park, S.K.; Park, C.S.; et al. Clinical Practice Guideline: Clinical Efficacy of Nasal Surgery in the Treatment of Obstructive Sleep Apnea. *Clin. Exp. Otorhinolaryngol.* **2023**, *16*, 201. [CrossRef]
9. Maniaci, A.; Lechien, J.R.; La Mantia, I.; Calvo-Henriquez, C.; Iannella, G.; Locatello, L.G.; Saibene, A.M.; Leigh, S.J.; Ingrassia, A.; Nocera, F.; et al. Effectiveness of submucosal turbinoplasty in refractory obstructive rhinitis: A prospective comparative trial. *Eur. Arch. Otorhinolaryngol.* **2022**, *279*, 4397–4406. [CrossRef]
10. Schoustra, E.; van Maanen, P.; den Haan, C.; Ravesloot, M.J.L.; de Vries, N. The Role of Isolated Nasal Surgery in Obstructive Sleep Apnea Therapy—A Systematic Review. *Brain Sci.* **2022**, *12*, 1446. [CrossRef]
11. Agarwal, S.S.; Datana, S.; Sahoo, N.K.; Bhandari, S.K. Correlating Nasal Patency with Obstructive Sleep Apnea in Obese Versus Non-Obese Patients: An Acoustic Rhinometry Study. *Indian J. Otolaryngol. Head Neck Surg.* **2022**, *74* (Suppl. S2), 1483–1491. [CrossRef] [PubMed]
12. Kemppainen, T.; Ruoppi, P.; Seppä, J.; Sahlman, J.; Peltonen, M.; Tukiainen, H.; Gylling, H.; Vanninen, E.; Tuomilehto, H. Effect of weight reduction on rhinometric measurements in overweight patients with obstructive sleep apnea. *Am. J. Rhinol.* **2008**, *22*, 410–415. [CrossRef]
13. Nascimento, J.A.; Genta, P.R.; Fernandes, P.H.; Barroso, L.P.; Carvalho, T.S.; Moriya, H.T.; Madeiro, F.; Lorenzi-Filho, G.; Nakagawa, N.K. Predictors of oronasal breathing among obstructive sleep apnea patients and controls. *J. Appl. Physiol.* **2019**, *127*, 1579–1585. [CrossRef] [PubMed]
14. Netzer, N.C.; Stoohs, R.A.; Netzer, C.M.; Clark, K.; Strohl, K.P. Using the Berlin Questionnaire to identify patients at risk for the sleep apnea syndrome. *Ann. Intern. Med.* **1999**, *131*, 485–491. [CrossRef] [PubMed]
15. Gaberino, C.; Rhee, J.S.; Garcia, G.J.M. Estimates of nasal airflow at the nasal cycle mid-point improve the correlation between objective and subjective measures of nasal patency. *Respir. Physiol. Neurobiol.* **2017**, *238*, 23–32. [CrossRef] [PubMed]
16. Teodorescu, M.; Polomis, D.A.; Teodorescu, M.C.; Gangnon, R.E.; Peterson, A.G.; Consens, F.B.; Chervin, R.D.; Jarjour, N.N. Association of obstructive sleep apnea risk with asthma control in adults. *Chest* **2010**, *138*, 543–550. [CrossRef]
17. Marin, J.M.; Carrizo, S.J.; Vicente, E.; Agusti, A.G. Long-term cardiovascular outcomes in men with obstructive sleep apnoea-hypopnoea with or without treatment with continuous positive airway pressure: An observational study. *Lancet* **2005**, *365*, 1046–1053. [CrossRef]
18. Cheung, Y.; Tai, B.; Loo, G.; Khoo, S.; Cheong, K.Y.; Barbe, F.; Lee, C. Screening for Obstructive Sleep Apnea in the Assessment of Coronary Risk. *Am. J. Cardiol.* **2017**, *119*, 996–1002. [CrossRef] [PubMed]
19. Ben-Noun, L.L.; Sohar, E.; Laor, A. Neck Circumference as a Simple Screening Measure for Identifying Overweight and Obese Patients. *Obes. Res.* **2001**, *9*, 470–477. [CrossRef]
20. Nitkiewicz, S.; Barański, R.; Kukwa, A.; Zając, A. Respiratory disorders–measuring method and equipment. *Metrol. Meas. Syst.* **2018**, *25*, 187–202. [CrossRef]
21. Ottaviano, G.; Fokkens, W.J. Measurements of nasal airflow and patency: A critical review with emphasis on the use of peak nasal inspiratory flow in daily practice. *Allergy* **2016**, *71*, 162–174. [CrossRef] [PubMed]
22. Giotakis, A.I.; Tomazic, P.V.; Riechelmann, H.; Vent, J. Objective Assessment of Nasal Patency. *Facial Plast. Surg.* **2017**, *33*, 378–387. [CrossRef] [PubMed]
23. Piromchai, P.; Netnoi, J.; Srirompotong, S.; Thanawirattananit, P. Comparison of nasal patency after nose-blowing between pinch versus no pinch method: A randomized controlled trial. *Sci. Rep.* **2021**, *11*, 22084. [CrossRef] [PubMed]
24. Casey, K.P.; Borojeni, A.A.T.; Koenig, L.J.; Rhee, J.S.; Garcia, G.J.M. Correlation between Subjective Nasal Patency and Intranasal Airflow Distribution. *Otolaryngol. Head Neck Surg.* **2017**, *156*, 741–750. [CrossRef] [PubMed]
25. Primov-Fever, A.; Zaretsky, U.; Elad, D.; Wolf, M. Evaluation of nasal airway patency by analysis of breathing sounds. *Acta Otolaryngol.* **2016**, *136*, 219–224. [CrossRef] [PubMed]
26. Verhoeven, S.; Schmelzer, B. Type and severity of septal deviation are not related with the degree of subjective nasal obstruction. *Rhinology* **2016**, *54*, 355–360. [CrossRef] [PubMed]
27. André, R.F.; Vuyk, H.D.; Ahmed, A.; Graamans, K.; Nolst Trenité, G.J. Correlation between subjective and objective evaluation of the nasal airway. A systematic review of the highest level of evidence. *Clin. Otolaryngol.* **2009**, *34*, 518–525. [CrossRef] [PubMed]
28. Naito, K.; Miyata, S.; Saito, S.; Sakurai, K.; Takeuchi, K. Comparison of perceptional nasal obstruction with rhinomanometric and acoustic rhinometric assessment. *Eur. Arch. Otorhinolaryngol.* **2001**, *258*, 505–508. [CrossRef] [PubMed]
29. Tompos, T.; Garai, T.; Zemplén, B.; Gerlinger, I. Sensation of nasal patency compared to rhinomanometric results after septoplasty. *Eur. Arch. Otorhinolaryngol.* **2010**, *267*, 1887–1891. [CrossRef]
30. Braun, T.; Rich, M.; Kramer, M.F. Correlation of three variables describing nasal patency (HD, MCA, NOSE score) in healthy subjects. *Braz. J. Otorhinolaryngol.* **2013**, *79*, 354–358. [CrossRef]
31. Lam, D.J.; James, K.T.; Weaver, E.M. Comparison of Anatomic, Physiological, and Subjective Measures of the Nasal Airway. *Am. J. Rhinol.* **2006**, *20*, 463–470. [CrossRef] [PubMed]

32. Tjahjono, R.; Singh, N. Correlation between nasal mucosal temperature change and the perception of nasal patency: A literature review. *J. Laryngol. Otol.* **2021**, *135*, 104–109. [CrossRef] [PubMed]
33. Zhao, K.; Jiang, J.; Blacker, K.; Lyman, B.; Dalton, P.; Cowart, B.J.; Pribitkin, E.A. Regional peak mucosal cooling predicts the perception of nasal patency. *Laryngoscope* **2014**, *124*, 589–595. [CrossRef] [PubMed]
34. La Mantia, I.; Grigaliute, E.; Ragusa, M.; Cocuzza, S.; Radulesco, T.; Saibene, A.M.; Calvo-Henriquez, C.; Fakhry, N.; Michel, J.; Maniaci, A. Effectiveness and rapidity on olfactory fuction recovery in CRS patients treated with Dupilumab: A real life prospective controlled study. *Eur. Arch. Otorhinolaryngol.* **2024**, *281*, 219–226. [CrossRef] [PubMed]
35. Nakata, S.; Miyazaki, S.; Ohki, M.; Morinaga, M.; Noda, A.; Sugiura, T.; Sugiura, M.; Teranishi, M.; Katayama, N.; Nakashima, T. Reduced nasal resistance after simple tonsillectomy in patients with obstructive sleep apnea. *Am. J. Rhinol.* **2007**, *21*, 192–195. [CrossRef]
36. Blomster, H.; Kemppainen, T.; Numminen, J.; Ruoppi, P.; Sahlman, J.; Peltonen, M.; Seppa, J.; Tuomilehto, H. Impaired nasal breathing may prevent the beneficial effect of weight loss in the treatment of OSA. *Rhinology* **2011**, *49*, 587–592. [CrossRef]
37. Leitzen, K.P.; Brietzke, S.E.; Lindsay, R.W. Correlation between nasal anatomy and objective obstructive sleep apnea severity. *Otolaryngol. Head Neck Surg.* **2014**, *150*, 325–331. [CrossRef]

Journal of
Clinical Medicine

MDPI

Article

Electrical Ear Canal Stimulation as a Therapeutic Approach for Tinnitus—A Proof of Concept Study

Jana Vater, Moritz Gröschel, Agnieszka J. Szczepek and Heidi Olze *

Department of Otorhinolaryngology, Head and Neck Surgery, Charité-Universitätsmedizin Berlin, Corporate Member of Freie Universität and Berlin Humboldt Universität zu Berlin, Charitéplatz 1, 10117 Berlin, Germany; jana.vater@charite.de (J.V.); moritz.groeschel@charite.de (M.G.); agnes.szczepek@charite.de (A.J.S.)
* Correspondence: heidi.olze@charite.de

Abstract: Background: Tinnitus—the perception of sound despite the absence of an external source—can be a debilitating condition for which there are currently no pharmacological remedies. Our proof of concept study focused on the immediate effects of non-invasive electrical stimulation through the ear canal on loudness and tinnitus-induced distress. In addition, we aimed to identify variables that may affect the simulation outcomes. **Methods:** Sixty-six patients (29 women and 37 men, mean age 54.4 ± 10.4) with chronic tinnitus were recruited to the tertiary referral hospital between December 2019 and December 2021. They underwent 10 min of electrical stimulation through the ear canal for three consecutive days. Visual analog scales measured loudness and tinnitus-induced distress immediately before and after stimulation. **Results**: After three days of electrical stimulation, tinnitus loudness decreased in 47% of patients, 45.5% reported no change, and 7.6% reported worsening. Tinnitus severity decreased in 36.4% of cases, 59.1% of patients reported no change, and 4.5% reported worsening. Women responded positively to therapy earlier than men. In addition, tinnitus distress decreased in patients with compensated tinnitus but not in those with uncompensated tinnitus. Finally, patients with bilateral tinnitus improved earlier than those with unilateral tinnitus, and the age of the patients did not influence the stimulation results. **Conclusions**: Our proof of concept study confirms the potential of non-invasive electrical stimulation of the ear as a promising screening approach to identifying patients for more advanced electrostimulation treatment, such as an extracochlear anti-tinnitus implant. These findings have practical implications for tinnitus management, offering hope for improved patient care.

Keywords: tinnitus; electrical stimulation; cochlea; extracochlear stimulation; anti-tinnitus implant

1. Introduction

Tinnitus is the subjective perception of a sound without an external source [1] and is a symptom that can be caused by various conditions (e.g., hearing loss, cardiovascular or neurological disease, thyroid disease, diabetes, or cancer). Several etiological factors were identified for tinnitus, such as peripheral differentiation and synaptopathy, spontaneous ascending activity, GABA-ergic deficiency, or cholinergic excess, all likely contributing to central plasticity [2]. However, in clinical settings, the cause of tinnitus frequently remains unknown, in which case tinnitus is idiopathic. There is currently no drug treatment available for this condition. Sometimes, causal treatments can effectively reduce or even eliminate tinnitus. A good example is auditory therapy, such as fitting hearing aids [3,4] or auditory rehabilitation with cochlear implants [5] in patients with tinnitus caused by hearing loss.

There are currently no FDA-approved pharmacologic treatments for tinnitus. Cognitive and multimodal behavioral therapies are used to reduce the psychological distress caused by tinnitus and to prevent or treat psychological complications. The need for such treatment is determined by the level of distress caused by tinnitus and existing or developing comorbidities. However, even with all therapeutic options, patients with high tinnitus burden may experience severe limitations in daily life and work ability [6,7]. In addition to decreased quality of life, tinnitus is associated with high socioeconomic costs [8]. Therefore, a reliable and effective treatment for tinnitus would be of significant medical and socioeconomic importance.

Therapeutic approaches using electrical stimulation of the cochlea to reduce tinnitus perception have been developed since the 1970s [9,10]. In addition, numerous studies that have analyzed the effects of cochlear implants (CI) on tinnitus have found them effective in reducing tinnitus loudness [11–14]. However, despite the evidence that CI can reduce tinnitus, it is unclear whether the reduction is achieved by counteracting peripheral deafferentation [15], electrical stimulation via an implanted electrode [16], or by the interaction of both. In addition, although several clinical studies have provided data on partial or complete reduction of tinnitus in patients with cochlear implants, it is not yet clear before implantation which patients will respond positively to tinnitus reduction after CI activation. Research suggests an association between a higher degree of hearing loss and a greater likelihood of tinnitus improvement after cochlear implantation [17]. Still, this is not a rule that always works.

The literature confirms the beneficial effects of cochlear implants on tinnitus in many CI users [11,13,18]. In addition, there is evidence that auditory rehabilitation with CI improves quality of life and reduces stress and psychological comorbidities [18]. Therefore, developing an extracochlear implant for tinnitus patients, regardless of the degree of hearing loss, is essential in clinical audiology. Hence, the need emerged to create a system that could electrically stimulate the inner ear in tinnitus sufferers without the necessity for irreversible tissue damage—for example, in the form of a micro-implant placed on the round window. As part of the "INTAKT" initiative funded by the German Federal Ministry of Education and Research and dedicated to designing implants to help resolve various physiological deficits, the current project focused on determining the feasibility and effectiveness of external electrical stimulation through the ear canal in reducing tinnitus. Another project goal was to identify factors that may influence the anti-tinnitus efficacy of electrical stimulation. Obtaining such information is critical to developing an extracochlear implant for treating tinnitus and is an essential contemporary topic in clinical audiology.

To address these issues, the current proof-of-principle feasibility study aimed to determine if electrical stimulation using an electrode placed in the ear canal could decrease loudness and tinnitus-induced distress in human subjects. In addition, the results were analyzed based on the type of stimulation, the subjects' gender, and the severity or laterality of the tinnitus.

2. Materials and Methods

2.1. Study Design

The Charité Universitätsmedizin Berlin Ethics Committee (permit number EA1/125/18 obtained on 15 January 2019) approved this prospective proof-of-principle study conducted between 2019 and 2021. The study design reflected the early investigation stage of research [19,20] and was uncontrolled. Because two different electrical stimulation schemes were used, the patients were randomly (single-blinding) assigned to each group (Stimulation Groups 1 or 2).

2.2. Sample Description

Inclusion criteria;

- Age 18 years or older;
- Diagnosis of chronic subjective idiopathic tinnitus;
- No physical pathologies affecting the auditory system (e.g., vestibular schwannoma, meningioma, vascular compression of the hearing nerve, vascular abnormalities in the CNS, multiple sclerosis);
- Willingness to participate and a signed informed consent;

Exclusion criteria;

- Age below 18 years;
- Diagnosis of acute idiopathic tinnitus;
- Diagnosis of objective tinnitus;
- Eardrum perforation;
- Diagnoses of cancer.

Sixty-six subjects diagnosed with chronic idiopathic tinnitus (minimum six-month duration) were included in the study based on the above inclusion-exclusion criteria. The sample characteristics are presented in Table 1. During the pre-study diagnostic process in the specialized outpatient unit, the patients underwent a detailed psychoneurological examination, including magnetic resonance imaging, to exclude possible organic causes for their tinnitus, such as schwannomas, meningiomas, or vascular malformations. The age difference between the sex groups was not statistically significant (Mood's Median Test $X^2 = 0.696$; $p = 0.406$). None of the patients had diabetes; 26 had cardiovascular and 12 had thyroid gland conditions. The patients with moderate and moderately severe hearing loss were fitted with hearing aids.

Table 1. Sample characteristics.

sex	women men	$n = 29$ $n = 37$	43.9% 45.1%
age	mean 54.4 years (SD ± 10.4)	(min 26–max 80 years)	
hearing loss	normal hearing (better than 20 dB *) mild (20–34 dB) moderate (35–49 dB) moderately severe (50–64 dB)	$n = 10$ $n = 43$ $n = 6$ $n = 7$	15.2% 65.2% 9.1% 10.6%
tinnitus laterality	unilateral bilateral	$n = 12$ $n = 54$	18.2% 81.8%
Duration of tinnitus in months ($n = 32$)	mean 28.13 (SD ± 19.18)	(min 6–max 48 or more)	
Tinnitus Questionnaire score at admission ($n = 59$)	mean 41.59 (SD ± 17.56)	(min 11–max 81)	
cardiovascular disease		$n = 26$	39.4%
thyroid disease		$n = 12$	18.2%

SD, standard deviation; n, number of patients; *, grading according to the updated WHO definition [21], the values consider the pure tone average in the better ear for 500, 1000, 2000, and 4000 Hz.

2.3. Electrical Stimulation Conditions

The appointments were scheduled on three consecutive days (Figure 1). They were conducted in an outpatient audiology clinic where patients underwent 10 min of stimulation with an ear canal electrode by a physician and an audiologist. In preparation for stimulation, patients were asked to lie on their backs and turn their heads to the side to comfortably insert the electrode into the ear canal. The electrode carrier constructed in the Department of ORL consisted of two flexible arms inserted into the ear canal. The arms unfolded in the ear canal and stabilized over the opposite ear canal walls. The electrode did not touch the ear canal tissues or the eardrum. Sterile saline (Freka Drainjet, cat. # 1313041, Fresenius Kabi Deutschland GmbH, Bad Homburg, Germany) was dripped into the ear canal to allow the current to flow.

Electrical stimulation was applied to one ear only in patients with unilateral tinnitus on the affected side and patients with bilateral tinnitus on the side subjectively perceived as "worse". The stimulation gold electrode was inserted 1–1.5 cm into the ear canal and secured to the outer ear with a clip. The neutral electrode was placed on the forehead and fixed with a sterile surgical patch. During the gradual increase in current intensity, patients were asked to report possible side effects of the stimulation. These included burning or pain on the forehead where the neutral electrode was placed. In such cases, the current intensity was immediately reduced.

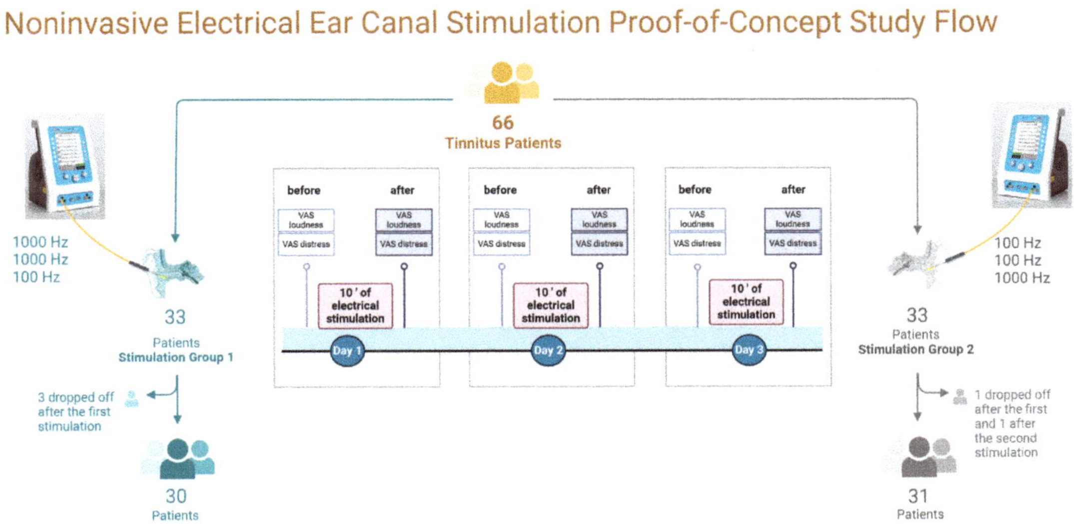

Figure 1. Schematic presentation of the study flow. Sixty-six tinnitus patients were randomly assigned to two stimulation groups. Both groups underwent ten minutes of electrical stimulation in the ear canal on three consecutive days. In the Stimulation Group 1, 1000 Hz was applied on two days and 100 Hz on the third day. In the Stimulation Group 2, 100 Hz was applied on two days and 1000 Hz on the third day. Immediately before and after stimulation, patients were asked to rate their subjective tinnitus loudness and tinnitus-related distress on a visual analog scale (VAS). Created with Biorender.com.

The C2 XTEND generator (inomed Medizintechnik GmbH, Emmendingen, Germany) randomly applied electrical stimulation with either 100 Hz or 1000 Hz frequency on the first two stimulation days (see Table 2 for details). The other frequency was used on the third stimulation day. This created two stimulation groups. Group 1 received stimulation at 1000 Hz for the first two sessions and 100 Hz for the third session. Group 2 received stimulation at 100 Hz during the first two sessions and at 1000 Hz during the third session.

Table 2. The parameters used for each of the stimulation programs.

	100 Hz	1000 Hz
Mode	continuous	continuous
Modulation frequency	1 Hz	5 Hz
Polarity	biphasic 50	biphasic 50
Puls width	1000 µs	400 µs
Interstimulus interval	10 ms	1 ms
Carrier frequency	100 Hz	1000 Hz
Initial current value	0.01 mA	0.01 mA
Maximal current value	3.0 mA	3.0 mA

The initial stimulation current intensity was 0.01 mA, gradually increasing to 3.0 mA. The average current used was 1.5 mA.

2.4. Assessment of Tinnitus Severity, Loudness, and Tinnitus-Induced Distress

Tinnitus severity level was assessed at admission using the Tinnitus Questionnaire (TQ). TQ was initially developed by Hallam et al. [22], and here, its validated German version was used [23]. The TQ measures the degree of tinnitus-induced distress, and its scores can range from 0 to 84. A clinically relevant system for tinnitus classification based on the total TQ score was developed, in which the TQ cutoff score of 47 is used to differentiate between habituated/compensated (below 47 points) and unhabituated/decompensated tinnitus (47 points and above). Because of technical reasons, the TQ scores were available only for 59 patients.

Patients rated tinnitus loudness and tinnitus-induced distress using the Visual Analog Scale (VAS), where 1 = very quiet, 10 = very loud, 1 = not bothersome, and 10 = very bothersome, just before and immediately after stimulation.

2.5. Dropouts

Five patients did not complete this study (Figure 1). Two patients from Stimulation Group 1 experienced worsening tinnitus loudness and distress immediately after the first stimulation, and one from Stimulation Group 2 after the second stimulation. They did not attend the consecutive appointments. One patient (Stimulation Group 1) with no changes after the first stimulation missed the other two appointments. One patient (Stimulation Group 2) experienced total suppression of tinnitus loudness and distress during the first stimulation and discontinued the stimulation.

2.6. Statistics

Statistical calculations were performed using IBM SPSS version 29.0 (IBM Deutschland GmbH, Ehningen, Germany). Because the data were not normally distributed, nonparametric statistical tests were performed.

3. Results

3.1. Electrostimulation-Induced Changes in Tinnitus Loudness and Tinnitus Distress

We first analyzed the data regarding the benefit of electrical stimulation for individual patients. When comparing the VAS score from before the first stimulation to those reported after the third stimulation, 31 (47%) patients reported improvement, 30 (45.5%) no change, and 5 (7.6%) subjective worsening of tinnitus loudness (Figure 2A). VAS scores for tinnitus-induced distress indicated improvement in 24 (36.4%) cases, no change in 39 (59.1%), and worsening in 3 patients (4.5%) (Figure 2B).

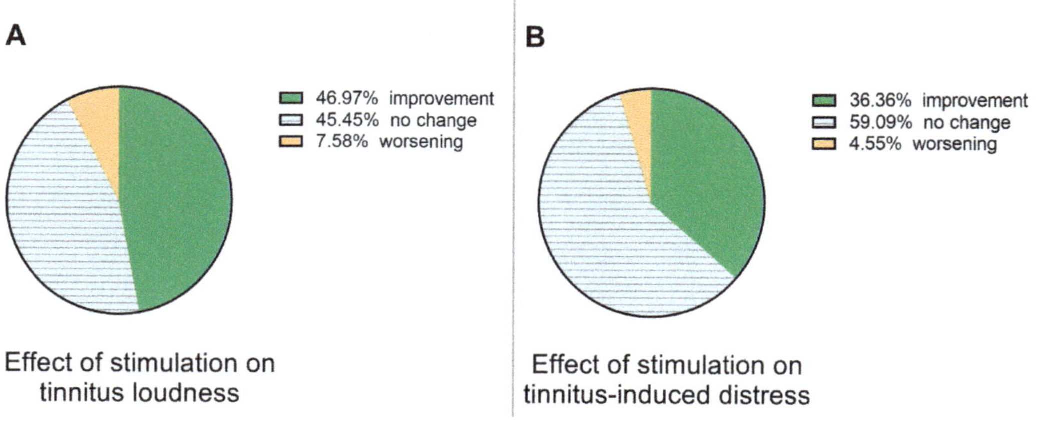

Figure 2. Effectiveness of electrical stimulation therapy in individual patients concerning tinnitus loudness (**A**) and tinnitus-induced distress (**B**).

There were statistically significant differences between the VAS scores before and after the stimulation for the entire cohort regarding tinnitus loudness and tinnitus-induced distress. A Wilcoxon matched-pairs signed rank test showed that the subjective tinnitus loudness decreased (Figure 3A) when measured immediately after the first stimulation ($Z = -2.918$, $p = 0.028$), after the second stimulation ($Z = -4.424$, $p < 0.001$), and after the third stimulation ($Z = -4.192$, $p < 0.001$). There was also a significant decrease in loudness measured between before the first and after the last stimulation ($Z = -4.839$, $p < 0.001$).

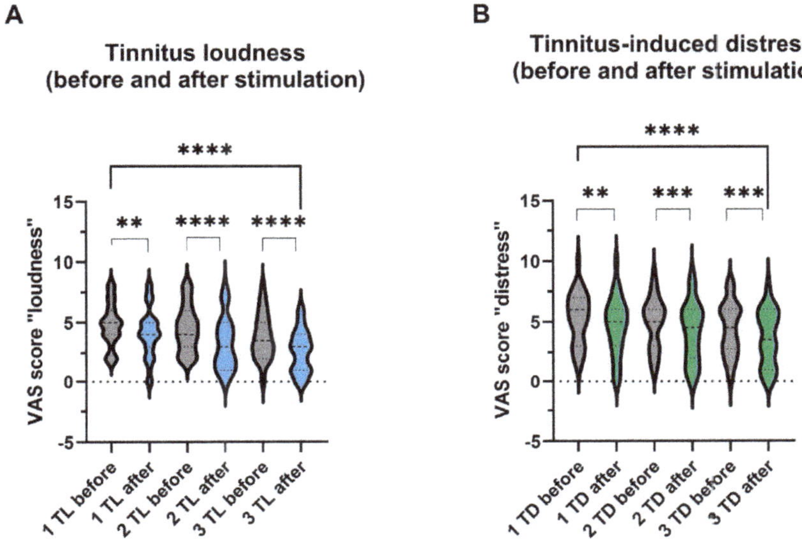

Figure 3. Changes in tinnitus loudness and distress after each stimulation session were registered in patients who reported improvement after stimulation ($n = 31$). Mean values of visual analog scale (VAS) scores reflecting subjective tinnitus loudness (**A**) and tinnitus-induced distress (**B**) for the entire cohort are shown as violin plots. The Wilcoxon matched-pairs signed rank test measured the significance of differences before and after stimulation; TL, tinnitus loudness, TD, tinnitus-induced distress, 1, 2, and 3 refer to the stimulation days; ** $p < 0.05$, *** $p < 0.01$, **** $p < 0.001$, ns—not significant.

Similarly to tinnitus loudness, changes in the tinnitus-induced distress were significant after the first stimulation ($Z = -2.859$, $p < 0.05$) and after the second ($Z = -3.114$, $p < 0.01$) and third stimulation ($Z = -3.241$, $p < 0.001$). There was also a significant difference in tinnitus-induced distress measured between the first and after the last stimulation ($Z = -4.086$, $p < 0.001$) (Figure 3B).

3.2. Lack of Difference in Outcome between the Stimulation Groups

The results of the two stimulation groups were compared to determine whether the sequence of stimulation frequencies (100 or 1000 Hz) influences the loudness or distress of tinnitus. The comparison of the VAS before and after the third stimulation showed a statistically significant improvement for both measured parameters and no significant differences between the groups. A Mann–Whitney U test was performed to evaluate whether VAS scores for tinnitus loudness and distress differed by stimulation group (Figure 4). The results indicated no significant difference between the VAS scores before or after stimulation in stimulation group 1 and stimulation group 2. These results suggest that the order of electrical stimulation (first 100 Hz and then 1000 Hz, or vice versa) is irrelevant to the outcome.

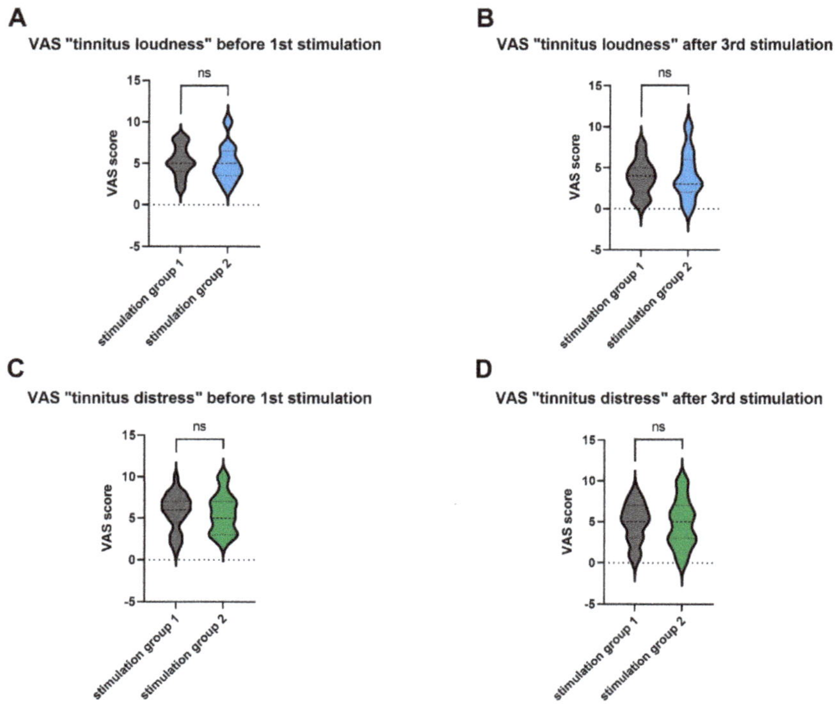

Figure 4. Visual analog scale (VAS) scores indicating tinnitus loudness or distress were compared between stimulation groups 1 and 2 (n = 66). The VAS scores indicating "tinnitus loudness" were measured immediately before the first stimulation (**A**) or immediately after the third stimulation (**B**). The VAS scores indicating "tinnitus distress" were measured immediately before the first stimulation (**C**) or immediately after the third stimulation (**D**). The scores are shown separately for each stimulation group. Using the Mann–Whitney U test, no significant differences were found between the groups, either at baseline (Figure 3A,C) or at the end of the study (Figure 3B,D). ns—not significant.

3.3. Positive Response to Electrical Stimulation Is Observed Earlier in Women than in Men

The comparison between the VAS before the first stimulation and the VAS after the third stimulation with a sex split showed a statistically significant improvement in both measured parameters for both sexes.

The difference in VAS scores between the gender groups concerning the beginning of the study (VAS tinnitus loudness Mood's Median Test $X^2 = 0.679$; $p = 0.410$; VAS tinnitus distress Mood's Median Test $X^2 = 0.097$; $p = 0.905$) or study endpoint (VAS Tinnitus Loudness Mood's Median Test $X^2 = 0.295$; $p = 0.587$; VAS Tinnitus Distress Mood's Median Test $X^2 = 0.208$; $p = 0.648$) was not statistically significant.

There was a difference in the timing of response to electrical stimulation between the sexes. Women reported reduced tinnitus loudness immediately after the first ear stimulation (and after subsequent sessions), whereas men responded positively only after the second and third electrical stimulations (Table 3).

Table 3. The significance of changes in tinnitus loudness measured with VAS after the first, second, and third stimulation, as well as before the first and after the third simulation, was calculated using the Wilcoxon test. Two-sided asymptotic significance (p-value) indicated that women rated the tinnitus loudness after the first stimulation as significantly decreasing, whereas men did not.

	Men		Women	
	Z	p	Z	p
Tinnitus loudness first stimulation	−0.681	0.496	−2.121	0.034
Tinnitus loudness second stimulation	−3.211	0.001	−3.218	0.001
Tinnitus loudness, third stimulation	−3.176	0.001	−3.220	0.001
Tinnitus loudness delta first—third stimulation	−3.071	0.002	−3.657	0.001

3.4. Stimulation Results Vary between Groups with Different Levels of Tinnitus Severity

The breakdown of subjects by TQ score showed 37 patients with compensated (habituated) tinnitus (56.1%) and 22 patients with decompensated (unhabituated) tinnitus (33.3%). No TQ score was available for seven patients (10.6%). The Wilcoxon-matched pairs signed ranks test with stratification based on compensation/habituation criteria showed differences in the outcome of electrical stimulation between the groups. Patients with compensated (habituated) tinnitus benefited from stimulation therapy, as measured by both VAS domains (tinnitus loudness and tinnitus-induced annoyance). Patients with decompensated tinnitus benefited from the treatment concerning tinnitus loudness but not tinnitus-induced distress (Table 4).

Table 4. The significance of changes in tinnitus loudness and tinnitus-induced distress after the first, second, and third stimulations, as well as before the first and third simulations, was calculated using the Wilcoxon test. The sample was split based on tinnitus compensation (habituation). Two-sided asymptotic significance (p-value) indicated that both groups rated the loudness of tinnitus as significantly decreasing after the second and third stimulations. Only the compensated (habituated) group rated the tinnitus-induced distress as significantly decreasing after the second and third stimulations.

	Compensated (Habituated) Group		Decompensated (Unhabituated) Group	
	Z	p	Z	p
Tinnitus loudness first stimulation	−1.342	0.180	−1.065	0.287
Tinnitus loudness second stimulation	−3.286	0.001	−2.695	0.007
Tinnitus loudness, third stimulation	−3.256	0.001	−2.699	0.007
Tinnitus loudness delta first—third stimulation	−3.781	0.001	−2.590	0.010
Tinnitus-induced distress first stimulation	−1.455	0.146	−0.447	0.655
Tinnitus-induced distress second stimulation	−2.585	0.010	−1.897	0.058
Tinnitus-induced distress third stimulation	−2.716	0.007	−1.841	0.066
Tinnitus-induced distress delta first—third stimulation	−3.400	0.001	−1.781	0.075

3.5. Stimulation Results Vary between Patients with Unilateral and Bilateral Tinnitus

When the sample was analyzed according to the laterality of the tinnitus, no difference was found between the groups' median TQ or VAS scores (before the first stimulation). However, there was a significant difference in stimulation outcome. The Wilcoxon matched-pairs signed rank test showed that in the unilateral tinnitus group, a significant reduction in loudness was observed only after the third stimulation ($Z = -2.121$, $p = 0.034$). In contrast, in the bilateral tinnitus group, a significant improvement was observed after the first ($Z = -2.498$, $p = 0.012$) as well as after the second ($Z = -4.283$, $p < 0.001$) and third stimulation ($Z = -3.992$, $p < 0.001$). We found a significant overall improvement in both groups when comparing the VAS scores before the first stimulation with those after the third stimulation.

Similar results were obtained regarding tinnitus-induced distress. The Wilcoxon matched-pairs signed rank test indicated significant improvement in patients with bilateral tinnitus after the first ($Z = -2.088$, $p = 0.037$), second ($Z = -3.114$, $p = 0.002$), and third ($Z = -2.971$, $p < 0.001$) stimulation. Patients with unilateral tinnitus improved significantly after the third stimulation ($Z = -2.000$, $p = 0.046$). Only the group with bilateral tinnitus significantly improved when comparing the VAS scores before the first and after the third stimulation.

3.6. Age, Duration of Tinnitus and the Degree of the Hearing Loss Do Not Affect the Stimulation Outcome

We calculated Spearman's rank-order correlation to determine if the stimulation outcome (effect on tinnitus loudness and tinnitus-induced distress) is influenced by the patient's age, duration of tinnitus, or hearing loss. None of the variables tested (age, tinnitus duration, grade of hearing loss, or TQ score at admission) influenced the outcome (Table 5). The grade of hearing loss was correlated with the patient's age and TQ score at admission.

Table 5. Spearman's rank-order correlation was run to determine the relationship between tinnitus duration, patient's age, TQ score, or the grade of the hearing loss, and the effectiveness of electrical stimulation on tinnitus loudness or tinnitus-induced distress. The significant correlations are shown in bold and identified with an asterisk.

		Tinnitus Duration in Months	Effectiveness Regarding Tinnitus Loudness	Effectiveness Regarding Tinnitus-Induced Distress	Age	TQ Score at Admission	Grade of Hearing Loss
Tinnitus duration in months	Correlation Coefficient	--					
	Sig. (2-tailed)						
	n	32					
Effectiveness regarding tinnitus loudness	Correlation Coefficient	0.212	--				
	Sig. (2-tailed)	0.245					
	n	32	66				
Effectiveness regarding tinnitus-induced distress	Correlation Coefficient	−0.142	**0.662 ***	--			
	Sig. (2-tailed)	0.438	**0.000**				
	n	32	66	66			
Age	Correlation Coefficient	0.201	0.135	0.033	--		
	Sig. (2-tailed)	0.270	0.280	0.795			
	n	32	66	66	66		
TQ score at admission	Correlation Coefficient	0.196	−0.012	−0.106	0.245	--	
	Sig. (2-tailed)	0.282	0.929	0.426	0.062		
	n	32	59	59	59	59	
Grade of hearing loss	Correlation Coefficient	0.113	−0.108	−0.130	**0.383 ***	**0.425 ***	--
	Sig. (2-tailed)	0.538	0.389	0.298	**0.002**	**0.001**	
	n	32	66	66	66	59	66

4. Discussion

In the current proof-of-concept study, we wanted to determine if non-invasive electrical stimulation through the ear canal can suppress loudness and tinnitus-induced distress. Moreover, we sought to determine the factors influencing the suppressing effect. The study was designed to deliver proof of concept and demonstrate the feasibility of electrical stimulation in reducing tinnitus loudness and distress. The factors tested included the frequency of current used for stimulation, the sequence of application of different stimulation currents, tinnitus grade at admission, tinnitus laterality, sex, and age of the patients. Some intermediate results obtained during this project have already been reported in the literature [20] to satisfy the funding agency's requirements.

Analysis of the electrical stimulation results showed that 47% of patients in our study experienced a statistically significant reduction in tinnitus loudness. Other studies using a similar electrical stimulation system to reduce tinnitus have had mixed results. Mielczarek et al. performed two studies. The first included six patients who received unilateral stimulation, after which improvement was noted in 83.3% of the ears and no change in 16.7% [24]. In the second study, the ears of 28 patients with tinnitus were tested individually, and a reduction in tinnitus intensity was found in 75%, no change in 18%, and worsening in 7% [25]. The study by Zeng et al. [26] included ten patients with tinnitus, four of whom received non-invasive stimulation via the outer ear. Two patients reported no change during or after stimulation. The other two reported a slight reduction in tinnitus during stimulation, and one found its complete disappearance after stimulation. Finally, a study by Suh et al. [27] in 14 tinnitus patients showed an average 22% reduction in tinnitus when stimulated through the ear canal. There are fundamental differences between our current study and those conducted by other researchers. The first difference is in the number of patients, which were 66 in our study, 6 and 28 in Mielczarek's study, 4 in Zeng's study, and 14 in Suh's study. Not only the number but also the age of the patients varied (mean 54.4 ± 10.44 years in our study, 53.4 ± 15.6 and 58.5 ± 11.83 years in Mielczarek's study, 61.5 ± 9.25 years in Zeng's study, and 44 years in Suh's study with no SD mentioned).

Other differences are the parameters used for stimulation, such as frequency (100 or 1000 Hz for us, 250 Hz [24], or 0.25, 1, 2, 3, 4, 5, 6, 7, and 8 kHz [25] for Mielczarek, 10 to 10,000 Hz for Zeng and 0.01 to 10 kHz for Suh), as well as stimulation duration (10 min for us, not specified for Mielczarek, 2–3 min and sometimes longer for Zeng, and 3 min or longer for Suh). In addition, due to a lack of suitable commercially available equipment, we and other groups used homemade stimulation devices, which could have also contributed to differences in the results.

The frequency of the current used (100 Hz or 1000 Hz) and the sequence of its application did not produce significant differences in reducing tinnitus loudness or distress under the applied conditions. The subjective loudness of the tinnitus measured in the entire group had already decreased significantly on the first day after the 10-min stimulation and on the second and third days. In contrast, tinnitus distress did not decrease significantly until the second and third days of stimulation.

Women reported reduced tinnitus loudness after the first, second, and third stimulation. In contrast, men reported a reduction after the second and third stimulation. Gender differences in sensory reactivity to external electrical stimulation are known to explain the greater sensitivity to pain in women [28,29], likely due to differences in body fat or water content [30]. This type of study has not yet been conducted in audiological research. Still, the physical factors affecting women's greater sensitivity to electrical stimulation could likely be universal, explaining the results of our study.

We also found that patients with compensated/habituated and decompensated/unhabituated tinnitus reported significantly reduced loudness after the second and third stimulations. Despite this, only patients with compensated/habituated tinnitus experienced a significant reduction in tinnitus distress after the 3 days of electrical stimulation. No comparable data are available in published research; however, it is known that the emotional status of patients affects both loudness and tinnitus-induced distress [31,32] and can be subject to fluctuations [33]. We hypothesize that the patients with decompensated/unhabituated tinnitus may have negative valence and emotional status that contribute to tinnitus-induced distress but are not a target of electrical stimulation. However, since the emotional status of the patients was not the subject of our study, we cannot confirm or reject such a hypothesis.

There were differences in stimulation efficacy between patients with unilateral and bilateral tinnitus. The latter group reported a reduction in tinnitus loudness after the first stimulation as well as the second and third stimulations. In contrast, patients with unilateral tinnitus improved only after the third stimulation. We thought this result could be attributed to possible differences in tinnitus habituation between the groups. Still, the proportion of compensated/habituated cases within the two groups (7 cases (58.3%) in the unilateral group and 30 (55.6%) in the bilateral group) were comparable and cannot explain the effect seen. However, our sample was relatively small, and no data were available on compensation for three patients with unilateral tinnitus (25% of the group) and four patients in a bilateral group (7.4%). Different results were obtained by Genitsaridi et al. [34]

and Song et al. [35], who suggested that unilateral tinnitus is more distressing than bilateral. Nevertheless, our observations are consistent with those made by Aazh et al. [36], who used a large sample of patients (n = 311) with unilateral and bilateral tinnitus for the comparative analysis and did not find differences in tinnitus severity between the two groups by Tinnitus Handicap Inventory THI. Furthermore, sex distribution was similar within the groups (W/M 33%/67% in unilateral and 46%/54% in bilateral group), therefore unlikely accounting for the effect seen. We also sought to explain the differences in the efficacy of electrical stimulation on tinnitus-induced distress in terms of audiological parameters. Using degrees of hearing loss in the comparative analysis, we found no explanation for the observed differences, which agrees with the study of Yang et al. [37]. Aazh et al. pointed out the importance of interaural asymmetry in unilateral but not bilateral tinnitus patients [36]. That aspect should be studied in the future in electrical stimulation. Moreover, neuropsychological differences between the patients with unilateral and bilateral tinnitus suggest significant deficits in the auditory memory and attention of the unilateral and not bilateral group [34], highlighting the disparity between unilateral and bilateral tinnitus.

Spearman's rank-order correlation confirmed the long-known association between hearing loss and tinnitus grade [38] or age and degree of hearing loss [39]. Still, it did not reveal any association between the electrical stimulation results and the patient's age, duration of tinnitus, degree of tinnitus, or hearing loss, suggesting complex mechanisms underlying the efficacy of stimulation.

The information gathered during this study fulfilled the expectations of the INTAKT project by providing parameters relevant to extracochlear electrical stimulation for tinnitus. This knowledge will be helpful in the future development of a tinnitus implant. In addition, the results should help select patients for cochlear implantation and may help predict tinnitus reduction after CI.

Our study is not without limitations. The first is the relatively small sample size, which should be increased. Initially, at least 100 patients were supposed to be included. However, because we conducted the study during the pandemic period (from the end of 2019 to the end of 2021), we were limited by patient access to the hospital, national and internal regulations governing the clinical research activities of tertiary healthcare centers during the pandemic, as well as the high incidence of COVID-19 among staff. The second limitation is the lack of a control group, which agrees with the proof-of-concept design but leaves questions about the placebo effect open. Future randomized controlled trials should include control, sham-stimulated tinnitus patients, who would be informed that the stimulation begins when, in fact, the equipment would be switched off. A final pitfall of our research is the insufficient audiometric information on matched tinnitus loudness and frequency and possible comorbid psychological conditions. It is recommended that such information be collected in future studies.

We envision a twofold future for this project. First, continuing the stimulation scheme described here would be essential to determine if stimulation on four or more consecutive days could extinguish or decrease the tinnitus sound and distress, as it did in one patient in our sample. It would also be essential to know how long the positive effect of electrical stimulation lasts. Second, this project was designed as a pilot one in preparation for the design of an extracochlear anti-tinnitus implant. The information gained during this study should help draw a blueprint for such a device in the near future.

5. Conclusions

The results of electrical stimulation through the ear canal in tinnitus patients presented in the current paper demonstrate the feasibility of such a procedure in a hospital setting and confirm the results of a few studies by other groups showing that almost half of the patients benefit from this type of therapy. The novel information provided by our research is that women respond more quickly to electrical stimulation than men, that the severity of tinnitus negatively affects the outcome of stimulation in terms of tinnitus distress but not in terms of loudness, and that the laterality of the tinnitus also contributes to the final outcome. In conclusion, non-invasive electrical stimulation through the ear canal seems to be a promising treatment for tinnitus. The results of our study suggest that further development of this type of therapy towards extracochlear tinnitus implants is warranted, as it may become a valuable therapeutic approach. Despite the benefits of the electrical stimulation provided by intracochlear stimulation with a CI, many tinnitus patients do not qualify for such surgery because they have no or only mild hearing loss. An extracochlear implant would be extremely valuable for these patients by directly eliminating the perception of tinnitus and leaving their hearing abilities intact.

Author Contributions: Conceptualization, H.O.; methodology, H.O. and J.V.; validation, J.V., M.G. and A.J.S.; formal analysis, J.V., H.O. and A.J.S.; investigation, J.V. and H.O.; resources, H.O.; data curation, J.V. and A.J.S.; writing—original draft preparation, J.V.; writing—review and editing, J.V., M.G., A.J.S. and H.O.; visualization, A.J.S.; supervision, H.O.; project administration, J.V.; funding acquisition, H.O. All authors have read and agreed to the published version of the manuscript.

Funding: This research was funded by The German Federal Ministry of Education and Research, grant number 16SV7875.

Institutional Review Board Statement: The study was conducted in accordance with the Declaration of Helsinki, and approved by the Institutional Ethics Committee of the Charité Universitätsmedizin Berlin (EA1/125/18, date of approval 15 January 2019).

Informed Consent Statement: Informed consent was obtained from all subjects involved in the study.

Data Availability Statement: The data presented in this study are available on request from the corresponding author due to ethical reasons.

Acknowledgments: The authors acknowledge the valuable contribution of Stefan Gräbel.

Conflicts of Interest: The authors declare no conflicts of interests.

Abbreviations

CI	cochlear implant
CNS	central nervous system
dB	decibel
FDA	Federal Drug Administration
Hz	Hertz
p	probability
SD	standard deviation
TQ	Tinnitus Questionnaire
VAS	visual analog scale
WHO	World Health Organization
Z	a difference in the median pre- vs. post-test rank score

References

1. Baguley, D.; McFerran, D.; Hall, D. Tinnitus. *Lancet* **2013**, *382*, 1600–1607. [CrossRef] [PubMed]
2. Haider, H.F.; Bojić, T.; Ribeiro, S.F.; Paço, J.; Hall, D.A.; Szczepek, A.J. Pathophysiology of subjective tinnitus: Triggers and maintenance. *Front. Neurosci.* **2018**, *12*, 866. [CrossRef] [PubMed]
3. Lee, H.J.; Kang, D.W.; Yeo, S.G.; Kim, S.H. Hearing aid effects and satisfaction in patients with tinnitus. *J. Clin. Med.* **2022**, *11*, 1096. [CrossRef] [PubMed]
4. Shapiro, S.B.; Noij, K.S.; Naples, J.G.; Samy, R.N. Hearing loss and tinnitus. *Med. Clin. N. Am.* **2021**, *105*, 799–811. [CrossRef] [PubMed]
5. Peter, N.; Liyanage, N.; Pfiffner, F.; Huber, A.; Kleinjung, T. The influence of cochlear implantation on tinnitus in patients with single-sided deafness: A systematic review. *Otolaryngol. Head Neck Surg.* **2019**, *161*, 576–588. [CrossRef] [PubMed]
6. Friberg, E.; Rosenhall, U.; Alexanderson, K. Sickness absence and disability pension due to otoaudiological diagnoses: Risk of premature death—A nationwide prospective cohort study. *BMC Public Health* **2014**, *14*, 137. [CrossRef] [PubMed]
7. Zeman, F.; Koller, M.; Langguth, B.; Landgrebe, M. Which tinnitus-related aspects are relevant for quality of life and depression: Results from a large international multicentre sample. *Health Qual. Life Outcomes* **2014**, *12*, 7. [CrossRef] [PubMed]

8. Trochidis, I.; Lugo, A.; Borroni, E.; Cederroth, C.R.; Cima, R.; Kikidis, D.; Langguth, B.; Schlee, W.; Gallus, S. Systematic review on healthcare and societal costs of tinnitus. *Int. J. Environ. Res. Public Health* **2021**, *18*, 6881. [CrossRef]
9. Portmann, M.; Cazals, Y.; Negrevergne, M.; Aran, J.M. Temporary tinnitus suppression in man through electrical stimulation of the cochlea. *Acta Otolaryngol.* **1979**, *87*, 294–299. [CrossRef]
10. Graham, J.M.; Hazell, J.W. Electrical stimulation of the human cochlea using a transtympanic electrode. *Br. J. Audiol.* **1977**, *11*, 59–62. [CrossRef]
11. Arts, R.A.; George, E.L.; Stokroos, R.J.; Vermeire, K. Review: Cochlear implants as a treatment of tinnitus in single-sided deafness. *Curr. Opin. Otolaryngol. Head Neck Surg.* **2012**, *20*, 398–403. [CrossRef] [PubMed]
12. Quaranta, N.; Wagstaff, S.; Baguley, D.M. Tinnitus and cochlear implantation. *Int. J. Audiol.* **2004**, *43*, 245–251. [CrossRef] [PubMed]
13. Borges, A.L.F.; Duarte, P.; Almeida, R.B.S.; Ledesma, A.L.L.; Azevedo, Y.J.; Pereira, L.V.; Bahmad, F., Jr. Cochlear implant and tinnitus-a meta-analysis. *Braz. J. Otorhinolaryngol.* **2021**, *87*, 353–365. [CrossRef]
14. Bahmad, F., Jr.; Carasek, N.; Lamounier, P. Cochlear implant in tinnitus management. *Curr. Opin. Otolaryngol. Head Neck Surg.* **2023**, *31*, 155–157. [CrossRef] [PubMed]
15. Song, J.J.; Kim, K.; Sunwoo, W.; Mertens, G.; Van de Heyning, P.; De Ridder, D.; Vanneste, S.; Lee, S.Y.; Park, K.J.; Choi, H.; et al. A quantitative electroencephalography study on cochlear implant-induced cortical changes in single-sided deafness with tinnitus. *Front. Hum. Neurosci.* **2017**, *11*, 210. [CrossRef] [PubMed]
16. Zeng, F.G.; Tang, Q.; Dimitrijevic, A.; Starr, A.; Larky, J.; Blevins, N.H. Tinnitus suppression by low-rate electric stimulation and its electrophysiological mechanisms. *Hear. Res.* **2011**, *277*, 61–66. [CrossRef] [PubMed]
17. Dixon, P.R.; Crowson, M.; Shipp, D.; Smilsky, K.; Lin, V.Y.; Le, T.; Chen, J.M. Predicting reduced tinnitus burden after cochlear implantation in adults. *Otol. Neurotol.* **2020**, *41*, 196–201. [CrossRef] [PubMed]
18. Olze, H.; Ketterer, M.C.; Péus, D.; Häußler, S.M.; Hildebrandt, L.; Gräbel, S.; Szczepek, A.J. Effects of auditory rehabilitation with cochlear implant on tinnitus prevalence and distress, health-related quality of life, subjective hearing and psychological comorbidities: Comparative analysis of patients with asymmetric hearing loss (ahl), double-sided (bilateral) deafness (dsd), and single-sided (unilateral) deafness (ssd). *Front. Neurol.* **2022**, *13*, 1089610. [PubMed]
19. Spiering, W.; Williams, B.; Van der Heyden, J.; van Kleef, M.; Lo, R.; Versmissen, J.; Moelker, A.; Kroon, A.; Reuter, H.; Ansel, G.; et al. Endovascular baroreflex amplification for resistant hypertension: A safety and proof-of-principle clinical study. *Lancet* **2017**, *390*, 2655–2661. [CrossRef]
20. Schmidt, B. Proof of principle studies. *Epilepsy Res.* **2006**, *68*, 48–52. [CrossRef]
21. Stevens, G.; Flaxman, S.; Brunskill, E.; Mascarenhas, M.; Mathers, C.D.; Finucane, M. Global and regional hearing impairment prevalence: An analysis of 42 studies in 29 countries. *Eur. J. Public Health* **2013**, *23*, 146–152. [CrossRef] [PubMed]
22. Hallam, R.S.; Jakes, S.C.; Hinchcliffe, R. Cognitive variables in tinnitus annoyance. *Br. J. Clin. Psychol.* **1988**, *27*, 213–222. [CrossRef]
23. Goebel, G.; Hiller, W. The tinnitus questionnaire. A standard instrument for grading the degree of tinnitus. Results of a multicenter study with the tinnitus questionnaire. *HNO* **1994**, *42*, 166–172.
24. Mielczarek, M.; Michalska, J.; Polatynska, K.; Olszewski, J. An increase in alpha band frequency in resting state eeg after electrical stimulation of the ear in tinnitus patients—A pilot study. *Front. Neurosci.* **2016**, *10*, 453. [CrossRef] [PubMed]
25. Mielczarek, M.; Norena, A.; Schlee, W.; Olszewski, J. Excitation of the auditory system as a result of non-invasive extra-cochlear stimulation in normal subjects and tinnitus patients. *Front. Neurosci.* **2018**, *12*, 146. [CrossRef] [PubMed]
26. Zeng, F.G.; Richardson, M.; Tran, P.; Lin, H.; Djalilian, H. Tinnitus treatment using noninvasive and minimally invasive electric stimulation: Experimental design and feasibility. *Trends Hear.* **2019**, *23*, 2331216518821449. [CrossRef] [PubMed]
27. Suh, M.W.; Tran, P.; Richardson, M.; Sun, S.; Xu, Y.; Djalilian, H.R.; Lin, H.W.; Zeng, F.G. Electric hearing and tinnitus suppression by noninvasive ear stimulation. *Hear. Res.* **2022**, *415*, 108431. [CrossRef]
28. Maffiuletti, N.A.; Herrero, A.J.; Jubeau, M.; Impellizzeri, F.M.; Bizzini, M. Differences in electrical stimulation thresholds between men and women. *Ann. Neurol.* **2008**, *63*, 507–512. [CrossRef] [PubMed]
29. Lund, I.; Lundeberg, T.; Kowalski, J.; Svensson, E. Gender differences in electrical pain threshold responses to transcutaneous electrical nerve stimulation (tens). *Neurosci. Lett.* **2005**, *375*, 75–80. [CrossRef]
30. Seno, S.-I.; Shimazu, H.; Kogure, E.; Watanabe, A.; Kobayashi, H. Factors affecting and adjustments for sex differences in current perception threshold with transcutaneous electrical stimulation in healthy subjects. *Neuromodulation* **2019**, *22*, 573–579. [CrossRef]
31. Probst, T.; Pryss, R.; Langguth, B.; Schlee, W. Emotional states as mediators between tinnitus loudness and tinnitus distress in daily life: Results from the "trackyourtinnitus" application. *Sci. Rep.* **2016**, *6*, 20382. [CrossRef] [PubMed]
32. Mazurek, B.; Haupt, H.; Olze, H.; Szczepek, A. Stress and tinnitus—From bedside to bench and back. *Front. Syst. Neurosci.* **2012**, *6*, 47. [CrossRef] [PubMed]
33. Simoes, J.; Bulla, J.; Neff, P.; Pryss, R.; Marcrum, S.C.; Langguth, B.; Schlee, W. Daily contributors of tinnitus loudness and distress: An ecological momentary assessment study. *Front. Neurosci.* **2022**, *16*, 883665. [CrossRef] [PubMed]
34. Genitsaridi, E.; Kypraios, T.; Edvall, N.K.; Trpchevska, N.; Canlon, B.; Hoare, D.J.; Cederroth, C.R.; Hall, D.A. The spatial percept of tinnitus is associated with hearing asymmetry: Subgroup comparisons. *Prog. Brain Res.* **2021**, *263*, 59–80. [PubMed]
35. Song, K.; Shin, S.A.; Chang, D.S.; Lee, H.Y. Audiometric profiles in patients with normal hearing and bilateral or unilateral tinnitus. *Otol. Neurotol.* **2018**, *39*, e416–e421. [CrossRef]

36. Aazh, H.; McFerran, D.; Danesh, A.A.; Louw, C.; Moore, B.C.J. A comparison of interaural asymmetry, audiogram slope, and psychometric measures of tinnitus, hyperacusis, anxiety and depression for patients with unilateral and bilateral tinnitus. *Int. J. Audiol.* **2023**, 1–7. [CrossRef]
37. Yang, C.W.; Jung, J.; Kim, S.H.; Byun, J.Y.; Park, M.S.; Yeo, S.G. Comparison of clinical characteristics in patients with bilateral and unilateral tinnitus. *Acta Otolaryngol.* **2015**, *135*, 1128–1131.
38. Mazurek, B.; Olze, H.; Haupt, H.; Szczepek, A.J. The more the worse: The grade of noise-induced hearing loss associates with the severity of tinnitus. *Int. J. Environ. Res. Public Health* **2010**, *7*, 3071–3079. [CrossRef]
39. Gates, G.A.; Mills, J.H. Presbycusis. *Lancet* **2005**, *366*, 1111–1120. [CrossRef]

Journal of
Clinical Medicine

MDPI

Systematic Review

Adverse Events with Hypoglossal Nerve Stimulation in the Treatment of Obstructive Sleep Apnea—A Systematic Review of Clinical Trials and Real-World Data

Mathias Wollny [1], Clemens Heiser [2,3,4], Ulrich Sommer [2,3], Christoph Schöbel [5,6] and Marcel Braun [5,6,*]

1 MedImbursement, 27412 Tarmstedt, Germany
2 Department of Otorhinolaryngology/Head and Neck Surgery, Klinikum rechts der Isar, Technical University of Munich, 80539 München, Germany
3 ENT-Center Mangfall-Inn, 83043 Bad Aibling, Germany
4 Translational Neurosciences, Faculty of Medicine and Health Sciences, University of Antwerp, 2610 Antwerp, Belgium
5 Department of Pneumology, University Medicine Essen—Ruhrlandklinik, West German Lung Center, University Duisburg-Essen, 45141 Essen, Germany
6 Faculty of Sleep and Telemedicine, University Medicine Essen—Ruhrlandklinik, West German Lung Center, University Duisburg-Essen, 45141 Essen, Germany
* Correspondence: marcelbraun@mac.com

Abstract: Background/Objectives: Hypoglossal nerve stimulation (HNS) emerged as an alternative treatment for patients with obstructive sleep apnea (OSA) a decade ago. Long-term clinical trials and real-world data show that HNS treatment provides significant and sustained improvements in both OSA disease control and quality-of-life measures over time. Given the nature of HNS treatment, with the requirement of using an implantable neurostimulation system, patient safety is a critical domain in the assessment of this technology. The objective of this review was to evaluate adverse events (AEs) and complications with HNS therapy in a systematic review of published evidence. **Methods:** Medline, Cochrane, and Web of Science were systematically searched to identify randomized controlled and real-world observational studies reporting relevant outcomes with HNS therapy for treatment of OSA that included procedure-, device-, and treatment-related AEs. **Results:** Out of 418 articles screened, 27 were reviewed for eligibility, and 17 studies, the majority found to have low-to-moderate risk of bias, with data on 1962 patients were included for further analysis. Across included studies, reporting of AEs was heterogeneous with regard to the classifications used and the extent of reporting. Over an average follow-up duration of 17.5 ± 16.9 months, the pooled mortality rate was 0.01% (95% CI = 0.0 to 0.2%), with all reported deaths being unrelated to HNS treatment. The HNS system survival probability over the follow-up time of 60 months was 0.9834 (95% CI = 0.9768 to 0.9882), with infections and request for removal by patients being the most common indications. The pooled surgical revision rate was 0.08% (95% CI 0.0 to 0.2%). Most reported treatment-related side effects were transient stimulation-related discomfort (0.08%, 95% CI = 0.0 to 0.2%) and tongue abrasions (0.07%, 95% CI = 0.0 to 0.2%). Based on the systematic review, a standardized set of endpoints was defined, aiming to harmonize safety data relevant to HNS therapy. **Conclusions:** In this systematic review, HNS therapy for treatment of OSA is associated with a positive patient safety profile. AEs occur mainly at device implantation and during the treatment acclimatization period. Due to a lack of available evidence, partially implantable HNS systems are underrepresented in this review, which limits the generalizability of the results. Significant heterogeneity was found for adverse event reporting. A framework for reporting HNS outcomes that includes AEs and side effects is proposed to facilitate comparability of the reported data.

Keywords: neurostimulation; sleep apnea; complications; patient experience

1. Introduction

Obstructive sleep apnea (OSA) is a multifaceted disorder characterized by repeated upper-airway collapse during sleep, leading to intermittent hypoxia and frequent awakenings. It is associated with various symptoms and accompanying health conditions such as excessive daytime sleepiness, cognitive impairment, and an increased risk of traffic accidents [1]. Moreover, OSA is strongly linked to cardiovascular problems such as hypertension, coronary artery disease, and stroke, making it the most common modifiable cause of hypertension [2–5].

Over the decades, there have been significant advancements in understanding its prevalence, diagnostic methods, and treatment options. Initially defined in 1965, OSA treatment options were limited to surgical interventions like tracheotomy tube placement for bypassing airway obstruction or uvulopalatopharyngoplasty (UPPP), first proposed by Ikematsu, which became more popular in the same decade [6–8]. With the introduction of continuous positive airway pressure therapy (CPAP) in 1981, a crucial breakthrough in non-surgical management of OSA was marked [9]. Conservative medical measures, such as lifestyle changes, or physiological supports like CPAP or mandibular advancement devices (MADs) often have a slower onset of action, with potential side effects and complications becoming apparent as treatment progresses [10]. This is because they typically aim to treat the underlying cause of the problem and support or heal the body naturally, such as pneumatic splinting with CPAP therapy or mandibular advancement with an MAD. Because these approaches often take time to become fully effective, potential complications may develop gradually. This is especially true if the treatment does not have the desired effect or if there are unwanted side effects, such as pressure sores due to the need to fix the masks on the face, dry eyes due to air leakage, and so on. This requires longer and closer follow-up, not only to monitor that the desired positive effects of the therapy are achieved but also to avoid adverse events. On the other hand, complications or adverse events often occur earlier with interventional/surgical procedures because they involve direct intervention in the body and may be associated with direct risks during the procedure and in the immediate postoperative period [11]. These may include infection, bleeding, or other traumatic or implant-related events. Because these procedures have a faster and more direct effect on the body, complications may manifest more quickly, requiring careful monitoring and possibly intervention closer to the initial procedure. This makes the risks of interventional/surgical procedures immediately apparent and often makes them seem higher. Overall, however, it is important to carefully weigh the pros and cons of each type of therapy and decide which treatment option is most appropriate on an individual basis and considering recent evidence, the patient's condition, the severity of the problem, and other relevant factors. Interventional/surgical therapies should not be considered inherently riskier.

This analysis aims to summarize and consolidate the best-available knowledge on the safety and adverse events of hypoglossal nerve stimulation for the treatment of OSA and provide a standardized format to display the evidence and allow for alternative interpretations.

2. Materials and Methods

2.1. Systematic Review

The research question was defined utilizing the PICO (Population, intervention, comparator, outcomes) format, centering on adult patients diagnosed with obstructive sleep apnea (OSA) who underwent hypoglossal nerve stimulation (HNS) therapy. The primary outcomes of interest encompassed the documented rates of adverse events and complications associated with HNS therapy, specifically focusing on the following clinical scenarios: all-cause mortality, HNS system explantation or replacement, re-operation or revision, bleeding or hematoma, postoperative pain, tongue abrasion, neuropraxia, and discomfort related to stimulation.

To identify pertinent publications, a comprehensive search strategy was developed, covering databases such as Medline, Embase, Cochrane, and Google Scholar (Table 1). The search was conducted up to 19 December 2023, and Rayyan software facilitated electronic data collection and screening [12].

Table 1. Search strategy for identification of relevant literature.

Keywords	Publication Date	Inclusion Criteria
Obstructive sleep apnea [Title/Abstract] AND (Implantable nerve stimulator [Title/Abstract] OR hypoglossal [Title/Abstract] OR Inspire implant [Title/Abstract])	January 2000–December 2023	• Publication in English language • Reporting a follow-up period of at least six months after implantation • Reporting follow-up data of at least ten subjects • All-cause mortality, HNS system explantation or replacement, re-operation or revision, bleeding or hematoma, postoperative pain, tongue abrasion, neuropraxia, and discomfort related to stimulation.

Two researchers (MW and MB) independently conducted initial screening using a blinded approach to mitigate identification bias. Inclusion criteria encompassed studies with at least ten subjects published between January 2000 and December 2023, written in English, with a follow-up period of at least six months after implantation of the stimulation system, and reporting outcomes of interest as defined above. Exclusion criteria included review articles, case reports, animal or in vitro studies, editorials, abstracts, publications involving pediatric populations, and non-English language articles. Discrepancies in screening were resolved through discussion and documented following the Preferred Reporting Items for Systematic Review and Meta-Analysis (PRISMA) framework [13].

Full texts were reviewed to determine study eligibility guided by the PICO framework, which allowed the inclusion of both randomized controlled trials and observational cohort studies. Quality assessment employed the *Cochrane Handbook for Systematic Reviews of Interventions*, using the ROBINS-I tool for observational and case–control studies [14].

Upon identification of the final set of eligible articles, data on adverse events and complications were systematically extracted to an MS Excel database. Extracted information included details such as reported outcomes, number of subjects, reported follow-up period, study type, and device type used.

2.2. Statistical Analysis

Reported event rates, expressed as proportions of the study population affected by the respective events, were entered into RevMan 5.4 for meta-analysis. Pooled effect sizes were calculated from weighted average means with 95% confidence intervals. Heterogeneity among studies was assessed using the chi-squared test and Higgins and Thompson's I2 statistics. Statistical significance was considered at an alpha level of 0.05 for two-tailed z-tests.

2.3. Standardized Definition of Clinical Endpoints

Based on the systematic review and identified clinical endpoints relevant to the safety profile of HNS therapy, a standardized set of therapy-related adverse events and side effects is proposed.

3. Results

3.1. Study Selection

Out of 418 articles initially screened, 27 underwent a thorough review for eligibility. A total of 384 studies were removed for various reasons, and 10 had to be excluded from further analysis after full-text review for eligibility, mainly due to reporting of study data already considered in other publications. Subsequently, 17 studies, collectively comprising data from 1962 patients and covering an average follow-up duration of 17.5 ± 16.9 months, met the inclusion criteria for further analysis (Figure 1). Most of these studies were found to have a low-to-moderate risk of bias (Table 2). Reporting of adverse events (AEs) across the included studies demonstrated notable heterogeneity, both in the utilized classifications or definitions, as well as the extent of reporting. Standardized reporting guidelines for AEs and complications with HNS therapy have not yet been established to the authors' knowledge.

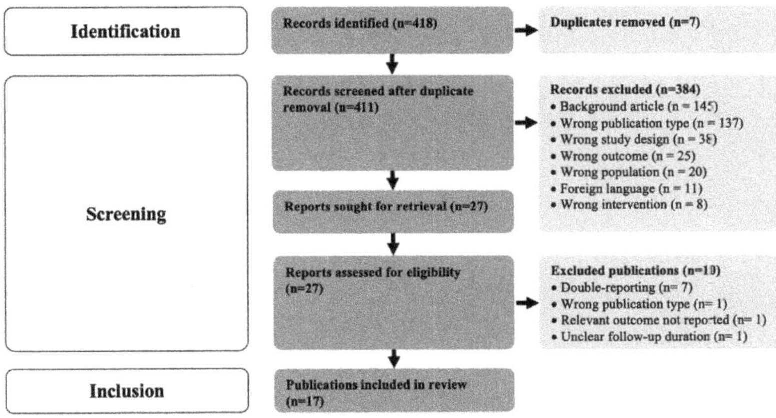

Figure 1. PRISMA flowchart of systematic literature search and review of identified studies.

3.2. All-Cause Mortality

The all-cause mortality rate of patients receiving HNS therapy, calculated over a mean follow-up duration of 17.5 ± 16.9 months, was low, with a weighted average of 0.01% (95% CI = 0.00 to 0.2%). Further analysis revealed that reasons for death during therapy were cancer (n = 3), cardiac events (n = 3), and homicide (n = 1), and none was considered by the reporting researchers as related to HNS treatment.

3.3. HNS System Survival

A Kaplan–Meier analysis was conducted to evaluate device survival over the follow-up reported in included studies, which included all 1962 patients in the studies identified (Figure 2 and Table 3). At a median follow-up duration of 12.0 months, the system survival probability was 0.9890 (95% CI = 0.9833 to 0.9927) and 0.9834 at the maximum follow-up duration of 60 months (95% CI = 0.9768 to 0.9882.). The most common reasons for device explantation were infection in the implant area of the HNS system and patient request for various reasons.

3.4. Device- or Implantation-Related and Treatment-Related Adverse Events and Side Effects

Rates of adverse events and side effects identified from the included studies and the respective 95% confidence intervals are presented in Figure 3. The pooled rate of surgical revision or re-operation was observed to be 0.08% (95% CI = 0.0 to 0.21%). Reasons identified encompassed revisions of hematoma or seroma, scar corrections, or repositioning of device components due to discomfort or technical dysfunction. Bleeding was defined as an event occurring either during surgery or leading to additional surgical measures, and occurred at a weighted average rate of 0.01% (95% CI = 0.00 to 0.07%). Neuropraxia was reported at a weighted average rate of 0.004% (95% CI = 0.00 to 0.02%), while postoperative pain was present at a rate of 0.07% (95% CI = 0.00 to 0.19%).

Table 2. Included studies, study characteristics, and risk-of-bias assessment using the ROBINS-I tool [14].

Study	Year	Sample Size	Follow-Up (Months)	Death	Explant/Replacement	Re-Operation/Revision	Bleeding	Post-Op Pain	Tongue Abrasion	Neuropraxia	Discomfort	Study Design	Device Type	Overall Bias	Reference
Ali NS et al.	2023	215	60	X	X	X	X	X	X	X	X	Observational cohort study	Fully implantable	critical	[15]
Eastwood PR et al.	2011	21	6	X	X	X	X	X	X	X	X	Observational cohort study	Fully implantable	serious	[16]
Eastwood PR et al.	2019	27	6	X	X	X	X	-	X	-	X	Observational cohort study	Partially implantable	moderate	[17]
Friedman M et al.	2016	43	6	X	X	X	X	X	X	X	X	Observational cohort study	Fully implantable	moderate	[18]
Heiser C et al.	2017	31	12	X	X	X	X	X	X	X	X	Observational cohort study	Fully implantable	moderate	[19]
Hinder D et al.	2022	50	12	X	X	X	-	-	-	-	-	Observational cohort study	Fully implantable	moderate	[20]
Kezirian EJ et al.	2014	32	12	X	X	X	X	X	X	X	X	Observational cohort study	Fully implantable	moderate	[21]
Mwenge GB et al.	2013	14	12	X	X	X	X	-	-	-	-	Observational cohort study	Fully implantable	moderate	[22]
Patil R et al.	2021	53	12	X	X	X	X	X	X	X	X	Observational cohort study	Fully implantable	moderate	[23]
Sarber KM et al.	2020	18	6	X	X	X	X	X	X	X	X	Observational cohort study	Fully implantable	serious	[24]
Schwartz AR et al.	2023	138	15	X	X	X	X	X	X	X	X	Randomized-controlled study	Fully implantable	moderate	[25]
Steffen A et al.	2019	60	36	X	X	X	X	X	X	X	X	Observational cohort study	Fully implantable	moderate	[26]
Suurna M et al.	2021	1019	12	X	X	X	X	-	X	-	X	Observational cohort study	Fully implantable	moderate	[27]
Van de Heyning PH et al.	2012	28	6	X	X	X	X	X	X	X	X	Observational cohort study	Fully implantable	moderate	[28]
Veugen CCAM et al.	2023	25	12	X	X	X	X	X	X	X	X	Observational cohort study	Fully implantable	low	[29]
Woodson BT et al.	2018	126	36	X	X	X	X	X	X	X	X	Observational cohort study	Fully implantable	low	[30]
Zhu Z et al.	2018	62	12	X	X	X	X	X	X	X	X	Observational cohort study	Fully implantable	moderate	[31]

Table 3. HNS system survival probability over follow-up time of included studies (SE = standard error of survival probability, CI = confidence interval of survival probability).

Month	Explantation Events	Subjects at Risk (n)	Censored Subjects at End of Period	Survival Probability (S_t)	SE	Lower 95% CI	Upper 95% CI
0	0	1962	0	1.0000	0.0000	1.0000	1.0000
6	9	1962	137	0.9950	0.0016	0.9907	0.9973
12	12	1825	1286	0.9890	0.0023	0.9833	0.9927
15	1	539	138	0.9885	0.0024	0.9827	0.9923
36	3	401	60	0.9870	0.0025	0.9809	0.9911
60	7	342	341	0.9834	0.0029	0.9768	0.9882

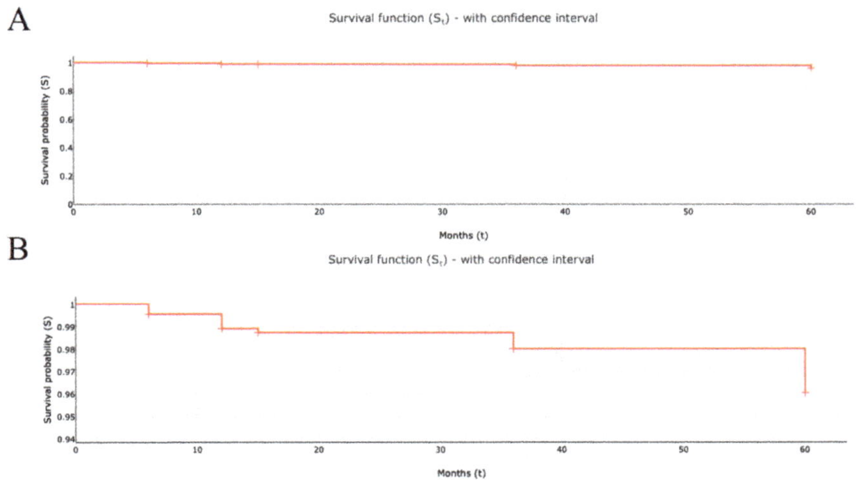

Figure 2. HNS system survival probability over follow-up time of included studies (S_t with 95% confidence interval): (**A**) = survival probability scaled from 0.0 to 1.0; (**B**) = survival probability scaled from 0.94 to 0.99.

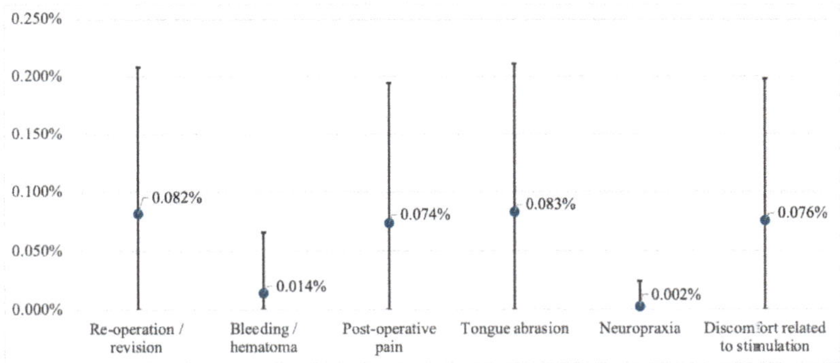

Figure 3. Weighted average rates and 95% confidence intervals of adverse events and side effects identified from included studies.

Most treatment-related side effects were reported as transient in the studies identified, and occurred primarily during the acclimatization period, while stimulation settings were being optimized over a period of three to six months after the implantation procedure. Discomfort related to stimulation was reported at a pooled rate of 0.08% (95% CI = 0.00 to 0.20%), while tongue abrasions were reported at a rate of 0.08% (95% CI = 0.00 to 0.21%).

3.5. Proposed Standardized Safety Endpoints for HNS Outcome Research

As a result of this systematic review, the absence of a standardized set of safety endpoints to be reported in clinical research on the outcomes of HNS therapy became apparent. This represents a significant gap, which complicates aggregation of results and makes comparability of outcomes difficult. To support future research and facilitate standardized data reporting, a set of relevant clinical endpoints are proposed and defined (Table 4). These endpoints shall be reported aside from the common objective and subjective efficacy and effectiveness endpoints relevant to the changes in OSA severity.

Table 4. Proposed standardized clinical endpoints for safety data in HNS therapy outcome research.

Proposed Clinical Endpoint	Timing/Definition
1. HNS system survival	End of study follow-up period • A: Initially implanted HNS system in situ • B: HNS system explanted upon patient request
2. Re-operation/revision	1. Re-operation or surgical revision in the index admission or ≤30 days of the index procedure • A: Re-operation or surgical revision due to bleeding, hematoma, or seroma • B: Re-operation or surgical revision related to any component of HNS system • C: Re-operation or surgical revision not related to any component of HNS system (hard- or software) 2. Re-operation or surgical revision > 30 days after the index procedure • A: Re-operation or surgical revision due to bleeding, hematoma, or seroma • B: Re-operation or surgical revision related to any component of HNS system • C: Re-operation or surgical revision not related to any component of HNS system (hard- or software)
3. Postoperative infections	Intervention due to infections ≤ 60 days of the index procedure • A: Re-operation or surgical revision due to infection in the implant area • B: Explant of any component of HNS system due to infection in the implant area
4. Neuropraxia or swallowing difficulties	Neuropraxia or swallowing difficulties presenting after the implantation procedure • A: Resolving without sequelae within 3 days after implantation procedure • B: Resolving without sequelae within 7 days after implantation procedure • C: Resolving without sequelae within 14 days after implantation procedure • D: Adverse event with sequelae or presenting > day 14
5. Post-operative pain	Post-operative pain related to any medical measure related to the implantation procedure • A: Pain requiring NSAR or other non-opioid pain-medication • B: Pain requiring oral opioids • C: Pain requiring intravenous pain medications • D: Pain requiring re-operation or surgical revision
6. Discomfort related to stimulation	1. Discomfort related to HNS stimulation occurring ≤ 30 days after system activation • A: Discomfort not impacting HNS adherence • B: Discomfort impacting HNS adherence 2. Discomfort related to HNS stimulation occurring > 30 days after system activation • A: Discomfort not impacting HNS adherence • B: Discomfort impacting HNS adherence

4. Discussion

To the best of the authors' knowledge, this is the first study to report aggregated data on the safety profile of HNS therapy for the treatment of OSA in adults. Overall, adverse events and side effects with HNS treatment are occurring at relatively low frequencies and severe complications are rare. Given the invasive nature of HNS therapy, which requires surgical implantation of a neurostimulation system that can consist of different components that are placed on different parts of the body, the safety profile is positive.

Various studies have shown that HNS therapy is an effective treatment for moderate–severe OSA in selected adult patients who have difficulty accepting or adhering to CPAP treatment and leads to a high surgical success rate with reasonable long-term complication rate related to the implanted device [32]. Besides the effectiveness in reducing OSA disease severity, the treatment leads to substantial and sustained improvement in quality of life and is associated with a positive patient experience [33,34]. As with any other medical treatment, HNS is not free from adverse events or complications, as shown in this research. Earlier studies reported different causes of adverse events related to HNS treatment, which include sensor lead malfunction, with reports of pain and malfunction due to sensor tip separation and migration of implant components [35]. Additionally, adverse events such as pneumothorax and pleural effusion have been reported during HNS implantation, especially in patients with comorbidities [36]. Explantations of HNS systems have been rare, with reasons including necessity for an MRI at a time when the device was not compatible, cosmetic reasons, and device-related infections. These findings highlight the importance of considering potential complications and risks associated with HNS therapy when managing patients with OSA and underlines the importance of standardized reporting of surgical interventions for the treatment of OSA to allow informed decision-making.

Importantly, the overall mortality with HNS therapy is very low, and no deaths in the included studies were related to the treatment. Since OSA itself is associated with significant long-term mortality, the aggregated rate reported here is quite low. Since current practice often excludes patients with significant comorbidities from HNS therapy, this might have contributed. On the other hand, effective OSA treatment with HNS may a have a positive effect on overall mortality. With a follow-up time of 60 months, the included studies will likely be too short to document such an effect. In addition, none of the studies was powered to detect any effects on this endpoint.

A recent study by Moroco et al. evaluated device-related revision and explantation rates with HNS implants, using post-market surveillance data to calculate event rates and risks [37]. Overall, 20,881 HNS treatments included, explantation and revision rates within the first year were 0.7% and 1.5%, respectively. In this real-world data set, the most common indication for explantation procedures was infection (0.4%) and surgical correction for revision procedures (0.7%). For HNS system with three-year follow-up data post-implantation (n = 5820), the explantation rate was 2.7% and the revision rate was 3.5%. Elective removal was the most common indication for explantation during this period (1.5%), while surgical correction was the most common reason for revision (1.1%). This study concluded that HNS demonstrates efficacy comparable to clinical trial data, with low rates of explantation and revision, indicating a satisfactory safety profile for this technology in real-world settings.

Thaler and Schwab reported on their experience implementing an HNS program at a tertiary care center [38]. They emphasized the importance of a team-based approach to patient flow, which requires close collaboration between sleep physicians and surgeons. The process included steps such as patient selection, preoperative evaluation, device implantation and activation, and long-term follow-up. The authors also discussed the challenges of patient selection for HNS treatment and emphasized the importance of thorough training and surgical planning. Another study from Murphy et al. found that surgical time for HNS implantation decreased significantly after the first five implants and then stabilized [39]. The average surgical time reduced by 27% from the first to the fifth implant, but the study did not determine when the learning curve reached a plateau. Adverse events were mostly resolved without intervention, and there were no serious complications related to the procedure. Interestingly, in this evaluation, surgeon experience did not significantly decrease the rate of surgical complications, possibly due to the low overall rate of serious complications and the limited number of implants at some centers.

Researchers at Virginia Commonwealth University conducted a study in 2022 to compare the safety of different surgical procedures for OSA based on real-world data from a federal health record database of sleep surgery outcomes [40]. One of the main findings from that study was that HNS statistically had a much lower complication rate (2–3%) compared to palatal surgery (20%) and multilevel surgery (21%) and lower readmission rates in the immediate postoperative period. The 90-day readmission rate was lowest in the HNS cohort, with 4% compared to palatal surgery alone (11%) and multilevel surgery (12%). The most common reasons for complications after traditional sleep surgery were bleeding, infection, wound dehiscence, respiratory compromise, myocardial infarction, stroke, deep vein thrombosis, renal failure, and pneumonia for palatal surgery. Specific complications reported for HNS procedures included the need for device revision, tongue weakness, difficulty speaking or swallowing, and device-related pain.

A potential explanation for the low rate of adverse events and complications from HNS therapy is the extent of standardization of patient pathways and surgical technique, which were optimized during clinical validation. Those were implemented in a relatively consistent approach, for example, via educational measures. In Germany, for example, a position paper from the German Society of Oto-Rhino-Laryngology, Head and Neck Surgery defines requirements for provider infrastructure and processes to ensure outcome quality and minimize complications, as well as minimal reporting standards to document treatment outcomes [41].

HNS therapy has been established as a viable alternative for the treatment of OSA over the past decade, offering significant and sustained improvements in disease control and quality of life. This systematic review underscores the favorable safety profile of HNS, highlighting its potential as a reliable treatment option. The findings have several important implications for clinical practice. Though the overall rate of complications and adverse events is low, patients should be thoroughly informed about the nature of HNS therapy, including the surgical procedure, potential risks, and benefits. Emphasis should be placed on discussing the possibility of temporary stimulation-related discomfort during acclimatization and other minor side effects during treatment initiation. While the surgical revision rate is low, clinicians should be prepared and trained to address any complications that may arise, such as device-related infections or explantation. For patient care after implantation, strategies should be developed to manage common side effects like tongue abrasions and stimulation-related discomfort, ensuring long-term patient comfort and sustainable therapy adherence.

Limitations

This study, though performed to high methodological standards and conducted with scientific rigor, is not free from limitations. It is important to underline that the extent of reporting adverse events among the identified research is low. After completion of the literature search process, a few relevant studies were published, which shed more light on this topic and confirm the findings from this analysis. Additionally, a high heterogeneity in reporting was found in published research on HNS outcomes. As such, among the 17 studies included, each varied with regard to the clinical endpoints reported. A set of standardized clinical safety endpoints as proposed in this article may help to increase the extent and consistency of reporting and improve comparability of outcomes. It is further important to note that most included studies reported data on a unilateral, breathing-synchronized HNS device, which may limit the generalizability of the results to other stimulation methods.

Furthermore, it is important to acknowledge that only two studies included were found to have low overall bias. As such, multiple confounders and biases could be present in the underlying data, which may have an impact of the findings presented in this study. Given the heterogeneity in reporting mentioned before, it was not possible to correct aggregated data, e.g., for device settings, medical service-procedures, and other parameters, related to the care context. For the endpoints we report here, such as explantation or re-operation, we believe that the data included are strong enough to conclude that HNS is overall a relatively safe surgical treatment option.

The findings of this study highlight the different types of adverse events and complications and the rate at which they can occur. The study also sheds light on the relatively high degree of heterogeneity in reporting these events in clinical studies and the need for standardization of endpoints. Given the high rates of complications and the irreversibility of traditional OSA surgery, this may also be relevant to this segment of OSA treatments. Improving reporting of adverse events will ultimately lead to a better understanding of potential risks related to surgical treatment for OSA, which will enable providers and patients to make informed decisions that consider individual characteristics and preferences of the patient. The set of endpoints related to adverse events and complications with HNS therapy proposed in this article may help to improve the database for this treatment and allow comparability of results from different care settings and across the spectrum of surgical interventions for OSA.

5. Conclusions

This review summarizes patient safety in the surgical intervention of HNS treatment that involves using an implantable neurostimulation system. The pooled mortality rate associated with HNS therapy was 0.01%, with reported deaths unrelated to the treatment. The HNS system safety profile was positive, with a device survival probability of 0.9834 (95% CI = 0.9768 to 0.9882) over a follow-up time of 60 months and a pooled surgical revision rate of only 0.08%. Common treatment-related side effects included transient stimulation-related discomfort and tongue abrasions, which mainly occurred during the acclimatization phase. Heterogeneity in reporting safety-related events was high across the included studies, which led to the development of a standardized set of endpoints, which is proposed in this article to harmonize safety data related to HNS therapy.

Author Contributions: Conceptualization: M.B., M.W., C.S., U.S. and C.H.; methodology: M.B. and M.W.; data curation: M.B., M.W. and C.H.; writing—original draft preparation: M.B., M.W. and C.H.; writing—critical review and editing: M.B., M.W., C.S., U.S. and C.H. All authors have read and agreed to the published version of the manuscript.

Funding: This research received no external funding.

Institutional Review Board Statement: Not applicable due to secondary analysis of published data.

Data Availability Statement: The data that support the findings of this study are not openly available due to reasons of sensitivity and are available from the corresponding author upon reasonable request.

Conflicts of Interest: M.W. is a consultant for SI-BONE (United States), a company unrelated to the research topic of this study, and reports personal fees from Inspire Medical Systems (United States). C.H. was a consultant for Inspire Medical Systems (United States) and has received personal fees from Neuwirth Medical Products (Germany) and research grants from Sutter Medizintechnik (Germany), Löwenstein Medical (Germany), Nyxoah (Belgium), and Inspire Medical Systems (United States). U.S. has received personal fees from Inspire Medical Systems (United States) and Neuwirth Medical Products (Germany) and research grants from Sutter Medizintechnik (Germany), Löwenstein Medical (Germany), Nyxoah (Belgium), and Inspire Medical Systems (United States). C.S. has received no personal fees, but reports institutional fees for lectures, advisory tasks and/or scientific projects from AstraZeneca (Germany), Bayer (Germany), Bioprojet, Bristol Myers Squibb, Idorsia, Inspire Medical Systems (United States), Jazz Pharmaceuticals (United States), Mementor, ResMed (Australia), Sleepiz (Switzerland), Zoll (Australia). M.B. has received personal fees from Onera Health (The Netherlands) and is a consultant for Astra Zeneca (Germany) and MLI SAS (France).

References

1. Olaithe, M.; Bucks, R.S. Executive dysfunction in OSA before and after treatment: A meta-analysis. *Sleep* **2013**, *36*, 1297–1305. [CrossRef] [PubMed]
2. Grote, L.; Hedner, J.; Peter, J.H. Sleep-related breathing disorder is an independent risk factor for uncontrolled hypertension. *J. Hypertens.* **2000**, *18*, 679–685. [CrossRef] [PubMed]
3. Peker, Y.; Carlson, J.; Hedner, J. Increased incidence of coronary artery disease in sleep apnoea: A long-term follow-up. *Eur. Respir. J.* **2006**, *28*, 596–602. [CrossRef] [PubMed]
4. Redline, S.; Yenokyan, G.; Gottlieb, D.J.; Shahar, E.; O'Connor, G.T.; Resnick, H.E.; Diener-West, M.; Sanders, M.H.; Wolf, P.A.; Geraghty, E.M.; et al. Obstructive sleep apnea-hypopnea and incident stroke: The sleep heart health study. *Am. J. Respir. Crit. Care Med.* **2010**, *182*, 269–277. [CrossRef] [PubMed]
5. Parati, G.; Lombardi, C.; Hedner, J.; Bonsignore, M.R.; Grote, L.; Tkacova, R.; Levy, P.; Riha, R.; Bassetti, C.; Narkiewicz, K.; et al. Position paper on the management of patients with obstructive sleep apnea and hypertension: Joint recommendations by the European Society of Hypertension, by the European Respiratory Society and by the members of European COST (COoperation

in Scientific and Technological research) ACTION B26 on obstructive sleep apnea. *J. Hypertens.* **2012**, *30*, 633–646. [CrossRef] [PubMed]
6. Gastaut, H.; Tassinari, C.A.; Duron, B. Polygraphic study of the episodic diurnal and nocturnal (hypnic and respiratory) manifestations of the Pickwick syndrome. *Brain Res.* **1966**, *1*, 167–186. [CrossRef] [PubMed]
7. Jung, R.; Kuhlo, W. Neurophysiological Studies of Abnormal Night Sleep and the Pickwickian Syndrome. *Prog. Brain Res.* **1965**, *18*, 140–159. [PubMed]
8. Ikematsu, A.; Yaku, Y.; Niho, M. The Ikematsu System for the Diagnosis of Snoring: A Review of 39 Years of Clinical Studies. In *Sleep Apnea and Rhonchopathy: 3rd World Congress, Tokyo, September 1991*; Karger Publishers: Berlin, German, 1993. [CrossRef]
9. Sullivan, C.E.; Issa, F.G.; Berthon-Jones, M.; Eves, L. Reversal of obstructive sleep apnoea by continuous positive airway pressure applied through the nares. *Lancet* **1981**, *1*, 862–865. [CrossRef] [PubMed]
10. Hoffmann, T.C.; Del Mar, C. Patients' expectations of the benefits and harms of treatments, screening, and tests: A systematic review. *JAMA Intern. Med.* **2015**, *175*, 274–286. [CrossRef]
11. Chan, A.-W.; Tetzlaff, J.M.; Altman, D.G.; Laupacis, A.; Gøtzsche, P.C.; Krleža-Jerić, K.; Hróbjartsson, A.; Mann, H.; Dickersin, K.; Berlin, J.A.; et al. SPIRIT 2013 Statement: Defining Standard Protocol Items for Clinical Trials. *Ann. Intern. Med.* **2013**, *158*, 200–207. [CrossRef]
12. Ouzzani, M.; Hammady, H.; Fedorowicz, Z.; Elmagarmid, A. Rayyan—A web and mobile app for systematic reviews. *Syst. Rev.* **2016**, *5*, 210. [CrossRef] [PubMed]
13. The PRISMA 2020 Statement: An Updated Guideline for Reporting Systematic Reviews | The BMJ. Available online: https://www.bmj.com/content/372/bmj.n71 (accessed on 20 October 2022).
14. ROBINS-I: A Tool for Assessing Risk of Bias in Non-Randomised Studies of Interventions | The BMJ. Available online: https://www.bmj.com/content/355/bmj.i4919 (accessed on 21 October 2022).
15. Ali, N.S.; Fitzpatrick IV, T.H.; Islam, A.S.; Nord, R.S. Mitigating Infection Risk in Upper Airway Stimulation. *Ann. Otol. Rhinol. Laryngol.* **2024**, *133*, 277–283. [CrossRef] [PubMed]
16. Eastwood, P.R.; Barnes, M.; Walsh, J.H.; Maddison, K.J.; Hee, G.; Schwartz, A.R.; Smith, P.L.; Malhotra, A.; McEvoy, R.D.; Wheatley, J.R.; et al. Treating obstructive sleep apnea with hypoglossal nerve stimulation. *Sleep* **2011**, *34*, 1479–1486. [CrossRef] [PubMed]
17. Eastwood, P.R.; Barnes, M.; MacKay, S.G.; Wheatley, J.R.; Hillman, D.R.; Nguyen, X.-L.; Lewis, R.; Campbell, M.C.; Petelle, B.; Walsh, J.H.; et al. Bilateral Hypoglossal Nerve Stimulation for Treatment of Adult Obstructive Sleep Apnea. *Eur. Respir. J.* **2019**, *55*, 1901320. [CrossRef]
18. Friedman, M.; Jacobowitz, O.; Hwang, M.S.; Bergler, W.; Fietze, I.; Rombaux, P.; Mwenge, G.B.; Yalamanchali, S.; Campana, J.; Maurer, J.T. Targeted hypoglossal nerve stimulation for the treatment of obstructive sleep apnea: Six-month results. *Laryngoscope* **2016**, *126*, 2618–2623. [CrossRef] [PubMed]
19. Heiser, C.; Knopf, A.; Bas, M.; Gahleitner, C.; Hofauer, B. Selective upper airway stimulation for obstructive sleep apnea: A single center clinical experience. *Eur. Arch. Otorhinolaryngol.* **2017**, *274*, 1727–1734. [CrossRef]
20. Hinder, D.; Schams, S.C.; Knaus, C.; Tschopp, K. Home sleep apnea testing with peripheral arterial tonometry to assess outcome in upper airway stimulation. *J. Clin. Sleep. Med.* **2022**, *18*, 2197–2205. [CrossRef] [PubMed]
21. Kezirian, E.J.; Goding, G.S.J.; Malhotra, A.; O'Donoghue, F.J.; Zammit, G.; Wheatley, J.R.; Catcheside, P.G.; Smith, P.L.; Schwartz, A.R.; Walsh, J.H.; et al. Hypoglossal nerve stimulation improves obstructive sleep apnea: 12-month outcomes. *J. Sleep. Res.* **2014**, *23*, 77–83. [CrossRef]
22. Mwenge, G.B.; Rombaux, P.; Dury, M.; Lengele, B.; Rodenstein, D. Targeted hypoglossal neurostimulation for obstructive sleep apnoea: A 1-year pilot study. *Eur. Respir. J.* **2013**, *41*, 360–367. [CrossRef]
23. Dhanda Patil, R.; Hong, M.P.; Ishman, S.L. Hypoglossal Nerve Stimulation in Veterans With Comorbid Insomnia and Sleep Apnea. *Otolaryngol. Head Neck Surg.* **2021**, *164*, 1345–1353. [CrossRef]
24. Sarber, K.M.; Chang, K.W.; Ishman, S.L.; Epperson, M.V.; Patil, R.D. Hypoglossal Nerve Stimulator Outcomes for Patients Outside the U.S. FDA Recommendations. *Laryngoscope* **2020**, *130*, 866–872. [CrossRef] [PubMed]
25. Schwartz, A.R.; Jacobowitz, O.; Eisele, D.W.; Mickelson, S.A.; Miller, M.B.; Oliven, A.; Certal, V.; Hopp, M.L.; Winslow, D.H.; Huntley, T.C.; et al. Targeted Hypoglossal Nerve Stimulation for Patients With Obstructive Sleep Apnea: A Randomized Clinical Trial. *JAMA Otolaryngol.–Head. Neck Surg.* **2023**, *149*, 512–520. [CrossRef] [PubMed]
26. Steffen, A.; Sommer, U.J.; Maurer, J.T.; Abrams, N.; Hofauer, B.; Heiser, C. Long-term follow-up of the German post-market study for upper airway stimulation for obstructive sleep apnea. *Sleep Breath* **2019**, *24*, 979–984. [CrossRef]
27. Suurna, M.V.; Steffen, A.; Boon, M.; Chio, E.; Copper, M.; Patil, R.D.; Green, K.; Hanson, R.; Heiser, C.; Huntley, C.; et al. Impact of Body Mass Index and Discomfort on Upper Airway Stimulation: ADHERE Registry 2020 Update. *Laryngoscope* **2021**, *131*, 2616–2624. [CrossRef] [PubMed]
28. Van de Heyning, P.H.; Badr, M.S.; Baskin, J.Z.; Cramer Bornemann, M.A.; De Backer, W.A.; Dotan, Y.; Hohenhorst, W.; Knaack, L.; Lin, H.-S.; Maurer, J.T.; et al. Implanted upper airway stimulation device for obstructive sleep apnea. *Laryngoscope* **2012**, *122*, 1626–1633. [CrossRef] [PubMed]
29. Veugen, C.C.A.F.M.; Dieleman, E.; Hardeman, J.A.; Stokroos, R.J.; Copper, M.P. Upper Airway Stimulation in Patients with Obstructive Sleep Apnea: Long-Term Surgical Success, Respiratory Outcomes, and Patient Experience. *Int. Arch. Otorhinolaryngol.* **2023**, *27*, e43–e49. [CrossRef] [PubMed]

30. Woodson, B.T.; Strohl, K.P.; Soose, R.J.; Gillespie, M.B.; Maurer, J.T.; de Vries, N.; Padhya, T.A.; Badr, M.S.; Lin, H.; Vanderveken, O.M.; et al. Upper Airway Stimulation for Obstructive Sleep Apnea: 5-Year Outcomes. *Otolaryngol.–Head. Neck Surg.* **2018**, *159*, 194–202. [CrossRef]
31. Zhu, Z.; Hofauer, B.; Wirth, M.; Frohnhofen, H.; Heiser, C. Selective upper airway stimulation in older patients. *Respir. Med.* **2018**, *140*, 77–81. [CrossRef] [PubMed]
32. Costantino, A.; Rinaldi, V.; Moffa, A.; Luccarelli, V.; Bressi, F.; Cassano, M.; Casale, M.; Baptista, P. Hypoglossal nerve stimulation long-term clinical outcomes: A systematic review and meta-analysis. *Sleep Breath* **2019**, *24*, 399–411. [CrossRef]
33. Braun, M.; Stoerzel, M.; Wollny, M.; Schoebel, C.; Ulrich Sommer, J.; Heiser, C. Patient-reported outcomes with hypoglossal nerve stimulation for treatment of obstructive sleep apnea: A systematic review and meta-analysis. *Eur. Arch. Otorhinolaryngol.* **2023**, *280*, 4627–4639. [CrossRef]
34. Braun, M.; Wollny, M.; Schoebel, C.; Sommer, J.U.; Heiser, C. Patient-reported experience with hypoglossal nerve stimulation in the treatment of obstructive sleep apnea. *Sleep Breath* **2024**, *28*, 221–230. [CrossRef] [PubMed]
35. Bellamkonda, N.; Shiba, T.; Mendelsohn, A.H. Adverse Events in Hypoglossal Nerve Stimulator Implantation: 5-Year Analysis of the FDA MAUDE Database. *Otolaryngol. Head Neck Surg.* **2021**, *164*, 443–447. [CrossRef] [PubMed]
36. Lorenz, F.J.; Goyal, N. Iatrogenic Pneumothorax During Hypoglossal Nerve Stimulator Implantation: A Large Database Analysis. *Otolaryngol. Head Neck Surg.* **2023**, *168*, 876–880. [CrossRef] [PubMed]
37. Moroco, A.E.; Wei, Z.; Byrd, I.; Rasmussen, A.; Chio, E.G.; Soose, R.J.; Huyett, P.; Steffen, A.; Heiser, C.; Boon, M.S.; et al. Device-related outcomes following hypoglossal nerve stimulator implantation. *J. Clin. Sleep. Med.* **2024**, *ahead of print*. [CrossRef]
38. Thaler, E.R.; Schwab, R.J. Single-institution experience and learning curve with upper airway stimulation. *Laryngoscope* **2016**, *126* (Suppl. S7), S17–S19. [CrossRef] [PubMed]
39. Murphey, A.W.; Baker, A.B.; Soose, R.J.; Padyha, T.A.; Nguyen, S.A.; Xiao, C.C.; Gillespie, M.B. Upper airway stimulation for obstructive sleep apnea: The surgical learning curve. *Laryngoscope* **2016**, *126*, 501–506. [CrossRef] [PubMed]
40. Nord, R.; Fitzpatrick, T.; DeShazo, J.P.; Reiter, E.R. Comparison of readmission and complication rates between traditional sleep surgery and hypoglossal nerve stimulation. *Laryngoscope Investig. Otolaryngol.* **2022**, *7*, 1659–1666. [CrossRef] [PubMed]
41. Steffen, A.; Heiser, C.; Galetke, W.; Herkenrath, S.-D.; Maurer, J.T.; Günther, E.; Stuck, B.A.; Woehrle, H.; Löhler, J.; Randerath, W. Hypoglossal nerve stimulation for obstructive sleep apnea: Updated position paper of the German Society of Oto-Rhino-Laryngology, Head and Neck Surgery. *Eur. Arch. Otorhinolaryngol.* **2021**, *279*, 61–66. [CrossRef] [PubMed]

Journal of
Clinical Medicine

MDPI

Article

Esophageal Dysmotility in Multiple System Atrophy: A Retrospective Cross-Sectional Study

Rumi Ueha [1,2,*], Misaki Koyama [2], Akiko Seto [3], Taku Sato [2], Takao Goto [2], Kenta Orimo [3], Jun Mitsui [3] and Tatsuya Yamasoba [2]

1 Swallowing Center, The University of Tokyo Hospital, Tokyo 113-8655, Japan
2 Department of Otolaryngology and Head and Neck Surgery, Faculty of Medicine, The University of Tokyo, Tokyo 113-8655, Japan; m.sekiguchi.tymc9@gmail.com (M.K.); taku.koro.z@gmail.com (T.S.); gottytakao@gmail.com (T.G.); tyamasoba-tky@umin.ac.jp (T.Y.)
3 Department of Neurology, Faculty of Medicine, The University of Tokyo, Tokyo 113-8655, Japan; seto-ngs@umin.ac.jp (A.S.); gokudogunma@gmail.com (K.O.); mituij-tky@g.ecc.u-tokyo.ac.jp (J.M.)
* Correspondence: ruu1025@yahoo.co.jp or uehar-oto@h.u-tokyo.ac.jp; Tel.: +81-3-3815-5411

Abstract: Background/Objective: Multiple system atrophy (MSA) is often associated with dysphagia and esophageal dysmotility (ED). However, ED in patients with MSA is poorly understood. To assess the relationship between ED, dysphagia, and other clinical findings in such patients and investigate the details of ED in MSA using high-resolution manometry (HRM). **Methods:** Patients from The University of Tokyo Hospital with MSA who underwent swallowing examinations, esophagography, and HRM between 2017 and 2022 were enrolled. A retrospective chart review of patients' backgrounds, swallowing function, and esophageal motility was performed. ED was evaluated using the Chicago Classification version 4.0. **Results:** Seventy-four patients with MSA were identified. The median age was 64 years, 48 patients (65%) were male, and the cerebellar variant type was predominant (69%). Abnormal upper esophageal sphincter (UES) resting pressure was observed in 34 patients (46%) and intraesophageal stasis in 65 (88%). High-severity MSA was a risk factor for developing dysphagia, vocal fold movement impairment, and abnormal UES function ($p < 0.05$). However, no overt clinical risk factors for ED were identified. Various types of ED were detected using HRM, and ineffective esophageal motility was the most frequent disorder. **Conclusions:** ED is a common occurrence in patients with MSA. Although a high-severity MSA may be a risk factor for developing dysphagia and vocal fold motion impairment, ED can occur regardless of clinical severity. Since ED is rarely detected based on subjective symptoms, careful evaluation of esophageal motility by esophagography or HRM is warranted in patients with MSA.

Keywords: multiple system atrophy; esophageal motility disorders; upper esophageal sphincter; high-resolution manometry; Chicago Classification

1. Introduction

Multiple system atrophy (MSA) is a rare and progressive neurodegenerative disorder characterized by its impact on various areas of the nervous system, encompassing both the brain and autonomic nervous systems. MSA is classified into parkinsonian (MSA-P) and cerebellar (MSA-C) variants [1]. Progressive degeneration of nerve cells and loss of nerve fibers can lead to various symptoms, including problems with movement and coordination, bladder control, and sexual function; tremors; speech difficulties; and issues with swallowing and breathing [2,3]. There is no established treatment for MSA; treatment is primarily supportive care aimed at managing symptoms and improving patients' quality of life [3,4]. Respiratory infections and sudden death during sleep are well-known causes of death in MSA [5,6], and studies have speculated that food and fluid regurgitation during sleep may induce respiratory compromise [7–9].

Esophageal motility is governed by the vagus nerve, and the vagal afferent pathway is essential for the central regulation of peristalsis [10,11]. Considering the involvement of the autonomic system in MSA [12], patients with MSA may experience esophageal dysmotility (ED) because of changes in pressure and motility within the esophagus. Only few studies have reported esophageal involvement in patients with MSA [8,9]. Our group has previously reported a high incidence of ED, abnormal upper esophageal sphincter (UES) resting pressure, and abnormal deglutitive proximal esophageal contraction (ADPEC) in pharyngeal high-resolution manometry (pHRM) [9,13], and a high prevalence of intraesophageal stasis (IES) and intraesophageal reflux (IER) in videofluorographic esophagrams (VFEs) in patients with MSA [9]. However, the relationship between ED, dysphagia, and other clinical findings in patients with MSA remains poorly understood.

VFEs are a commonly used method to evaluate esophageal motility. However, detailed dynamic assessment of esophageal motility disorders using HRM has recently become increasingly common [14]. Both these tests are recommended when assessing esophageal motility because the pathologies evaluated using VFEs and HRM differ. The Chicago Classification is commonly used in the gastroenterology field [15] for esophageal motility assessment using esophageal HRM (eHRM), and it is currently in its fourth edition (2020) [16]. This classification provides a standardized approach for the analysis and categorization of ED and divides ED into two types: "disorders of the esophagogastric junction outflow" and "disorders of peristalsis". Disorders of the esophagogastric junction outflow can be further classified into four types: types 1–3 achalasia and esophagogastric junction outflow obstruction. Peristaltic disorders include absent contractility, distal esophageal spasms, hypercontractile esophagus, and ineffective esophageal motility (IEM) [16]. There have been several reports regarding ED in patients with MSA in VFEs [8,9], but none have used eHRM.

This study aimed to assess how prevalent ED is in patients with MSA and investigate the impact of clinical factors, including disease severity, vocal fold motion impairment (VFMI), and swallowing dysfunction. Then, we examined details of ED in MSA using eHRM.

2. Materials and Methods

2.1. Patients and Ethics

Only patients diagnosed with MSA at the Department of Neurology and referred to the Department of Otolaryngology at The University of Tokyo Hospital for a swallowing evaluation between 2017 and 2022 were included, as were those who underwent all swallowing examinations, VFEs, and HRM (pharyngeal or esophageal) (Figure 1). Patient diagnoses were confirmed according to the consensus statement of the diagnostic criteria and excluded based on Gilman's criteria [1]. The Human Ethics Committee of The University of Tokyo (2487 and 2022179NI) approved this study. All patients provided written informed consent, and their anonymity was preserved. This study was conducted following the ethical guidelines established by the 1964 Declaration of Helsinki and its subsequent amendments.

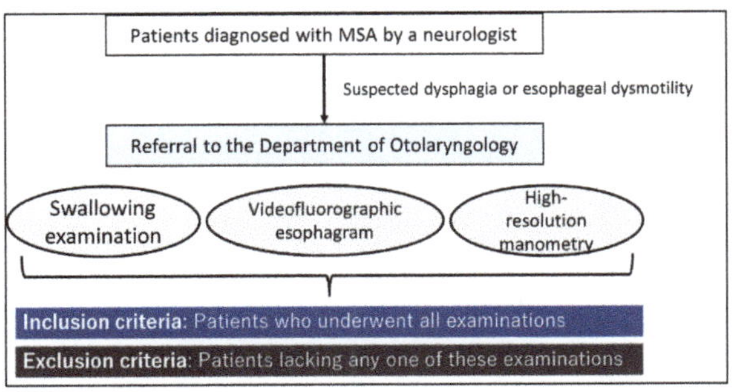

Figure 1. Inclusion and exclusion criteria.

2.2. Methodology

This study was a retrospective, single-center analysis based on medical charts from a hospital database. First, the analysis focused on clinical and demographic details, such as age, sex, and type of disease (MSA-C or MSA-P), disease duration, the severity level of MSA [17], use of prokinetic agents, the presence of VFMI, the presence of tracheostoma, the penetration–aspiration scale (PAS) score [18] on thin liquid (10 mPa·s, 5 mL), the functional oral intake scale (FOIS) [19], HRM parameters, and VFE findings. At our institution, VFEs and HRM are performed within one week of the swallowing endoscopic evaluation. Clinical findings were evaluated from medical charts at time points within 1 month before and after these examinations. The severity of MSA was assessed on a scale of 1 to 5 using the unified multiple system atrophy rating scale (UMSARS) part IV [20] (Table 1). Resting UES, impaired UES opening during swallowing, and ADPEC were examined as HRM parameters [9,13]. VFE findings such as IES, IER, and gastroesophageal reflux (GER) were evaluated [8,21]. Using the PAS [18] and FOIS [19], scores of 1–8 (most severe score: 8) and levels of 1–7 (normal level: 7) were assigned, respectively (Table 1).

Table 1. Patients' demographic details of severity levels of multiple system atrophy (unified multiple system atrophy rating scale, part IV) [20], penetration–aspiration scale [18], functional oral intake scale [19], and grading of intraesophageal stasis of contrast agent [21].

	Unified multiple system atrophy rating scale, part IV: global disability scale
Scale 1	Completely independent. Able to do all chores with minimal difficulty or impairment. Essentially normal. Unaware of any difficulty.
Scale 2	Not completely independent. Needs help with some chores.
Scale 3	More dependent. Help with half of chores. Spends a large part of the day with chores.
Scale 4	Very dependent. Now and then does a few chores alone or begins alone. Much help needed.
Scale 5	Totally dependent and helpless. Bedridden.
	Penetration–aspiration scale
Score 1	Material does not enter the airway.
Score 2	Material enters the airway, remains above the vocal folds, and is ejected from the airway.
Score 3	Material enters the airway, remains above the vocal folds, and is not ejected from the airway.
Score 4	Material enters the airway, contacts the vocal folds, and is ejected from the airway.
Score 5	Material enters the airway, contacts the vocal folds, and is not ejected from the airway.
Score 6	Material enters the airway, passes below the vocal folds, and is ejected into the larynx or out of the airway.
Score 7	Material enters the airway, passes below the vocal folds, and is not ejected from the trachea despite effort.
Score 8	Material enters the airway, passes below the vocal folds, and no effort is made to eject.
	Functional oral intake scale
Level 1	No oral intake.
Level 2	Tube dependent with minimal/inconsistent oral intake.
Level 3	Tube supplements with consistent oral intake.
Level 4	Total oral intake of a single consistency.
Level 5	Total oral intake of multiple consistencies requiring special preparation.
Level 6	Total oral intake with no special preparation but must avoid specific foods or liquid items.
Level 7	Total oral intake with no restrictions.
	Grading of intraesophageal stasis of contrast agent
Grade 0	Absence of intraesophageal stasis.
Grade 1	A minimal amount of contrast agent stagnation or a coating of contrast agent.
Grade 2	Stagnation with contrast agent that completely filled the lumen of the esophagus.

Second, partial correlations between the clinical profiles (age, sex, MSA type, disease severity, PAS scores, VFMI, IES, resting UES, impaired UES opening, and ADPEC) were statistically evaluated. Then, we statistically validated involvement of clinical factors in each of the abnormal esophageal findings, such as abnormal resting UES pressure, impaired UES opening during the swallow, ADPEC, and severe IES (grade ≥ 2) in HRM.

Finally, the type and frequency of esophageal motility disorders, based on the Chicago Classification version 4.0 [16], were investigated in patients whose esophageal motility was evaluated using eHRM.

2.3. HRM Study

As previously reported [9,13], HRM studies were performed on all patients in the upright position. An HRM catheter (Unisensor, Portsmouth, NH, USA) was lubricated with 4% viscous lidocaine, inserted transnasally, and positioned from the oropharynx to the esophagus (Starlet; Star Medical, Tokyo, Japan). The manometric catheter had an outer diameter of 4 mm, and 20 (for pHRM) or 36 (for eHRM) circumferential pressure sensors were spaced 1 cm apart. A videofluoroscopic swallowing study (VFSS) was simultaneously carried out in the lateral view. The study protocol included a 5 min baseline recording, followed by 3 dry swallows and 3 wet swallows for pHRM or 3 dry swallows and 10 wet swallows for eHRM using 5 mL of contrast agent (iohexol: Omnipaque®, Daiichi-Sankyo, Tokyo, Japan). pHRM was implemented from 2017 to 2019, and eHRM was implemented starting in 2020 at our facility. Although the catheter for pHRM was too short to evaluate the entire esophagus, HRM values of proximal esophageal measures, such as resting UES pressure, UES opening duration during swallowing, and the proximal esophageal contraction integral, were obtained for all patients using either pHRM or eHRM (Figure 2A).

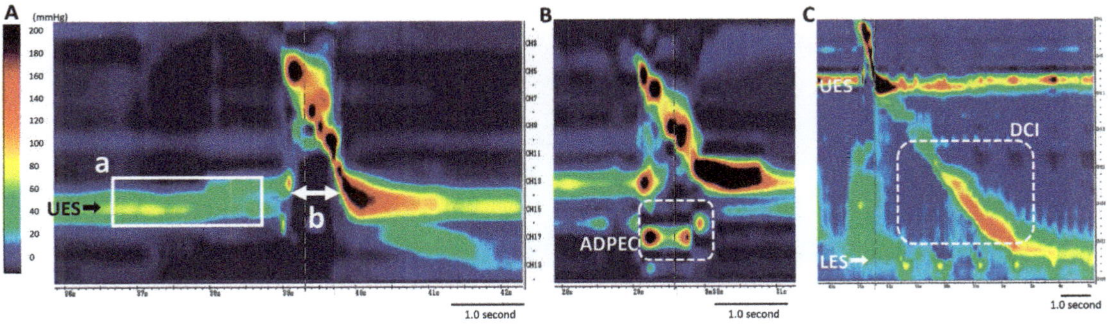

Figure 2. (**A**) Pharyngeal high-resolution manometry. a: resting upper esophageal sphincter (UES) pressure. b: UES opening during swallowing. (**B**) Abnormal hypertensive and discoordinated proximal esophageal contraction during swallowing (ADPEC). (**C**) Esophageal high-resolution manometry. DCI, distal contractile integral; LES, lower esophageal sphincter.

Abnormal HRM metrics in the UES and proximal esophagus were identified using the following criteria: abnormal resting UES pressure, hypertensive resting UES pressure (>104 mmHg), hypotensive resting UES pressure (<34 mmHg), and impaired UES relaxation pressure/duration (relaxation pressure > 12 mmHg/< 0.45 s) [13,22,23]. ADPEC was previously defined as abnormal hypertensive and discoordinated proximal esophageal contractions during swallowing as assessed by HRM [13]. In addition, a proximal esophageal contraction integral above 0 mmHg during UES opening was defined as abnormal (ADPEC) (Figure 2B). eHRM can evaluate lumen pressure from the hypopharynx to the lower esophagus (Figure 2C), and esophageal measures by eHRM were used to classify esophageal motility disorders according to the Chicago Classification version 4.0.

2.4. Videofluorographic Study

Videofluorographic studies were performed in the lateral and anteroposterior views. First, 3 swallows of 5 mL of thin liquid (10 mPa·s) were administered in the lateral view, and then the PAS score was evaluated. Next, a VFE was performed in the anteroposterior view with 3 swallows of 5 mL liquid. Swallowing was induced after the previous intraesophageal stasis was cleared during the second and third examinations. The presence and location of IES, IER, and GER were assessed.

The esophagus was anatomically divided into three sections based on fluoroscopic imaging according to previous reports [8,9,21]: (1) the cervical esophagus, proximal to the clavicles; (2) the aortic esophagus, from the clavicles distal to the aortic arch; and (3) the thoracic esophagus, from the bottom of the aortic arch to the lower esophageal sphincter (Figure 3a). IES was determined when the contrast agent failed to pass through any portion of the esophagus after the initial swallow, and after the completion of the primary peristaltic wave. The amount of contrast agent stagnation was quantified on a scale of 0 to 2: grade 0, absence of IES; grade 1, coating of contrast agent or minimal amount of contrast agent stagnation; and grade 2, stasis with a retained contrast agent that filled the lumen of the esophagus [21]. IER was present if any portion of the contrast agent traveled to a more proximal anatomical division of the esophagus [9,21]. GER is defined as any bolus that passes through the gastroesophageal junction and returns to the esophagus [9,21]. Two independent investigators performed all measurements. All patients were classified into two groups based on normal or abnormal resting UES pressure, normal or impaired UES opening during swallowing, the absence or presence of ADPEC, and IES grade (grades 0–1 or 2). Differences in the clinical features between the two groups were evaluated.

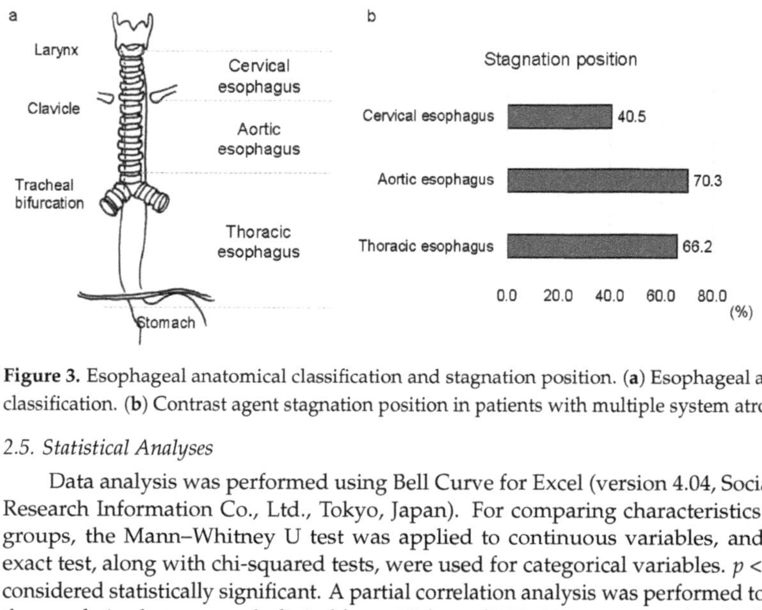

Figure 3. Esophageal anatomical classification and stagnation position. (**a**) Esophageal anatomical classification. (**b**) Contrast agent stagnation position in patients with multiple system atrophy.

2.5. Statistical Analyses

Data analysis was performed using Bell Curve for Excel (version 4.04, Social Survey Research Information Co., Ltd., Tokyo, Japan). For comparing characteristics between groups, the Mann–Whitney U test was applied to continuous variables, and Fisher's exact test, along with chi-squared tests, were used for categorical variables. $p < 0.05$ was considered statistically significant. A partial correlation analysis was performed to examine the correlation between each clinical factor. Values of 0.25–0.50 were considered a fair degree of association; 0.50–0.75, moderate to fair relation; and >0.75, good to excellent relation.

3. Results

3.1. Demographic Data and Characteristics of Patients

The demographic details of the enrolled patients are shown in Table 2. We identified 74 patients with MSA who met the eligibility criteria. The median age was 64 (interquartile range [IQR], 58–70) years, and a predominance of male patients (65%) was observed. Among the patients, 51 of 74 (69%) were diagnosed with MSA-C. The remaining 23 patients (31%) were diagnosed with MSA-P. The median disease duration was 48 (IQR, 33–66) months, and the median disease severity level was 3 (IQR, 2–4). Only four patients (4.1%) were taking oral prokinetic agents. VFMI was observed in 39 patients with MSA (53%), and tracheostomy was performed in 8 patients (11%). The median PAS score for patients with MSA was 2 (IQR, 1–5), and the median FOIS score was 7 (IQR, 5–7).

Table 2. Demographic and clinical data.

Characteristic	
Patients-no.	74
Age-years, median (IQR)	64 (58–70)
Men-no. (%)	48 (64.9)
MSA-C: MSA-P (no.)	51:23
MSA disease duration-mth. median (IQR)	48 (33–66)
Disease severity level	3 (2–4)
Use of prokinetic agents-no. (%)	4 (4.1)
Vocal fold motion impairment-no. (%)	39 (52.7)
Tracheostomy-no. (%)	8 (10.8)
PAS score. median (IQR)	2 (1–5)
FOIS score. median (IQR)	7 (5–7)

no., number; IQR, interquartile range; MSA, multiple system atrophy; MSA-C, cerebellar variant type of multiple system atrophy; MSA-P, parkinsonian variant type of multiple system atrophy; PAS, penetration–aspiration scale; FOIS, functional oral intake scale.

3.2. Esophageal Involvement in Patients with MSA

In patients with MSA, abnormal resting UES pressure was observed in 34 patients (46%); lower resting UES pressure was present in 29 patients (39%), whereas higher resting UES pressure was present in 5 patients (7%). Impaired UES opening during swallowing was found in 8 patients (11%), and ADPEC was detected in 26 patients (35%). IES was observed in 65 patients (88%): grade 0 in 9 patients (12%), grade 1 in 48 patients (65%), and grade 2 in 17 patients (23%). Regarding the location of contrast stasis, IES frequently occurred in the aortic esophagus (52 patients, 70%) and thoracic esophagus (49 patients, 66%) (Figure 3b). IER and GER were observed in 46 (62%) and 6 (8%) patients, respectively (Table 3).

Table 3. Esophageal involvement in all patients.

Esophageal Involvement		
Abnormal resting UES pressure-no. (%)		34 (45.9)
	Higher UES pressure	5 (5.8)
	Lower UES pressure	29 (39.2)
Impaired UES opening-no. (%)		8 (10.8)
ADPEC-no. (%)		26 (35.1)
Intraesophageal stasis	Grade median (IQR)	1 (1–1)
	Grade 0-no. (%)	9 (12.2)
	Grade 1-no. (%)	48 (64.9)
	Grade 2-no. (%)	17 (23.0)
Intraesophageal reflux-no. (%)		46 (62.2)
Gastroesophageal reflux-no. (%)		6 (8.1)

UES, upper esophageal sphincter; no., number; ADPEC, abnormal deglutitive proximal esophageal contraction; IQR, interquartile range.

3.3. Clinical Risk Factors for ED in Patients with MSA

Patients were classified into two groups according to the presence or absence and degree of abnormal findings related to ED to examine the clinical risk factors for ED in patients with MSA: abnormal resting UES pressure, impaired UES opening during swallowing, ADPEC, and IES grade (grades 0–1, or 2). The clinical factors listed in Table 4 were evaluated. MSA severity and penetration–aspiration were risk factors for abnormal UES function, including abnormal resting UES pressure and impaired UES opening during swallowing. MSA severity and VFMI were risk factors for ADPEC, whereas no overt clinical risk factors for IES were identified (Table 4).

Table 4. Clinical risk factors for esophageal dysmotility in patients with multiple system atrophy.

	Resting UES Pressure			UES Opening during Swallow		
	Normal	Abnormal	*p* Value	Normal	Impaired	*p* Value
Number (%)	40 (54.1)	34 (45.9)		66 (89.2)	8 (10.8)	
Age-years, median (IQR)	64 (55–69)	65 (60–71)	0.14	64 (58–70)	62 (55–67)	0.58
Men-no. (%)	19 (55.9)	29 (72.5)	0.14	44 (66.7)	4 (50.0)	0.35
MSA-C: MSA-P (no.)	C 20, P 14	C 31, P 9	0.08	C 47, P 19	C 4, P 4	0.22
Disease severity level	3 (2–4]	3 (3–4]	0.038 *	3 (2–4)	4 (4–5)	0.0013 **
Vocal fold motion impairment-no. (%)	20 (58.8)	19 (47.5)	0.33	33 (50.0)	6 (75.0)	0.18
PAS score. median (IQR)	1 (1–3)	3 (1–7)	0.034 *	1 (1–3)	8 (5–8)	<0.001 ***
	ADPEC			IES		
	Absent	Present	*p* Value	Grade 0–1	Grade 2	*p* Value
Number (%)	48 (64.9)	26 (35.1)		57 (77.0)	17 (23.0)	
Age-years, median (IQR)	66 (59–73)	63 (56–65)	0.047 *	63 (57–71)	67 (63–70)	0.28
Men-no. (%)	31 (64.6)	17 (65.4)	0.95	22 (61.4)	13 (76.5)	0.25
MSA-C: MSA-P (no.)	C 35, P 15	C 18, P 8	0.97	C 39, P 18	C 12, P 5	0.87
Disease severity level	3 (2–4)	3 (3–4)	0.0035 **	3 (2–4)	3 (3–4)	0.32
Vocal fold motion impairment-no. (%)	20 (41.7)	19 (73.1)	0.001 **	28 (49.1)	11 (64.7)	0.26
PAS score. median (IQR)	1 (1–5)	3 (1–6)	0.30	2 (1–5)	1 (1–6)	0.32

UES, upper esophageal sphincter; IQR, interquartile range; no., number; MSA-C, cerebellar variant type of multiple system atrophy; MSA-P, parkinsonian variant type of multiple system atrophy; PAS, penetration–aspiration scale; ADPEC, abnormal deglutitive proximal esophageal contraction; IES, intraesophageal stasis. *: $p < 0.05$; **: $p < 0.01$; ***: $p < 0.001$.

In addition, we investigated the correlation of each of the two factors among age, sex, MSA type, UMSARS part IV score, PAS score, VFMI, and esophageal movement disorder (abnormal resting UES pressure, UES opening disorder, and ADPEC) in patients with MSA. Partial correlation analysis was performed to determine the correlation between two variables after removing the effects of other variables. Positive correlations were observed between age and PAS, severity and VFMI, and severity and PAS, as well as between impaired UES opening during swallowing and PAS. However, no other clinical factors correlating with esophageal motility disorders were identified (Figure 4, Supplemental Table S1).

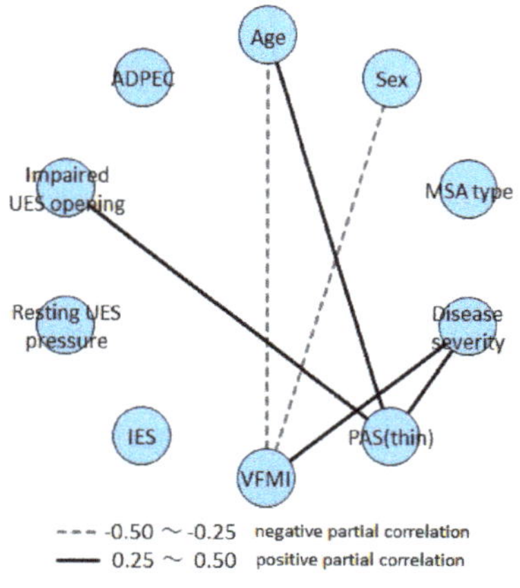

Figure 4. Partial correlation networks. PAS, penetration–aspiration scale; VFMI, vocal fold motion impairment; IES, intraesophageal stasis; UES, upper esophageal sphincter; ADPEC, abnormal deglutitive proximal esophageal contraction. −0.5 to −0.25: negative partial correlation, 0.25–0.5: positive partial correlation.

3.4. Various Esophageal Motility Disorders in Patients with MSA

Of the 74 patients with MSA, 38 were evaluated for esophageal motility using eHRM. eHRM revealed esophageal motility disorders in 31 patients (81.6%). According to the Chicago Classification version 4.0, 20 patients had IEM, 8 had achalasia (4 Type 1, 1 Type 2, and 3 Type 3), and 3 showed absent contractility. IEM was the most frequent disorder, and achalasia, which indicates impaired lower esophageal sphincter relaxation, was found in approximately 20% of the patients (Figure 5).

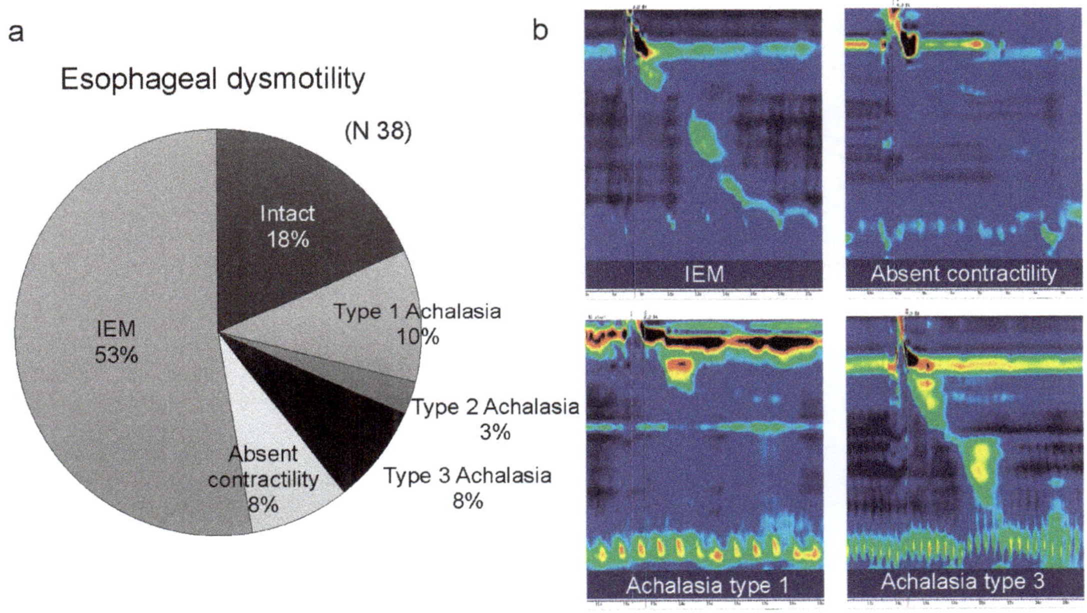

Figure 5. Various esophageal motility disorders in multiple system atrophy. (**a**) Proportion of various esophageal motility disorders. (**b**) Representative high-resolution manometric findings of various esophageal motility disorders. IEM, ineffective esophageal motility.

4. Discussion

MSA is a rare, progressive condition characterized by neurodegeneration that influences the autonomic nervous system and motor functions. Esophageal involvement in MSA has rarely been examined, although swallowing dysfunction, VFMI, and sleep apnea are frequent symptoms of MSA [24]. In this study, we identified a high prevalence of ED in patients with MSA. No clinical factors, including MSA severity, were correlated with ED, except for UES function, whereas MSA severity and aspiration were risk factors for abnormal UES function. In addition, we demonstrated that patients with MSA showed various types of esophageal motility disorders according to the Chicago Classification version 4.0.

The esophagus, a tube composed of fibrous and muscular tissue, facilitates the transport of food from the hypopharynx to the stomach via peristaltic contractions. The autonomic nervous system controls esophageal peristalsis and sphincter function with contributions from the parasympathetic and sympathetic divisions through the vagus nerve. Proximal regions, including the UES, are composed of striated muscle. Peristalsis in the striated muscle is controlled by somatic nerves with cell bodies located in the brainstem, specifically in a region of the rostral nucleus ambiguus. The sequential contractions of peristalsis are orchestrated by a pattern generator circuit in the brainstem, which incorporates the nucleus of the solitary tract and is modulated by vagal afferents. The distal esophageal regions, including the lower sphincter, are composed of smooth muscle, and the central and peripheral neural systems with intramural enteric circuitry control peristalsis. The myenteric plexus of the esophagus contains the peripheral neuronal elements that mediate the esophageal off-response, lower esophageal sphincter's relaxation, and hyperpolarization of the circular esophageal muscle cells [10,11,25]. Autonomic nervous system dysfunction leads to a decrease in the amplitude and frequency of esophageal contractions, resulting in delayed food transport from the pharynx to the stomach. This delay can cause food stagnation in the esophagus, leading to regurgitation and aspiration into the lungs. Since aging has been reported to be correlated with esophageal motor abnormalities [26], the high frequency of ED in MSA, which often occurs in middle-aged patients, should consider the influence of age.

Abnormal UES function in patients with MSA has been reported in several papers, with one reporting decreased UES pressure [27] and another reporting abnormally high UES pressure [28]. Since Parkinson's disease is associated with an abnormally increased UES resting pressure [29], it is not surprising to observe a higher UES resting pressure in patients with MSA-P, in which parkinsonism is predominant. In this study, both abnormally high and low UES pressures were observed in patients with MSA. However, lower UES pressures were observed more frequently, which may be attributed to the higher prevalence of patients with MSA-C compared with that of MSA-P patients in this study. In addition, similar to a previous report that patients with VFMI are more likely to have UES opening [30], this study showed that VFMI is a risk factor for impaired UES opening. This result is supported by the fact that the vagal nucleus governs both vocal fold movement and UES function.

Given that MSA leads to progressive neuronal degeneration in multiple brain regions, we speculated that patients with this condition could show various pathological esophageal motility issues. To the best of our knowledge, no previous study has evaluated esophageal motility using eHRM in patients with MSA, and this is the first report describing these findings. In this study, eHRM revealed that IEM was the most frequently observed, followed by types 1–3 achalasia, which indicates inadequate relaxation of the LES and no esophageal peristalsis, suggesting that MSA can cause various esophageal motility disorders. Furthermore, hypothesizing that clinical factors might contribute to esophageal motility disorders, we examined the partial correlation between ED and clinical factors, including age, sex, MSA type (P or C), and MSA severity. However, no significant associations were observed among them. Therefore, this means that patients with MSA, even those with mild MSA severity, should be aware of ED.

Patients with ED should be cautioned against nocturnal involuntary gastroesophageal regurgitation because sudden death is the most serious consequence of MSA [31] and has been reported to be the second most common cause of death in MSA [5]. The causes of sudden death include upper airway obstruction, central respiratory disturbance, or both [32], and the causes of upper airway obstruction include floppy epiglottis, VFMI, increased sputum because of dysphagia, and aspiration and suffocation secondary to food regurgitation during sleep [24,33,34]. A report [35] of a patient with MSA who had repeated aspiration pneumonia despite complete gastrostomy nutrition and no longer developed aspiration pneumonia after endoscopic jejunostomy feeding suggests caution against pneumonia because of aspiration of subclinical gastroesophageal regurgitation in patients with MSA. Generally, in MSA, ED can occur regardless of clinical severity. Thus, medical professionals must pay close attention to ED in these patients. The appropriate evaluation of esophageal motility may prevent or delay severe complications in patients with MSA because patients with ED do not necessarily report subjective symptoms. Suppose VFEs and HRM identify ED in patients with MSA. In that case, management options may involve treatments and recommendations such as medications to facilitate gastrointestinal motility, avoiding foods that are difficult to digest, and keeping an upright or semi-upright position for a few hours after meals to reduce the likelihood of food regurgitation. Looking ahead, it would be ideal to develop an artificial intelligence-driven diagnosis [36] of ED by deep learning from questionnaire scores (e.g., the FSSG questionnaire [37]) and other key clinical factors.

This study had several limitations. First, the study's retrospective nature is subject to selection bias, and longitudinal observations are required to elucidate the clinical significance of esophageal evaluation in patients with MSA. Second, an esophageal mucosal evaluation was not performed in most patients, although esophagitis may have influenced esophageal motility. Third, the amount of contrast agent used for the VFEs was small (5 mL), and the number of VFE evaluations was limited to reduce the potential aspiration risk. Future research on ED in patients with MSA should include longitudinal questionnaire surveys on esophageal symptoms, as well as prospective studies of esophageal evaluation, including upper gastrointestinal endoscopy, VFEs, and HRM.

5. Conclusions

ED is common among patients with MSA. Although a high severity of MSA may be a risk factor for developing dysphagia and VFMI, ED can occur regardless of clinical severity. Careful evaluation of esophageal motility by VFEs or HRM is warranted in patients with MSA, as subjective symptoms and physical examination rarely detect ED.

Supplementary Materials: The following supporting information can be downloaded at: https://www.mdpi.com/article/10.3390/jcm13175026/s1, Table S1. Partial correlation coefficient.

Author Contributions: R.U.: developed the concept, designed the study, collected and analyzed the data, and wrote the draft of the manuscript. M.K.: collected and analyzed the data, and reviewed the manuscript. A.S.: collected the data and reviewed the manuscript. T.S.: collected the data and reviewed the manuscript. T.G.: collected and analyzed the data, and reviewed the manuscript. A.S., K.O. and J.M.: collected the data and reviewed the manuscript. T.Y.: developed the concept and reviewed the manuscript. All authors: interpreted the data and contributed to the writing of the manuscript. All authors have read and agreed to the published version of the manuscript.

Funding: This work was supported by the Japanese Foundation for Research and Promotion of Endoscopy.

Institutional Review Board Statement: The study protocol was approved by the Human Ethics Committee of the University of Tokyo (No. 2487, 2022179NI, 31 October 2022) and complied with the tenets of the amended Declaration of Helsinki.

Informed Consent Statement: Written informed consent was obtained from every patient, and patient anonymity was preserved.

Data Availability Statement: The datasets used and analyzed during the current study are available from the corresponding author on reasonable request.

Conflicts of Interest: The authors declare that the research was conducted without any commercial or financial relationships that could be construed as a potential conflict of interest.

Abbreviations

MSA	multiple system atrophy
ED	esophageal dysmotility
HRM	high-resolution manometry
UES	upper esophageal sphincter
MSA-P	multiple system atrophy parkinsonian variant
MSA-C	multiple system atrophy cerebellar variant
ADPEC	abnormal deglutitive proximal esophageal contraction
pHRM	pharyngeal high-resolution manometry
VFE	videofluorographic esophagram
IES	intraesophageal stasis
IER	intraesophageal reflux
eHRM	esophageal high-resolution manometry

VFMI	vocal fold motion impairment
PAS	penetration–aspiration scale
FOIS	functional oral intake scale
UMSARS	unified multiple system atrophy rating scale
GER	gastroesophageal reflux
VFSS	videofluoroscopic swallowing study
IQR	interquartile range

References

1. Gilman, S.; Wenning, G.; Low, P.A.; Brooks, D.; Mathias, C.J.; Trojanowski, J.Q.; Wood, N.; Colosimo, C.; Durr, A.; Fowler, C.J.; et al. Second consensus statement on the diagnosis of multiple system atrophy. *Neurology* **2008**, *71*, 670–676. [CrossRef] [PubMed]
2. Fanciulli, A.; Wenning, G.K. Multiple-system atrophy. *N. Engl. J. Med.* **2015**, *372*, 249–263. [CrossRef]
3. Poewe, W.; Stankovic, I.; Halliday, G.; Meissner, W.G.; Wenning, G.K.; Pellecchia, M.T.; Seppi, K.; Palma, A.; Kaufmann, H. Multiple system atrophy. *Nat. Rev. Dis. Primers* **2022**, *8*, 56. [CrossRef] [PubMed]
4. Flabeau, O.; Meissner, W.G.; Tison, F. Multiple system atrophy: Current and future approaches to management. *Ther. Adv. Neurol. Disord.* **2010**, *3*, 249–263. [CrossRef]
5. Zhang, L.; Cao, B.; Zou, Y.; Wei, Q.-Q.; Ou, R.; Liu, W.; Zhao, B.; Yang, J.; Wu, Y.; Shang, H. Causes of death in Chinese patients with multiple system atrophy. *Aging Dis.* **2018**, *9*, 102–108. [CrossRef]
6. Papapetropoulos, S.; Tuchman, A.; Laufer, D.; Papatsoris, A.G.; Papapetropoulos, N.; Mash, D.C. Causes of death in multiple system atrophy. *J. Neurol. Neurosurg. Psychiatry* **2007**, *78*, 327–329. [CrossRef] [PubMed]
7. Davis, P.K.; Remick, D.G.; Parascandola, S.A.; Spangler, S.; Wise, R.K.; Martin, L.F. Intravascular plastic catheters potentiate tumor necrosis factor release and cardiac dysfunction secondary to infection. *Curr. Surg.* **1989**, *46*, 486–489.
8. Taniguchi, H.; Nakayama, H.; Hori, K.; Nishizawa, M.; Inoue, M.; Shimohata, T. Esophageal involvement in multiple system atrophy. *Dysphagia* **2015**, *30*, 669–673. [CrossRef]
9. Ueha, R.; Sato, T.; Goto, T.; Yamauchi, A.; Nativ-Zeltzer, N.; Mitsui, J.; Belafsky, P.C.; Yamasoba, T. Esophageal dysmotility is common in patients with multiple system atrophy. *Laryngoscope* **2021**, *131*, 832–838. [CrossRef] [PubMed]
10. Park, H.; Conklin, J.L. Neuromuscular control of esophageal peristalsis. *Curr. Gastroenterol. Rep.* **1999**, *1*, 186–197. [CrossRef]
11. Chen, J.H. Ineffective esophageal motility and the vagus: Current challenges and future prospects. *Clin. Exp. Gastroenterol.* **2016**, *9*, 291–299. [CrossRef] [PubMed]
12. Coon, E.A.; Cutsforth-Gregory, J.K.; Benarroch, E.E. Neuropathology of autonomic dysfunction in synucleinopathies. *Mov. Disord.* **2018**, *33*, 349–358. [CrossRef] [PubMed]
13. Ueha, R.; Goto, T.; Sato, T.; Nativ-Zeltzer, N.; Shen, S.C.; Nito, T.; Belafsky, P.C.; Yamasoba, T. High resolution manofluorographic study in patients with multiple system atrophy: Possible early detection of upper esophageal sphincter and proximal esophageal abnormality. *Front. Med.* **2018**, *5*, 286. [CrossRef]
14. Aspirot, A.; Faure, C. Esophageal dysmotility: Characterization and pathophysiology. *Dis. Esophagus* **2013**, *26*, 405–409. [CrossRef]
15. Bredenoord, A.J.; Fox, M.; Kahrilas, P.J.; Pandolfino, J.E.; Schwizer, W.; Smout, A.J.P.M.; International High Resolution Manometry Working Group. Chicago classification criteria of esophageal motility disorders defined in high resolution esophageal pressure topography. *Neurogastroenterol. Motil* **2012**, *24* (Suppl. S1), 57–65. [CrossRef] [PubMed]
16. Yadlapati, R.; Kahrilas, P.J.; Fox, M.R.; Bredenoord, A.J.; Prakash Gyawali, C.; Roman, S.; Babaei, A.; Mittal, R.K.; Rommel, N.; Savarino, E.; et al. Esophageal motility disorders on high-resolution manometry: Chicago classification version 4.0©. *Neurogastroenterol. Motil.* **2021**, *33*, e14058. [CrossRef] [PubMed]
17. Watanabe, H.; Saito, Y.; Terao, S.; Ando, T.; Kachi, T.; Mukai, E.; Aiba, I.; Abe, Y.; Tamakoshi, A.; Doyu, M.; et al. Progression and prognosis in multiple system atrophy: An analysis of 230 Japanese patients. *Brain* **2002**, *125*, 1070–1083. [CrossRef]
18. Rosenbek, J.C.; Robbins, J.A.; Roecker, E.B.; Coyle, J.L.; Wood, J.L. A penetration-aspiration scale. *Dysphagia* **1996**, *11*, 93–98. [CrossRef]
19. Crary, M.A.; Mann, G.D.C.; Groher, M.E. Initial psychometric assessment of a functional oral intake scale for dysphagia in stroke patients. *Arch. Phys. Med. Rehabilit.* **2005**, *86*, 1516–1520. [CrossRef]
20. Wenning, G.K.; Tison, F.; Seppi, K.; Sampaio, C.; Diem, A.; Yekhlef, F.; Ghorayeb, I.; Ory, F.; Galitzky, M.; Scaravilli, T.; et al. Development and validation of the Unified Multiple System Atrophy Rating Scale (UMSARS). *Mov. Disord.* **2004**, *19*, 1391–1402. [CrossRef]
21. Jou, J.; Radowsky, J.; Gangnon, R.; Sadowski, E.; Kays, S.; Hind, J.; Gaumnitz, E.; Taylor, A.; Robbins, J. Esophageal clearance patterns in normal older adults as documented with videofluoroscopic esophagram. *Gastroenterol. Res. Pract.* **2009**, *2009*, 965062. [CrossRef] [PubMed]
22. Mathews, S.C.; Ciarleglio, M.; Chavez, Y.H.; Clarke, J.O.; Stein, E.; Chander Roland, B. Upper esophageal sphincter abnormalities are strongly predictive of treatment response in patients with achalasia. *World J. Clin. Cases* **2014**, *2*, 448–454. [CrossRef]
23. Park, C.-H.; Lee, Y.-T.; Yi, Y.; Lee, J.-S.; Park, J.H.; Yoon, K.J. Ability of high-resolution manometry to determine feeding method and to predict aspiration pneumonia in patients with dysphagia. *Am. J. Gastroenterol.* **2017**, *112*, 1074–1083. [CrossRef] [PubMed]

24. Tsuchiya, K.; Ueha, R.; Suzuki, S.; Goto, T.; Sato, T.; Nito, T.; Yamasoba, T. Heightened risk of early vocal fold motion impairment onset and dysphagia in the parkinsonian variant of multiple system atrophy: A comparative study. *Clin. Park. Relat. Disord.* **2020**, *3*, 100037. [CrossRef] [PubMed]
25. Richards, W.G.; Sugarbaker, D.J. Neuronal control of esophageal function. *Chest Surg. Clin. N. Am.* **1995**, *5*, 157–171.
26. Gutschow, C.A.; Leers, J.M.; Schröder, W.; Prenzel, K.L.; Fuchs, H.; Bollschweiler, E.; Bludau, M.; Hölscher, A.H. Effect of aging on esophageal motility in patients with and without GERD. *Ger. Med. Sci.* **2011**, *9*, Doc22.
27. Park, H.W.; Jung, H.Y.; Lee, D.; Kim, D.H.; Jung, K.W.; Chung, J.W.; Choi, K.S.; Choi, K.D.; Song, H.J.; Kim, J.H. A case of multiple system atrophy presenting with esophageal dysphagia. *Korean J. Neurogastroenterol. Motil.* **2008**. *14*, 140–144.
28. Alfonsi, E.; Versino, M.; Merlo, I.M.; Pacchetti, C.; Martignoni, E.; Bertino, G.; Moglia, A.; Tassorelli, C.; Nappi, G. Electrophysiologic patterns of oral-pharyngeal swallowing in parkinsonian syndromes. *Neurology* **2007**, *68*, 583–589. [CrossRef]
29. Higo, R.; Tayama, N.; Watanabe, T.; Niimi, S. Abnormal elevation of resting pressure at the upper esophageal sphincter of Parkinson's disease patients. *Eur. Arch. Otorhinolaryngol.* **2001**, *258*, 552–556. [CrossRef]
30. Higo, R.; Tayama, N.; Watanabe, T.; Nitou, T.; Takeuchi, S. Vocal fold motion impairment in patients with multiple system atrophy: Evaluation of its relationship with swallowing function. *J. Neurol. Neurosurg. Psychiatry* **2003**, *74*, 982–984. [CrossRef]
31. Shimohata, T.; Aizawa, N.; Nakayama, H.; Taniguchi, H.; Ohshima, Y.; Okumura, H.; Takahashi, T.; Yokoseki, A.; Inoue, M.; Nishizawa, M. Mechanisms and prevention of sudden death in multiple system atrophy. *Park. Relat. Disord.* **2016**, *30*, 1–6. [CrossRef] [PubMed]
32. Ozawa, T.; Sekiya, K.; Aizawa, N.; Terajima, K.; Nishizawa, M. Laryngeal stridor in multiple system atrophy: Clinicopathological features and causal hypotheses. *J. Neurol. Sci.* **2016**, *361*, 243–249. [CrossRef]
33. Isozaki, E.; Naito, A.; Horiguchi, S.; Kawamura, R.; Hayashida, T.; Tanabe, H. Early diagnosis and stage classification of vocal cord abductor paralysis in patients with multiple system atrophy. *J. Neurol. Neurosurg. Psychiatry* **1996**, *60*, 399–402. [CrossRef] [PubMed]
34. Shepherd, K.; Hillman, D.; Eastwood, P. Symptoms of aerophagia are common in patients on continuous positive airway pressure therapy and are related to the presence of nighttime gastroesophageal reflux. *J. Clin. Sleep Med.* **2013**, *9*, 13–17. [CrossRef] [PubMed]
35. Ogawa, T.; Oodaira, H.; Suzuki, Y.; Hashimoto, R.; Kato, H. Successive application of percutaneous endoscopic gastrostomy with jejunal extension and percutaneous endoscopic jejunostomy in a case of multiple system atrophy. *Rinsho Shinkeigaku* **2009**, *49*, 370–373. (In Japanese) [CrossRef]
36. Taciuc, I.-A.; Dumitru, M.; Vrinceanu, D.; Gherghe, M.; Manole, F.; Marinescu, A.; Serboiu, C.; Neagos, A.; Costache, A. Applications and challenges of neural networks in otolaryngology (Review). *Biomed. Rep.* **2024**, *20*, 92. [CrossRef]
37. Kusano, M.; Shimoyama, Y.; Sugimoto, S.; Kawamura, O.; Maeda, M.; Minashi, K.; Kuribayashi, S.; Higuchi, T.; Zai, H.; Ino, K.; et al. Development and evaluation of FSSG: Frequency scale for the symptoms of GERD. *J. Gastroenterol.* **2004**, *39*, 888–891. [CrossRef]

Journal of
Clinical Medicine

MDPI

Article

Clinical, Histological, and HPV-Related Factors Associated to Diffuse Presentation of Exophytic Nasal Papillomas

Marta Fulla [1,2,*], Beatriz Quiros [3,4,5], Omar Clavero [3,4,5], Montse Gomà [2,6], Álvaro de Andrés-Pablo [3,4], Miquel Àngel Pavon [3,4,7], Anna Penella [1,2], Laia Alemany [3,4,7], Xavier González-Compta [1,2,8,†] and Marisa Mena [3,4,5,†]

1 Department of Otorhinolaryngology, Hospital Universitari Bellvitge, 08907 L'Hospitalet de Llobregat, Spain; apenella@bellvitgehospital.cat (A.P.); xgonzalez@bellvitgehospital.cat (X.G.-C.)
2 Program of Molecular Mechanisms and Experimental Therapy in Oncology, Bellvitge Biomedical Research Institute (IDIBELL), 08907 L'Hospitalet de Llobregat, Spain; mgoma@bellvitgehospital.cat
3 Cancer Epidemiology Research Program, Catalan Institute of Oncology (ICO), 08907 L'Hospitalet de Llobregat, Spain; bquiros@iconcologia.net (B.Q.); oclavero_ext@iconcologia.net (O.C.); adeandres@idibell.cat (Á.d.A.-P.); mpavon@iconcologia.net (M.À.P.); lalemany@iconcologia.net (L.A.)
4 Epidemiology, Public Health, Cancer Prevention and Palliative Care Program, Institut d'Investigació Biomèdica de Bellvitge (IDIBELL), 08907 L'Hospitalet de Llobregat, Spain
5 Centro de Investigación Biomédica en Red de Cáncer (CIBERONC), Instituto de Salud Carlos III, 28029 Madrid, Spain
6 Department of Pathology, Hospital Universitari Bellvitge, 08907 L'Hospitalet de Llobregat, Spain
7 Centro de Investigación Biomédica en Red de Epidemiología y Salud Pública (CIBERESP), Instituto de Salud Carlos III, 28029 Madrid, Spain
8 Faculty of Medicine, University of Barcelona, 08907 Barcelona, Spain
* Correspondence: mfulla@bellvitgehospital.cat; Tel.: +34-932-607-500; Fax: +34-932-607-533
† These authors contributed equally to this work.

Abstract: Background: Sinonasal exophytic papillomas (SNEP) are benign tumours arising from nasal mucosa. Human papillomavirus (HPV) infection seems to be related to the aetiology of a fraction of SNEP cases. SNEP presentation can be focal (FSNEP) or diffuse (DSNEP), but factors related to focal or diffuse presentation have not yet been well ascertained. This study aimed to analyse clinical, histological, and HPV-related differences between FSNEP and DSNEP. **Methods**: A retrospective cohort of 18 patients with SNEP from our centre were evaluated. Demographic, clinical and follow-up data were collected. All samples were subject to histopathological evaluation, DNA quality control, HPV-DNA detection, and viral load assessment. Univariate analyses were performed to evaluate differences between FSNEP and DSNEP. **Results**: Twelve SNEP patients were included in the final analysis. Seven patients had a diffuse nasal presentation, being younger than patients affected with FSNEP (42.7 years vs. 65.2 years, $p = 0.019$). The nasal septum was significantly more affected in DSNEP than in FSNEP (85.7% vs. 20%, $p = 0.029$). HPV-DNA was detected more frequently (100%) in DSNEP (HPV11 in six cases, HPV6 in one case) than in FSNEP (40%, $p = 0.045$, HPV6 in two cases). The median viral load among HPV6-positive samples was 626.8 virus/cell for FSNEP and 80.2 for DSNEP, and among HPV11-positive samples was 1673.7 for DSNEP. Recurrences were more frequent in the diffuse than in the focal group (85.7% vs. 20%, $p = 0.029$). **Conclusions**: The diffuse presentation of SNEP seems to be related to younger patients, nasal septum involvement, HPV infection, mostly HPV11, and a higher risk of recurrence.

Keywords: rhinology; surgery of the paranasal sinuses; clinical research; nose and paranasal sinuses; cohort study

1. Introduction

Sinonasal papillomas, a group of benign epithelial neoplasms located at the sinonasal tract, are classified as exophytic (SNEP), inverted, and oncocytic papillomas according to their histological characteristics (WHO classification of head and neck tumours 4th Edition 2017) [1]. All types may coexist [2].

SNEPs, also known as everted, fungiform, septal, or transitional papilloma, are the second most diagnosed subtype after sinonasal inverted papilloma. They represent 20–45% of all sinonasal papillomas with an incidence of 0.17 per 100.000 inhabitants per year [3–5]. They are more frequently diagnosed in males and in younger populations [6].

SNEPs usually manifest as progressive unilateral nasal obstructions, but in some cases, they can affect bilaterally or multifocally and may cause a complete nasal blockage. Less frequently, they can produce epistaxis or be diagnosed as a lesion emerging through the nostril. They mostly affect the anterior part of the nasal septum, but can also involve the lateral wall and the paranasal sinus [6,7]. They can be found as a localised or focal SNEP (FSNEP) or as a multifocal nasal pathology, although the latter is poorly described in the literature [8–10]. The diffuse or multifocal SNEP (DSNEP) has a different behaviour due to the wide involvement of the nasal mucosa and bilateral affectation. DSNEP often require multiple surgeries, given the high recurrence rate, and a closer follow-up [8]. The factors responsible for the diffuse presentation are not well ascertained due to the relative low prevalence of DSNEP. Recurrence rates in SNEP are around 22% [3,6], and previous publications observed recurrence in 83.3% of diffuse and bifocal SNEPs versus no recurrences in FSNEPs [8]. Malignant transformation is exceptional [11,12], with a single reported series of five SNEPs including two cases progressing to squamous cell carcinoma [13].

Histologically, an SNEP is composed of branching papillary structures covered by non-keratinizing squamous or transitional epithelium. Interspersed mucin-secreting cells and intraepithelial mucous cysts are often identified (Figure 1). The main differential diagnosis is the inverted sinonasal papilloma that shows a typically endophytic or inverted growth pattern and the cutaneous squamous papilloma of the nasal vestibular skin. Unlike SNEPs, a skin squamous papilloma entirely comprises squamous cells and lacks intraepithelial mucocytes [2,7,14].

SNEP treatment is endoscopic surgical resection. However, in the diffuse form with multiple recurrences, the use of adjuvant drugs may decrease the percentage of relapse. DSNEP has similarities to recurrent respiratory papillomatosis (RRP): both are benign lesions related to HPV in the respiratory tract tending to present multiple recurrences. The local injection of cidofovir in DSNEP has been published recently with promising outcomes, despite small sample size [15]. The rationale for the use of bevacizumab in DSNEP is based in the recent RRP-related literature [16,17]. Chen et al. concluded that a submucosal nasal injection of bevacizumab is a safe treatment in hereditary hemorrhagic telangiectasia patients [18].

SNEP aetiology has not been fully elucidated. Lately, different agents have been reported as implicated in the development of sinonasal papillomas such as chronic sinonasal inflammation, drug use, or smoking. In SNEP, no association with chronic rhinosinusitis has been reported [3,8]. In the last decades, several studies have explored the relationship between sinonasal papillomas and human papillomavirus (HPV), mostly in inverted subtype, without confirming an etiological implication [19–22]. Detection rates of HPV in SNEPs are estimated to be around 60%, despite the heterogeneity of the data in the world literature, with a predominance of low-risk HPV genotypes (HPV 6 and 11) [3,5,8,23–25].

To the best of our knowledge, there has not yet been evidence on the relationship between the presence of HPV infection and focal or diffuse SNEP clinical presentation.

The hypothesis of this study was that some clinical, histological, and HPV-related factors such as HPV-DNA prevalence, type distribution, and viral load could be related to the diffuse presentation of SNEP.

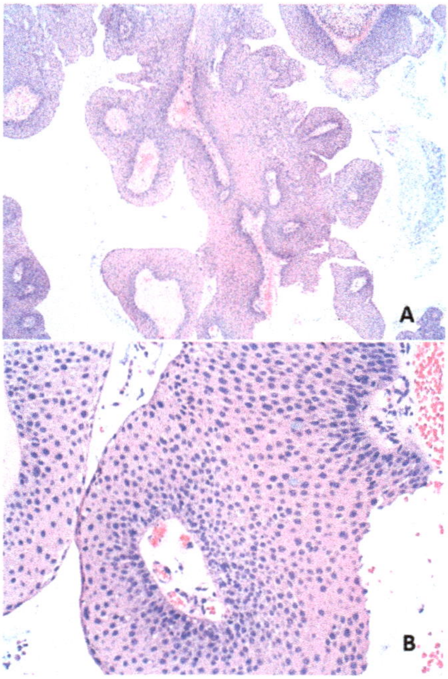

Figure 1. Sinonasal exophytic papilloma. (**A**) Squamous epithelium with exophytic growth pattern (hematoxylin-eosin 4×). (**B**) High power image shows non-keratinizing squamous epithelium and the presence of goblet cells with cytoplasmatic mucus (hematoxylin-eosin 20×).

2. Materials and Methods

2.1. Study Design

We conducted a retrospective study of a cohort of primary SNEPs consecutively diagnosed between 2013 and 2019 in our centre according to pathology department databases. Demographics and information about history of smoking, history of known HPV infection, immunosuppression, symptoms, localization in the nasal cavity, presentation (focal or diffuse), CT-scan findings, treatment, and follow-up were collected from medical records of otorhinolaryngology and pathology departments. We defined DSNEP as a multifocal lesion seen by nasal endoscopy and confirmed by biopsy. Unique lesions were classified as FSNEP. All cases were treated by endoscopic surgery using microdebrider and also, in DSNEP patients, with a local injection of bevacizumab. A complete resection without considering margins was performed in all cases.

Protocols were approved by our hospital ethics committee with the number PR413/20 and approval code ICO-VPH-PE-2020, which required informed consent to use archived samples, that were signed by the patients during the medical management and follow-up.

2.2. Formalin-Fixed, Paraffin-Embedded (FFPE) Blocks Processing and Histopathological Evaluation

FFPE blocks were processed under strict conditions to avoid contamination as previously described [26]. Briefly, four paraffin sections were selected for each FFPE block. Sections one and four were intended for histopathological evaluation after hematoxylin and eosin (H&E) staining and sections two and three for HPV testing and genotyping (sandwich method). Paraffin blocks were analysed under strict pre/post polymerase chain reaction (PCR) physical separation. To assess the DNA quality control, blank FFPE blocks were systematically processed in parallel as sentinels for contamination. Two pathologists designed a form specifically for the study (see Supplementary Material) for pathology review. The pathologists had no access to the original local diagnosis. After the first evaluation, a pre-established algorithm was used for diagnostic consensus concerning the two pathologists. All pathology slides were revised by a trained pathologist at ICO. The two pathologists reviewed the cases with discordant diagnosis and settled the diagnosis for a final evaluation.

2.3. Samples Further Processing and HPV Genotyping

FFPE-embedded samples were processed as previously described [27]. Total DNA was isolated using Maxwell® RSC DNA FFPE Kit (Promega, Madison, WI, USA), and HPV positivity and genotyping was tested before viral load determination using Anyplex™ II HPV28 Detection (Seegene Inc., Seoul, Republic of Korea) assay and following manufacturers' instructions. Anyplex™ II HPV28 Detection (Seegene Inc.) assay detects 28 HPV types including high-risk types and low-risk types (6, 11, 16, 18, 26, 31, 33, 35, 39, 40, 42, 43, 44, 45, 51, 52, 53, 54, 56, 58, 59, 61, 66, 68, 69, 70, 73, 82). All HPV11 or HPV6 positive samples were included in the viral load analysis.

2.4. HPV-DNA Detection, Genotyping, and Viral Load Determination

Custom TaqMan assays (Applied Biosystems) targeting HPV E6 gene of either HPV-6 or HPV-11, and previously designed by Forslund 2005 and Pan 2004 [24,25], respectively, were used to determine HPV copies. RNaseP TaqMan Copy number reference assay (applied biosystems) was used to determine the number of cells, assuming 2 copies of the *RPPH1* gene per cell.

HPV load was performed using the DNA leftover obtained for HPV testing and genotyping.

In total, 20 µL qPCR reactions containing 10 µL EagleTaq Master mix, 1 µL TaqMan assay, and 9 µL sample DNA were performed. DNA from 10^4 HaCaT cells was added to each qPCR reaction as background DNA. All qPCR reactions were carried out in triplicate in a CFX96 (Bio-Rad) as follows: 95 °C for 10 min, 45 cycles at 95 °C for 15 s, at 60 °C for 60 s, and at 72 °C for 1 s.

The number of copies of each target gene was obtained by linear interpolation from Cts and copy numbers obtained in regression standard curves. DNA from plasmids containing HPV-6 and HPV-11 genomes (ATCC-45150 and -45151, respectively) was used to obtain linear regression standard curves for absolute quantification of HPV-6 and HPV-11 copies. Viral load was described as HPV E6 copies per cell.

2.5. Statistical Analysis

Descriptive statistics were calculated for each of the variables studied. Fisher's exact tests were used for categorical variables to analyse statistically significant differences between DSNEP and FSNEP cases, and (Student's) *t*-test for continuous variables. Follow-up and time to recurrence were estimated. The statistical significance was established at p 0.05, adjusted by Bonferroni correction in case of characteristics with multiple choice options. The Cohen's D index was calculated for continuous variables and Cramér's V index for nominal variables to measure the effect size. All the analyses were performed with STATA 16.0 software.

3. Results

Eighteen SNEP patients diagnosed between 2013 and 2019 were selected and reviewed from the files of the pathology department in our centre. A total of 12 cases, from which FFPE samples were available, were included in the histopathological analysis and, finally, 12 were processed and tested (Figure 2).

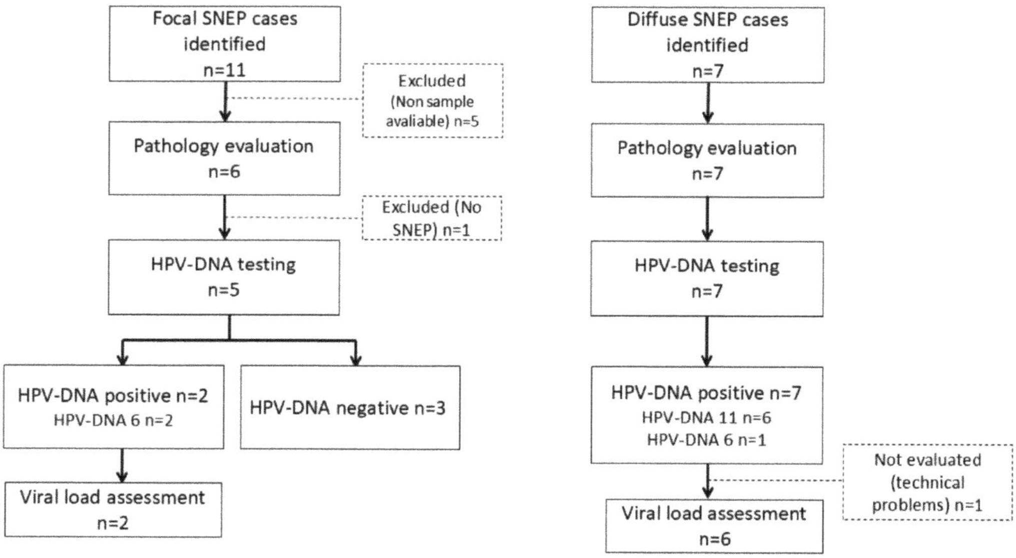

Figure 2. Flow chart of cases included in the study.

The characteristics of the patients are presented in Table 1. Most patients were males (83.3%) and ever-smokers (66.7%) with a mean age of 52.1 years and a median age of 48.5 years (range 30–92). None of them had a history of known HPV infection or immunosuppression. The majority of SNEP patients complained of nasal blockage at the diagnosis (75%) but others had rhinorrea (16.7%), epistaxis (16.7%), otitis media with effusion (8.3%), or no symptoms at all (8.3%). The most common localization of SNEP was in the septum (58.3%), followed by the inferior turbinate head (41.7%), the cupula of the nasal fossae (33.3%), and the lateral wall (33.3%). Less frequently, SNEP affected the floor of the nasal fossae and the middle turbinate head (two cases in each localization). Preoperative imaging was performed in 10 patients (83.3%) by CT scan. MRI was not used in any case. No imaging was performed in two patients (one FSNEP and one DSNEP) due to the small size of the lesions and its anterior location in the nasal fossae. CT scans showed swelling of the sinonasal mucosa (80%), sinus occupation (50%), and polipoid formation in the nasal fossae (40%). Diffuse nasal presentation were diagnosed in seven cases (58.3%). Seven patients (58.3%) had recurrence with a median time of recurrence of 5 months (range 1–67). The median time of follow-up was 46 months (range 4–100). No malignant transformation was detected during the follow-up. HPV-DNA prevalence was 75% (50% positive for HPV11, 25% positive for HPV6). Although histopathological evaluation confirmed that all 12 samples were exophytic nasal papillomas, minority foci of inverted papilloma were found in three cases.

Table 1. Demographic, clinical histological, and HPV characteristics of SNEP patients.

Characteristics	Cases (N = 12) n (%)	FSNEP (N = 5) n (%)	DSNEP (N = 7) n (%)	*p*-Value
Gender				
Male	10 (83.3)	3 (60.0)	7 (100.0)	0.152
Female	2 (16.7)	2 (40.0)	0	

Table 1. *Cont.*

Characteristics	Cases (N = 12) n (%)	FSNEP (N = 5) n (%)	DSNEP (N = 7) n (%)	p-Value
Age (years)				
Mean	52.1	65.2	42.7	
Rank	30–92	51–92	30–62	**0.019**
Median	48.5	54	42	
Smoking status				
Ever	8 (66.7)	2 (40.0)	6 (85.7)	0.152
Never	4 (33.3)	3 (60.0)	1 (14.3)	
Clinical symptoms *				
Nasal blockage	9 (75)	4 (80)	5 (71.4)	0.636 (1)
Rhinorrea	2 (16.7)	1 (20)	1 (14.3)	0.682 (1)
Epistaxis	2 (16.7)	1 (20)	1 (14.3)	0.682 (1)
Otitis media with effusion	1 (8.3)	1 (20)	0	0.417 (1)
No symptoms	1 (8.3)	0 (20)	1 (14.3)	0.583 (1)
Localization *				
Septum	7 (58.3)	1 (20.0)	6 (85.7)	0.045 (2)
Inferior turbinate head	5 (41.7)	1 (20.0)	4 (57.1)	0.179 (2)
Cupula/roof	4 (33.3)	2 (40.0)	2 (28.6)	0.576 (2)
Lateral wall	4 (33.3)	2 (40.0)	2 (28.6)	0.576 (2)
Floor	2 (16.7)	0	2 (28.6)	0.318 (2)
Middle turbinate head	2 (16.7)	0	2 (28.6)	0.318 (2)
Radiological characteristics *				
Swelling of sinonasal mucosa	8 (80)	3 (75)	5 (83.3)	0.576 (3)
Sinus occupation	5 (50)	2 (50)	3 (50)	0.689 (3)
Polipoid formation in the fossae	4 (40)	1 (25)	3 (50)	0.424 (3)
No CT scan	2 (16.7)	1 (20)	1 (14.3)	0.682 (3)
Behaviour				
Focal	5 (41.7)			
Diffuse	7 (58.3)			
Recurrence				
Yes	7 (58.3)	1 (20%)	6 (85.7)	0.045
No	5 (41.7)	4 (80%)	1 (14.3)	
Time to recurrence (months)				
Median	5	67	4	0.134
Rank	1–67	67	1–36	
Follow-up (months)				
Median	46	43	49	0.745
Rank	4–100	4–82	20–100	
HPV status				
Negative	3 (25.0)	3 (60.0)	0	**0.045**
Positive	9 (75.0)	2 (40.0)	7 (100.0)	
HPV genotype				
HPV11	6 (50.0)	0	6 (85.7)	**0.008 (4)**
HPV6	3 (25.0)	2 (40.0)	1 (14.3)	0.364 (4)
Negative	3 (25.0)	3 (60.0)	0	0.045 (4)
Histology				
Exophytic nasal papilloma	9 (75)	3 (60%)	6 (85.7)	0.364
Exophytic and inverted mixed papilloma	3 (25)	2 (40%)	1 (14.3)	

* Each case may fit in more than one item. In these cases, *p*-valor, to be considered for founding statistical differences, was adjusted with a Bonferroni correction: (1) $p = 0.01$; (2) $p = 0.008$; (3) $p = 0.013$; (4) $p = 0.017$. In bold, statistically significant differences. FSNEP: focal sinonasal exophytic papilloma, DSNEP: diffuse sinonasal exophytic papilloma.

Viral load of HPV6 positive cases ranged from 80.2 to 1169.9 copies/cell with a median of 83.9 copies/cell (mean of 444.6 copies/cell with a standard deviation of 627.9), and in HPV11 positive cases, ranged from 1058.7 to 3087.5 copies/cell with a median of 1673.7 copies/cell (mean of 1904.2 copies/cell and a standard deviation of 780.5). Viral loads were not evaluated due to technical problems in one HPV11 positive case (Table 2).

Table 2. HPV-DNA genotyping and viral load results.

Patient	Behaviour	HPV Genotype	Viral Load			
			Copies/Cell	Mean	Sdt	Median
1	FSNEP	Neg	NA	-	-	-
2	FSNEP	Neg	NA			
3	FSNEP	Neg	NA			
4	FSNEP	HPV-6	83.9	444.6	627.9	83.9
5	FNSEP	HPV-6	1169.9			
6	DSNEP	HPV-6	80.2			
7	DSNEP	HPV-11	1058.7	1904.2	780.5	1673.7
8	DSNEP	HPV-11	1488.4			
9	DSNEP	HPV-11	1673.7			
10	DSNEP	HPV-11	2212.9			
11	DSNEP	HPV-11	3087.5			
12	DSNEP	HPV-11	NE	NE	NE	NE

NA: not applicable. NE: not evaluated due to technical problems. FSNEP: focal sinonasal exophytic papilloma, DSNEP: diffuse sinonasal exophytic papilloma.

Statistically significant differences between patients affected by DSNEP and those affected by FSNEP were found for age (42.7 years vs. 65.2 years, respectively, $p = 0.019$). A strong association between age and focal/diffuse variables was observed (Cohen's D index value of 1.61). A higher proportion of males and ever-smokers in the DSNEP group was noticed; however, these were not statistically significant (100% vs. 60%, $p = 0.152$, and 85.7% vs. 40%, $p = 0.152$, respectively). No statistically significant differences were found between focal and diffuse presentation regarding clinical symptoms. The nasal septum was more affected in DSNEP (85.7% vs. 20%, $p = 0.029$), while FSNEP appeared more frequently in the lateral wall (40% vs. 28.6%, $p = 0.692$) and the cupula (40% vs. 28.6%, $p = 0.692$) of the nasal cavity, although these differences were not statistically significant. In FSNEP patients, CT-scan imaging showed swelling of the sinonasal mucosa in three cases (75%), an occupation of the maxillary or ethmoidal sinuses in two cases (50%), and polipoid formation in the nasal fossae in one case (25%); while in DSNEP, the CT scan revealed mucosal swelling in five cases (83.3%), sinus occupation in three cases (50%), and polipoid formation in three cases (50%). No statistically significant differences were detected. A higher incidence of recurrences in DSNEP was found and it was statistically significant (85.7% vs. 20%, $p = 0.045$) compared with the focal group. The median time of recurrence were 67 months for the focal single case and 4 months (range 1–36) for the diffuse group ($p = 0.134$). No statistically significant differences were found in the follow-up (median of 43 months vs. 49 months, $p = 0.745$).

There were statistically significant differences between diffuse and focal SNEP regarding HPV detection (100% vs. 40%, respectively, $p = 0.045$) and specifically in HPV11 detection (85.7% vs. 0%, respectively, $p = 0.008$). The strength of association between diffuse presentation and recurrence, HPV positivity, and HPV11 were analysed, obtaining Cramér V index values of 0.66, 0.68, and 0.85, respectively. In all three cases, a strong association was observed. Among HPV6-positive SNEPs, the median viral load was higher in FSNEP than in DSNEP (626.8 vs. 80.2 virus/cell) (Table 2), while all HPV11-positive SNEPs were diffuse. A higher proportion of exophytic and inverted mixed papillomas were found in the focal group (40% vs. 14.3%, $p = 0.364$) although the difference was not statistically significant.

4. Discussion

SNEP is a rare clinical entity, and its diffuse behaviour is poorly described in the literature [4,8,10,28,29]. Herein, we identified, included, and collected follow-up data of all DSNEP and FSNEP cases consecutively diagnosed and treated in our centre during the study period and assessed the differences between both groups. To our knowledge, no other studies have compared such sociodemographic and clinical variables between DSNEP and FSNEPs. Moreover, our study is the first to analyse HPV viral load in the SNEP setting.

Our results regarding age of SNEP presentation is similar to other published articles [2,3]. Diffuse presentation was more commonly found in younger SNEP patients in our series. Glâtre et al. [8] described the ages of SNEP patients at an individual level but did not analyse age differences between FSNEP and DSNEP.

Only one patient with FSNEP had a single recurrence (20%) while almost all DSNEP patients (85.7%) had recurrences. In the previous literature, the recurrence rate of focal SNEPs was estimated at around 22% [3,6], and Glâtre reported an 83.3% of recurrence in DNSEP and no recurrences in FSNEP [8]. Clinical symptoms and findings in CT scans in SNEPs were similar as those previously described [8], with no differences between focal and diffuse patterns. No histological differences between FSNEPs and DSNEPs were observed in our study.

The location of SNEPs in our study was in accordance with others' results [3,8,30]. In our series, DSNEPs were more frequently observed in the septum while FSNEPs affected mostly the lateral wall and the cupula of the nasal fossae. To the best of our knowledge, there is no information about nasal involvement in the literature.

Observed HPV prevalences (40% in FSNEP and 100% in DSNEP) are consistent with previous studies [4,23,24], although there is a wide variability present in the literature [3,5,8,25]. DSNEP seemed to be related to an increased HPV prevalence, mostly with HPV11 genotype. Glatre et al. [8] reported similar data, with 100% of HPV11 positivity in DSNEP and 50% of coinfection with HPV6. Previous reports showed that in other benign lesions associated to HPV, such as recurrent respiratory papillomatosis (RRP), HPV11 presence is related to worse prognosis [31,32], while others report that the HPV genotype does not influence the outcome [33–35]. No cases of coinfection were found in our series.

We observed a tendency of a higher viral load in FSNEP within the HPV6-positive subgroup, but we are comparing only three samples, and thus, it is not possible to conclude anything in this subject. Despite this, there are no previous studies in the literature on viral load results in SNEPs and this can be a precedent for further studies. In the RRP setting, some reports state that viral load decreased with each treatment until remission was achieved [36], while other studies suggested that viral load is not related to the severity of RRP [37,38]. We could hypothesize that the viral load may be an indicator of virus activity in SNEP and of a higher risk for presenting a more aggressive or diffuse lesion, but larger studies are needed to assess that. We did not analyse the viral load during all recurrences to check its evolution during the follow-up, as has been performed in RRP and anogenital wart studies [36,39].

Our study has several limitations, with the small sample size due to the low prevalence of this pathology being the most important one. However, the numbers are similar to previous articles [3,4,8,25] and reflect the reality of this pathology in our real-world setting. Therefore, the results observed could set the basis for other further studies including larger populations. Mixed SNEPs were not excluded because, in all cases, the exophytic component presented a clear predominance over the inverted one, and it is common to observe inverted areas in SNEPs. The outcomes of our analysis must be considered with caution because of the small sample size and, consequently, its limited statistical power.

Moreover, the number of recurrences may be determined because of the higher risk in interventions involving multiple lesions. P16 expression was not evaluated. However, for HPV6 or 11-positive and HPV-negative benign and premalignant lesions of the tonsil and larynx, p16 immunostaining is highly variable and is not thus recommended to predict HPV-presence. Our research can serve as a precedent for other studies to understand the physiopathology of DSNEP and to determine additional molecular factors that explain its behavior. Regarding DSNEP treatment, investigation into adjuvant drugs would be useful to reduce the number of surgeries needed and their side effects.

5. Conclusions

DSNEPs seem to be related to younger patients, the involvement of the nasal septum, the presence of HPV, mostly HPV11, and a higher risk of recurrence. Further research with larger numbers of cases is needed to unequivocally assess the risk factors associated with diffuse behaviour in the SNEP setting.

Supplementary Materials: The following supporting information can be downloaded at: https://www.mdpi.com/article/10.3390/jcm13226638/s1, Annex 1. Histological evaluation form.

Author Contributions: Conceptualization: M.F., L.A., X.G.-C. and M.M. Data curation: M.F. and A.P. Formal analysis: B.Q. Software: B.Q. Funding acquisition: L.A. and M.M. Investigation: Á.d.A.-P. and M.À.P. Methodology: B.Q., Á.d.A.-P., M.À.P., L.A., O.C. and M.G. Writing—original draft preparation: M.F., M.M. and A.P. Writing—review and editing: M.F., M.M., X.G.-C., B.Q., O.C., M.G., Á.d.A.-P., M.À.P. and L.A. All authors have read and agreed to the published version of the manuscript.

Funding: This research received no external funding.

Institutional Review Board Statement: This study was approved by the Comité de Ética de la Investigación del Hospital Universitari de Bellvitge (approval Code: PR413/20, approval Date: 24/01/2021).

Informed Consent Statement: Informed consent was obtained from all subjects involved in this study.

Data Availability Statement: The original contributions presented in the study are included in the article/supplementary material; further inquiries can be directed to the corresponding authors.

Acknowledgments: The authors deeply thank Manel Mañós for his expertise and guidance throughout this research. We want to particularly acknowledge patients and Biobank HUB-ICO-IDIBELL (PT20/00171) integrated in the ISCIII Biobanks and Biomodels Platform and Xarxa Banc de Tumors de Catalunya (XBTC) for their collaboration. We thank CERCA programme/Generalitat de Catalunya for institutional support.

Conflicts of Interest: Cancer Epidemiology Research Program (M.À.P., L.A., M.M., O.C., B.Q. and A.d.A.-P.) has received sponsorship for grants from Merck & Co., Roche, GSK, IDT, Hologic, and Seegene. These companies had no role in the design of the study; in the collection, analyses, or interpretation of data; in the writing of the manuscript; or in the decision to publish the results. The other authors have declared no conflicts of interest.

References

1. Slootweg, P.J.; El-Naggar, A.K. World Health Organization 4th edition of head and neck tumor classification: Insight into the consequential modifications. *Virchows Arch.* **2018**, *472*, 311–313. [CrossRef] [PubMed]
2. Bishop, J.A. OSPs and ESPs and ISPs, Oh My! An Update on Sinonasal (Schneiderian) Papillomas. *Head Neck Pathol.* **2017**, *11*, 269–277. [CrossRef] [PubMed]
3. Vorasubin, N.; Vira, D.; Suh, J.D.; Bhuta, S.; Wang, M.B. Schneiderian papillomas: Comparative review of exophytic, oncocytic, and inverted types. *Am. J. Rhinol. Allergy* **2013**, *27*, 287–292. [CrossRef] [PubMed]
4. Buchwald, C.; Franzmann, M.B.; Jacobsen, G.K.; Lindeberg, H. Human papillomavirus (HPV) in sinonasal papillomas: A study of 78 cases using in situ hybridization and polymerase chain reaction. *Laryngoscope* **1995**, *105*, 66–71. [CrossRef]
5. Beigh, A.; Rashi, R.; Junaid, S.; Khuroo, M.S.; Farook, S. Human Papilloma Virus (HPV) in Sinonasal Papillomas and Squamous Cell Carcinomas: A PCR-based Study of 60 cases. *Gulf J. Oncol.* **2018**, *1*, 37–42.
6. Hyams, V.J. Papillomas of the nasal cavity and paranasal sinuses. A clinicopathological study of 315 cases. *Ann. Otol. Rhinol. Laryngol.* **1971**, *80*, 192–206. [CrossRef]
7. Kim, S.J.; Byun, S.W.; Lee, S.S. Various tumors in the nasal vestibule. *Int. J. Clin. Exp. Pathol.* **2013**, *6*, 2713–2718.

8. Glâtre, R.; De Kermadec, H.; Alsamad, I.A.; Badoual, C.; Gauthier, A.; Brugel, L.; Parra, C.; Coste, A.; Prulière-Escabasse, V.; Bequignon, E. Exophytic sinonasal papillomas and nasal florid papillomatosis: A retrospective study. *Head Neck* **2018**, *40*, 740–746. [CrossRef]
9. Kumagai, M.; Endo, S.; Matsunaga, E.; Kida, A.; Sakata, H.; Yamamoto, M. Squamous papillomatosis of the bilateral nasal cavities. *Tohoku J. Exp. Med.* **2005**, *206*, 267–270. [CrossRef]
10. Bayne, K.; Joseph, D.O. A rare case and location of HPV 16 positive bilateral exophytic papilloma. *Otolaryngol. Case Rep.* **2019**, *13*, 100134. [CrossRef]
11. Norris, H.J. Papillary lesions of the nasal cavity and paranasal sinuses. I. Exophytic (squamous) papillomas. A study of 28 cases. *Laryngoscope* **1962**, *72*, 1784–1797. [CrossRef] [PubMed]
12. Terada, T. Malignant transformation of exophytic Schneiderian papilloma of the nasal cavity. *Pathol. Int.* **2012**, *62*, 199–203. [CrossRef] [PubMed]
13. Buchwald, C.; Lindeberg, H.; Pedersen, B.L.; Franzmann, M.B. Human papilloma virus and p53 expression in carcinomas associated with sinonasal papillomas: A Danish Epidemiological study 1980–1998. *Laryngoscope* **2001**, *111*, 1104–1110. [CrossRef]
14. Cardesa, A.; Alos, L.; Nadal, A. (Eds.) *Pathology of the Head and Neck*; Springer: Berlin/Heidelberg, Germany, 2016. [CrossRef]
15. Chatelet, F.; Vinciguerra, A.; Marc, M.; Herman, P.; Verillaud, B. Intralesional cidofovir injections for the treatment of multifocal exophytic sinonasal papilloma. *Int. Forum Allergy Rhinol.* **2024**. *Epub ahead of print*. [CrossRef] [PubMed]
16. Zeitels, S.M.; Barbu, A.M.; Landau-Zemer, T.; Lopez-Guerra, G.; Burns, J.A.; Fiedman, A.D.; Freeman, M.W.; Halvorsen, Y.D.; Hillman, R.E. Local injection of bevacizumab (Avastin) and angiolytic KTP laser treatment of recurrent respiratory papillomatosis of the vocal folds: A prospective study. *Ann. Otol. Rhinol. Laryngol.* **2011**, *120*, 627–634. [CrossRef]
17. Best, S.R.; Friedman, A.D.; Landau-Zemer, T.; Barbu, A.M.; Burns, J.A.; Freeman, M.W.; Halvorsen, Y.D.; Hillman, R.E.; Zeitels, S.M. Safety and dosing of bevacizumab (avastin) for the treatment of recurrent respiratory papillomatosis. *Ann. Otol. Rhinol Laryngol.* **2012**, *121*, 587–593. [CrossRef]
18. Chen, S., IV; Karnezis, T.; Davidson, T.M. Safety of intranasal Bevacizumab (Avastin) treatment in patients with hereditary hemorrhagic telangiectasia-associated epistaxis. *Laryngoscope* **2011**, *121*, 644–646. [CrossRef]
19. Fulla, M.; Szafarowski, T.; Frias-Gomez, J.; Quiros, B.; Clavero, O.; Gomà, M.; Pavon, M.A.; Jurek-Matusiak, O.; Lares, H.R.; Mañós, M.; et al. Human Papillomavirus and Factors Associated with Recurrence in Sinonasal Inverted Papillomas from Poland and Spain. *Head Neck Pathol.* **2020**, *14*, 758–767, Erratum in *Head Neck Pathol.* **2020**, *14*, 768–770. [CrossRef]
20. Vor der Holte, A.P.; Fangk, I.; Glombitza, S.; Wilkens, L.; Welkoborsky, H.J. Identification of Rare and Common HPV Genotypes in Sinonasal Papillomas. *Head Neck Pathol.* **2020**, *14*, 936–943. [CrossRef]
21. Mohajeri, S.; Lai, C.; Purgina, B.; Almutairi, D.; Baghai, T.; Dimitroulakos, J.; Kilty, S. Human papillomavirus: An unlikely etiologic factor in sinonasal inverted papilloma. *Laryngoscope* **2018**, *128*, 2443–2447. [CrossRef]
22. Justice, J.M.; Davis, K.M.; Saenz, D.A.; Lanza, D.C. Evidence that human papillomavirus causes inverted papilloma is sparse. *Int. Forum Allergy Rhinol.* **2014**, *4*, 995–1001. [CrossRef] [PubMed]
23. Lawson, W.; Schlecht, N.F.; Brandwein-Gensler, M. The role of the human papillomavirus in the pathogenesis of Schneiderian inverted papillomas: An analytic overview of the evidence. *Head Neck Pathol.* **2008**, *2*, 49–59. [CrossRef] [PubMed]
24. Syrjänen, K.; Syrjänen, S. Detection of human papillomavirus in sinonasal papillomas: Systematic review and meta-analysis. *Laryngoscope* **2013**, *123*, 181–192. [CrossRef]
25. Franzmann, M.B.; Buchwald, C.; Jacobsen, G.K.; Lindeberg, H. Expression of p53 in normal nasal mucosa and in sinonasal papillomas with and without associated carcinoma and the relation to human papillomavirus (HPV). *Cancer Lett.* **1998**, *128*, 161–164. [CrossRef]
26. Castellsagué, X.; Alemany, L.; Quer, M.; Halec, G.; Quirós, B.; Tous, S.; Clavero, O.; Alòs, L.; Biegner, T.; Szafarowski, T.; et al. HPV Involvement in Head and Neck Cancers: Comprehensive Assessment of Biomarkers in 3680 Patients. *J. Natl. Cancer Inst.* **2016**, *108*, djv403. [CrossRef]
27. de Sanjose, S.; Quint, W.G.; Alemany, L.; Geraets, D.T.; Klaustermeier, J.E.; Lloveras, B.; Tous, S.; Felix, A.; Bravo, L.E.; Shin, H.R.; et al. Human papillomavirus genotype attribution in invasive cervical cancer: A retrospective cross-sectional worldwide study. *Lancet Oncol.* **2010**, *11*, 1048–1056. [CrossRef]
28. Capaccio, P.; Ottaviani, F.; Cuccarini, V.; Corbellino, M.; Parravicini, C.; Menzo, S.; Schindler, A.; Pignataro, L. Surgery and topic cidofovir for nasal squamous papillomatosis in HIV+ patient. *Eur. Arch. Otorhinolaryngol.* **2009**, *266*, 937–939. [CrossRef]
29. Maithani, T.; Dey, D.; Pandey, A.; Chawla, N. Bilateral fungiform papilloma with synchronous verrucous carcinoma of the nasal septum: A rare presentation and a literature review. *J. Laryngol. Otol.* **2012**, *126*, 424–427. [CrossRef]
30. Perez-Ordoñez, B. Hamartomas, papillomas and adenocarcinomas of the sinonasal tract and nasopharynx. *J. Clin. Pathol.* **2009**, *62*, 1085–1095. [CrossRef]
31. Donne, A.J.; Hampson, L.; Homer, J.J.; Hampson, I.N. The role of HPV type in Recurrent Respiratory Papillomatosis. *Int. J. Pediatr. Otorhinolaryngol.* **2010**, *74*, 7–14. [CrossRef]
32. Li, J.; Zhang, T.Y.; Tan, L.T.; Wang, S.Y.; Chen, Y.Y.; Tian, J.Y.; Da, W.Y.; He, P.; Zhao, Y.M. Expression of human papillomavirus and prognosis of juvenile laryngeal papilloma. *Int. J. Clin. Exp. Med.* **2015**, *8*, 15521–15527. [PubMed]
33. Nogueira, R.L.; Küpper, D.S.; do Bonfim, C.M.; Aragon, D.C.; Damico, T.A.; Miura, C.S.; Passcs, I.M.; Nogueira, M.L.; Rahal, P.; Valera, F.C. HPV genotype is a prognosticator for recurrence of respiratory papillomatosis in children. *Clin. Otolaryngol.* **2021**, *46*, 181–188. [CrossRef] [PubMed]

34. Buchinsky, F.J.; Valentino, W.L.; Ruszkay, N.; Powell, E.; Derkay, C.S.; Seedat, R.Y.; Uloza, V.; Dikkers, F.G.; Tunkel, D.E.; Choi, S.S.; et al. Age at diagnosis, but not HPV type, is strongly associated with clinical course in recurrent respiratory papillomatosis. *PLoS ONE* **2019**, *14*, e0216697. [CrossRef] [PubMed]
35. Figueiredo, M.C.; Justino, M.C.; Delmonico, L.; Silvestre, R.T.; de Castro, T.L.; Dos Santos Moreira, A.; Macedo, J.M.B.; da Costa Carvalho, M.D.G.; Scherrer, L.; de Medeiros Lima, D.J.M.; et al. Prevalence and clinical implications of low-risk human papillomavirus among patients with recurrent respiratory papillomatosis in Rio de Janeiro, Brazil. *Auris Nasus Larynx* **2019**, *46*, 570–575. [CrossRef] [PubMed]
36. Deng, Z.; Ikegami, T.; Kiyuna, A.; Zhang, C.; Zhang, T.; Matayoshi, S.; Uehara, T.; Maeda, H.; Suzuki, M.; Ganaha, A. Methylation of CpG sites in the upstream regulatory region, physical status and mRNA expression of HPV-6 in adult-onset laryngeal papilloma. *Oncotarget* **2017**, *8*, 85368–85377. [CrossRef]
37. Yamada, S.; Itoh, T.; Ikegami, T.; Imai, A.; Mochizuki, D.; Nakanishi, H.; Ishikawa, R.; Kita, J.; Nakamura, Y.; Takizawa, Y.; et al. Association between human papillomavirus particle production and the severity of recurrent respiratory papillomatosis. *Sci. Rep.* **2023**, *13*, 5514. [CrossRef]
38. Ikegami, T.; Hirakawa, H.; Tsukahara, N.; Murakami, A.; Kise, N.; Kiyuna, A.; Kosugi, T.; Agena, S.; Kinjyo, H.; Hasegawa, N.; et al. Coordinated Expression of HPV-6 Genes with Predominant E4 and E5 Expression in Laryngeal Papilloma. *Microorganisms* **2021**, *9*, 520. [CrossRef]
39. Hu, Z.; Liu, L.; Zhang, W.; Liu, H.; Li, J.; Jiang, L.; Zeng, K. Dynamics of HPV viral loads reflect the treatment effect of photodynamic therapy in genital warts. *Photodiagn. Photodyn Ther.* **2018**, *21*, 86–90. [CrossRef]

Journal of
Clinical Medicine

MDPI

Article

Chronic Nasal Disease and Eustachian Tube Function: What Is the Role of Tubomanometry?

Sofia Anastasiadou [1,*], Polyzois Bountzis [2], Dimitrios-Evangelos Gkogkos [3], Petros Karkos [1], Jannis Constantinidis [1], Stefanos Triaridis [1] and George Psillas [1]

1 Department of Medicine, Achepa University Hospital of Thessaloniki, Aristotle University of Thessaloniki, 541 24 Thessaloniki, Greece; pkarkos@aol.com (P.K.); janconst@otenet.gr (J.C.); triaridis@hotmail.com (S.T.); psill@otenet.gr (G.P.)
2 Department of Mathematics and Physics, Universita della Campania "Luigi Vanvitelli", 81100 Caserta, Italy; pmpountzp@geo.auth.gr
3 Department of Applied Informatics, University of Macedonia, 546 36 Thessaloniki, Greece; dgkogkos@uom.edu.gr
* Correspondence: anastasiadousof23@gmail.com

Abstract: Background/objectives: Eustachian tube dysfunction (ETD) presents complex diagnostic challenges in otolaryngology, compounded by concurrent chronic nasal disease. Patient-reported outcome measures (PROMs) often assess ETD severity due to its elusive diagnosis. Tubomanometry (TMM) emerges as a promising diagnostic tool, yet its application alongside chronic nasal disease remains unclear. Our study aims to elucidate TMM's role in ETD diagnosis within the context of chronic nasal diseases, integrating subjective assessments, clinical examination, and TMM results. **Methods**: A prospective observational study was conducted with patients suffering from ETD and chronic nasal disease allocated in three different groups according to their nasal pathology. Clinical examination, PROMs in the form of ETDQ-7, and NOSE questionnaires as well as TMM were performed. Results of the above subjective and objective measurements were analysed and correlated statistically to determine the value of TMM in chronic nasal disease patients. **Results**: All recruited patients suffered from ETD and chronic nasal disease, with similarly affected ETDQ-7 scores across all groups, while NOSE scores differed significantly based on the underground nasal pathology. TMM values confirm the presence of ETD in all three groups, confirming the role of TMM within this cohort. Interestingly, TMM values can still confirm the presence of ETD in patients with chronic nasal disease but cannot discriminate among chronic nasal pathology patients, making TMM a diagnostic tool with uniformity among the chronic nasal pathologies. **Conclusions**: ETD in individuals with chronic nasal disease presents distinct complexities, requiring a tailored diagnostic approach. In this context, a thorough clinical assessment, integrating ETDQ-7 and NOSE questionnaires, supplemented by TMM where accessible, is crucial to confirm diagnosis. This study confirms that TMM can diagnose ETD in all nasal pathology patients without being influenced by the nature of the disease. This research endeavours to refine diagnostic strategies, enriching clinical decision-making, and enhancing ETD management in patients suffering with chronic nasal diseases.

Keywords: Eustachian tube dysfunction; chronic nasal disease; tubomanometry

1. Introduction

Eustachian tube dysfunction (ETD) stands as a multifaceted and intricate challenge within the realm of otolaryngology, posing difficulties in both understanding its underlying mechanisms and establishing precise diagnostic criteria [1]. Concurrent chronic nasal disease complicates the clinical picture as it adds more factors that contribute to similar symptoms. Chronic nasal disease significantly affects the nasopharynx as well as the ET orifices and plays a significant role in ETD presentation and symptoms. Patient reported outcome measures (PROMs) are usually used to assess the severity of ETD. Tubomanometry

(TMM) is a relatively novel objective diagnostic method of ETD and is the diagnostic tool of choice where it is available [2–4]. But what happens with TMM when there is concurrent chronic nasal disease remains vaguely unexplored. Similarly, which pathology to correct first, either the nasal disease or the ETD itself or even perform synchronous procedures, has not yet been discussed adequately in the literature. Our study aims to contribute valuable insights into the role of TMM in the diagnostic algorithm for ETD within the context of chronic nasal diseases. Integration of subjective symptom assessments, clinical examinations, and TMM results promises a comprehensive understanding of Eustachian tube function in this complex patient population.

Chronic nasal disease is multifaceted and can be expressed as chronic rhinitis, nasal septal deviation (NSD), as well as chronic rhinosinusitis (CRS). Based on the area of the nose affected, there are multiple different nasal pathologies, functional, structural, or inflammatory. In many cases, more than two pathologies co-exist with characteristics of both anatomical and inflammatory changes that contribute to the chronic nasal disease. It is occasionally challenging to discriminate between the two, and this represents one of the nuances in determining the relation between ETD and chronic nasal disease. This study aims to determine the reliability of TMM in patients with chronic nasal diseases and to identify if specific nasal pathologies, such as chronic rhinitis, NSD, or CRS with polyps, have a greater impact on TMM findings and thus on the diagnosis of ETD. Additionally, it seeks to correlate PROMs, specifically the Eustachian Tube Dysfunction Questionnaire-7 (ETDQ-7) and NOSE questionnaire scores [5], with TMM results to compare subjective and objective assessments of ETD in this particular patient population.

2. Methods

In this study, ear, nose, and throat (ENT) patients were recruited from outpatient or pre-operative assessment units that suffered with ETD and concurrent nasal pathology in Achepa University Hospital of Thessaloniki. They were provided with information leaflets, and the researchers had individual meetings with each patient to explain the process of the study. A consent form was signed by all patients after adequate discussion and information was provided. The data collection lasted 15 months and was also approved by the Committee of Bioethics and Deontology of the Hospital. The patients were allocated in three different groups according to their chronic nasal pathology. The first group presented with chronic rhinitis, the second one had NSD, and the third one chronic rhinosinusitis (CRS) with polyps. Patients in the septal deviation group were also subgrouped, taking into consideration the Baumann et al. six-type classification of septal deviation [6,7]. In the group with CRS with polyps, there were multiple polyps instead of one single polyp (e.g., antrochoanal polyp) and polyp location in the nose was documented as well. Each patient in every group had only one of these characteristic findings on examination, and there was no overlap of the chronic nasal pathologies.

The sample size was calculated based on the total population of chronic nasal disease patients that were reviewed in the outpatient department within a year, with a confidence interval of 90%, a standard deviation of 0.5%, and a margin of error within 5–7%. This is consistent with the current literature findings and ensures reliability of the results as well as represents a realistic sample size based on the overall population size in the outpatient department.

The presence of ETD and chronic nasal disease was established using both subjective and objective measurement tools. Patient reported outcome measures were utilised to recruit patients to the first phase of the trial. This involved a comprehensive evaluation employing the ETDQ-7 as well as the NOSE questionnaire [5]. A minimum score of 2.1 for ETDQ-7 and 4 for NOSE was required for a patient to be considered eligible for the study. It appears that the majority of the participants lie between 2.5 and 4.0 for ETDQ-7 and 5 and 20 for NOSE accordingly (Figures 1 and 2). According to the literature, this is the minimum score for each questionnaire to indicate pathology [5,8]. Inclusion criteria apart from the PROMs scores were the following: specific nasal pathology to be eligible for one of the three groups, examination findings of ETD, either retracted tympanic membrane or Type C tympanogram, age > 18 years, ETD symptoms for more than 12 weeks and for Group C only, middle meatal polyps [9]. Exclusion criteria were previous ENT operations; severe ear pathology such as ear drum perforation, tympanosclerosis, or cholesteatoma; adenoid hypertrophy; postnasal space lesions such as nasopharyngeal tumours; previous head and neck radiotherapy; congenital abnormalities; temporomandibular joint dysfunction; and various polyp locations for Group C. Temporomadibular joint dysfunction significantly mimics ETD symptoms, and patients in Group C had only polyps occupying their middle meatus. Inclusion and exclusion criteria as well as demographics can be found in Tables 1 and 2.

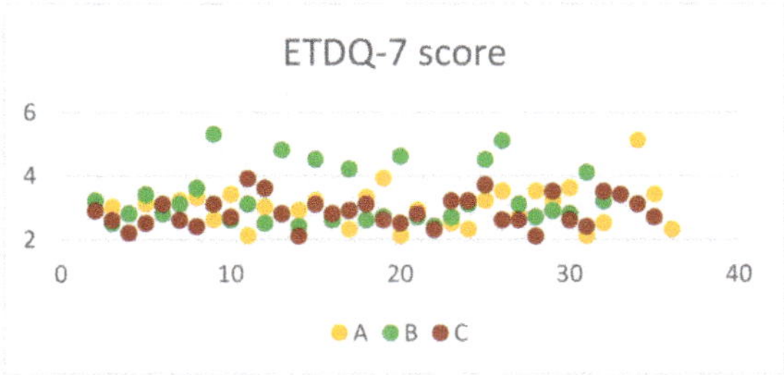

Figure 1. ETDQ7 score among groups.

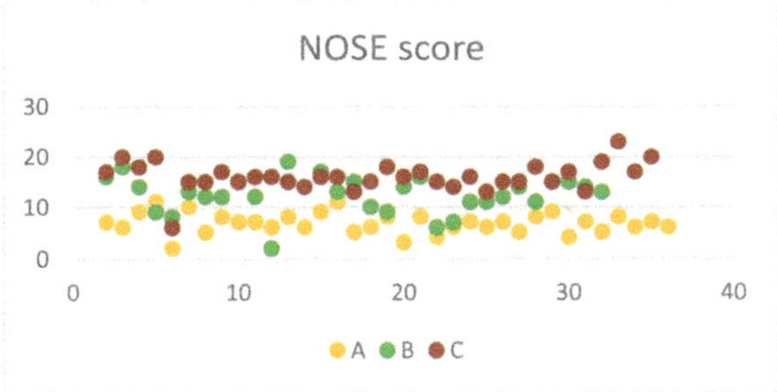

Figure 2. NOSE score among groups.

Table 1. Inclusion and exclusion criteria.

Inclusion Criteria	Exclusion Criteria
Age > 18 years old ETD symptoms > 12 weeks ETDQ-7 > 2.1 No ENT surgery previously No recent medication applied Retracted tympanic membrane and/or Type C tympanogram Chronic nasal disease	Previous ENT surgery Severe ear pathology (cholesteatoma, etc.) Adenoid hypertrophy Postnasal space lesion Previous H&N area radiotherapy

Table 2. Demographic characteristics among patient groups.

		Group A	Group B	Group C
Gender	M	40% (n = 14)	58.1% (n =18)	41.1% (n =15)
	F	60% (n = 21)	41.9% (n =13)	55.9% (n =19)
Age	Mean (SD)	41.2 (14.8)	36 (9.09)	48 (12.3)

Objective examination findings were utilised including otoscopy, anterior rhinoscopy, and flexible nasoendoscopy. These were used to determine whether they fulfil the inclusion criteria as well as which chronic nasal condition they suffer from. Tympanometry was also used as an adjunct to diagnose ETD. Either tympanometry or otoscopic findings of tympanic membrane retraction confirmed the ETDQ-7 score in order to progress to recruitment of the patients to the study.

Patients were divided in three groups, with 35 patients in the chronic rhinitis group (Group A), 31 patients in the NSD group (Group B), and 34 patients in the CRS group (Group C). Recruitment was stopped as an appropriate number for each group was reached, according to similar studies in the literature [10,11]. The patients allocated to Group A firstly presented with pathological NOSE scores that suggested chronic nasal obstruction. Subsequently, the patients underwent clinical examination to identify the cause of the pathological NOSE score. Chronic rhinitis was defined as nasal mucosa irritation mostly attributed to allergic rhinitis. The nose appeared congested with evidence of clear discharge and erythematous mucosa. The patients did not have any other significant pathology, no septal deviation, or nasal polyps. Group C patients were diagnosed with CRS with nasal polyps that were present in the middle meatus without causing complete nasal obstruction or fully occupying the inferior meatus. Patients underwent tubomanometry (TMM) to assess the severity of their ETD status. The R-value, a parameter derived from TMM, provides meaningful insights into ET function. An R-value ≤ 1 signifies a regular and timely opening of the ET, while an R-value > 1 indicates a delayed opening. The absence of a definable R-value suggests no detectable opening of the ET. Normal TMM findings are represented in Figures 3 and 4. This quantitative measure enhances the diagnostic precision in identifying chronic obstructive ET dysfunction. Finally, TMM scores were correlated to their specified nasal pathology as well as their PROMS, ETDQ-7, and NOSE scores.

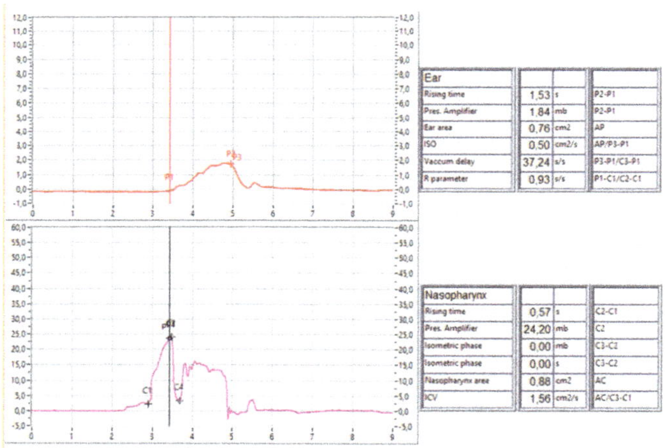

Figure 3. Normal TMM curves with measurements, right ear.

Statistical analysis was carried out using SPSS Statistics version XX software (IBM Corp., New York, NY, USA). The Spearman rank correlation coefficient was used, which is a non-parametric measure, to assess the strength and direction of the relationship between NOSE and ETDQ-7 scores with R, C2, and C2-C1. Values closer to 1 indicate strong positive correlation between the compared values, whereas values closer to -1 indicate strong negative correlation, respectively. We further performed the two-sided Spearman rank correlation test to explore statistically significant interactions among the variables. The comparisons among the groups were statistically analysed using the Kruskal–Wallis test. Dunn's post-hoc test was used to conduct pairwise comparisons between groups after finding a significant result from the Kruskal–Wallis test. A p-value < 0.05 was considered to indicate statistical significance.

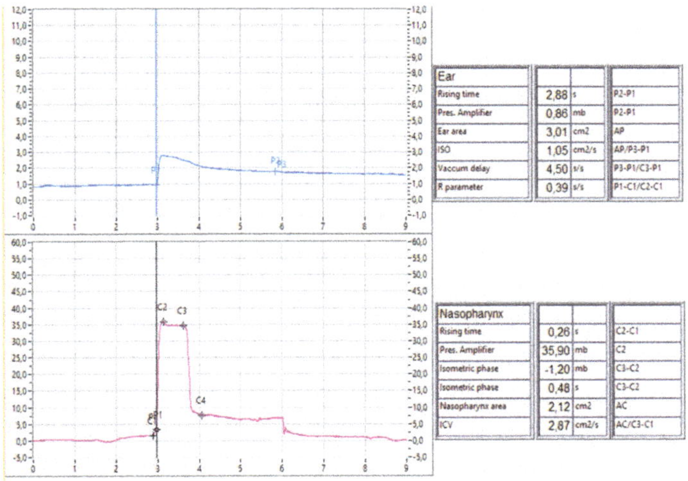

Figure 4. Normal TMM curves with measurements, left ear.

3. Results

From the 35 chronic rhinitis patients enrolled in Group A, 14 (40%) were males and 21 (60%) females. The mean (standard deviation) age of the enrolled patients was 41.2 (14.8) years old (Table 2). Clinical measures with otoscopy and rhinoscopy showed pathological outcomes with rhinetic swollen nasal mucosa and hypertrophic inferior turbinates with tympanic membrane retraction or tympanometry type C. The ETDQ-7 and NOSE scores were 3.14 and 6.77, respectively, which are both within the abnormal values (Table 3). TMM was therefore performed to assess Eustachian tube (ET) function bilaterally, with corresponding right and left R-scores equal to 1.15 (0.43) and 2.42 (4.49). Both these R scores indicate ETD with the ET to remain closed most of the time. TMM data are represented in Table 4 and are summarised in Figures 5–7. This confirms that TMM can correctly diagnose ETD in chronic rhinitis patients and also that TMM values correlate to clinical symptoms and PROMs.

Table 3. PROMs and TMM values among groups.

	Group A	Group B	Group C
		Mean (SD)	
ETDQ-7	3.14 (0.96)	3.30 (0.86)	2.85 (0.46)
NOSE	6.77 (2.03)	12.48 (3.63)	15.02 (2.84)
LR	2.42 (4.94)	1.08 (7.92)	0.99 (1.08)
RR	1.15 (0.43)	1.54 (10.28)	1.18 (0.59)
LC2	28.74 (5.48)	26.41 (7.92)	27.23 (4.23)
RC2	26.25 (7.43)	22.87 (10.28)	22.94 (9.22)

Table 4. Statistics of tubomanometry values for Group A.

	ETD-7	NOSE	RR	RC2	LR	LC2
Std. Deviation	1.0490	2.295	0.418261738030	7.2381	3.60317940615	5.7265
Variance	1.100	5.268	0.175	52.390	12.983	32.793
Range	5.1	10	1.990	24.9	21.869	26.3
Minimum	1.2	1	0.1100	11.0	0.030	10.5
Maximum	6.3	11	2.10	35.9	21.900	36.8

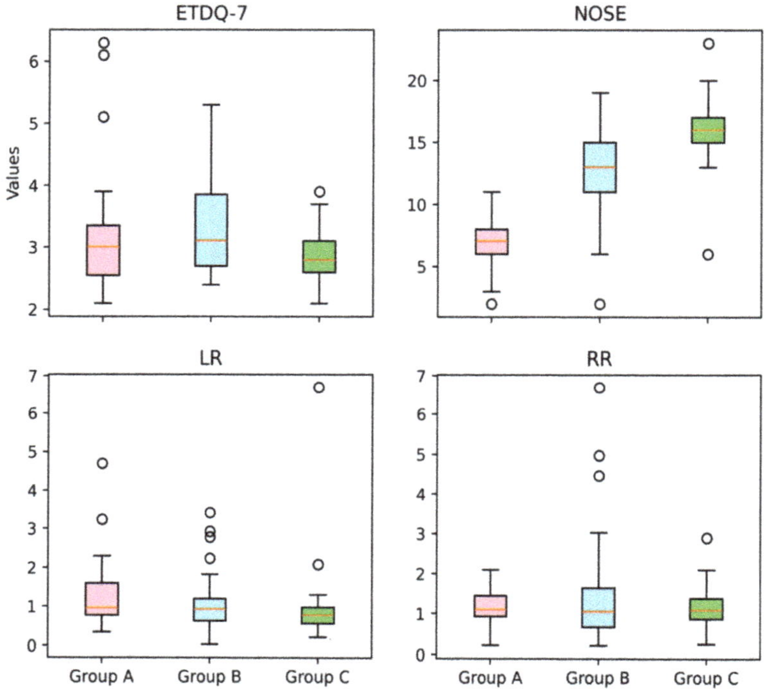

Figure 5. ETDQ-7, NOSE, LR, and RR scores among groups.

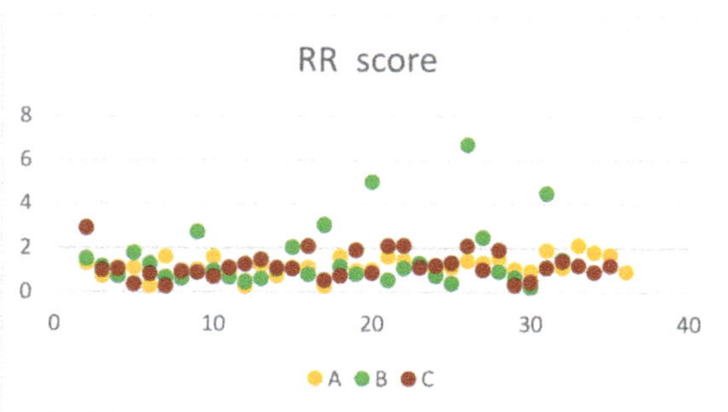

Figure 6. RR score among groups.

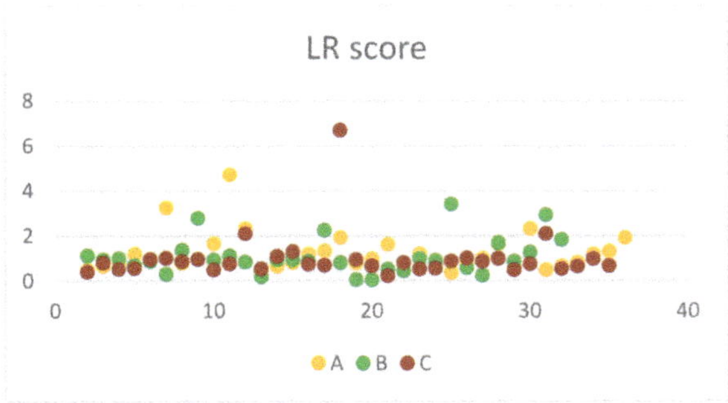

Figure 7. LR score among groups.

Similarly, in Group B, 31 patients with NSD were recruited, 18 (58.1%) were male and 13 (41.9) were females. The mean age of the group was 36 with a standard deviation of 9.09 (Table 2). Clinical examination with otoscopy and rhinoscopy showed NSD with associated tympanic membrane retraction or tympanometry type C. The ETDQ-7 score was 3.31 and NOSE score was 12.48, both indicating severe ET and nasal symptoms (Table 3). From a total of 31 patients, 11 patients had Type II as per Baumann et al. [6] NSD and 20 patients had type III. TMM values were right-sided R 1.54 and left-sided R score 1.08. The results also confirm that the side of the NSD corresponds to the most pathological R score as the contralateral side shows a milder ETD with a lower R score closer to 1. This also reflects to what the patient reported as the most heavily congested side of the nose. TMM data are represented in Table 5 and are summarised in Figures 5–7. Therefore, TMM can be reliably used in NSD patients and can also be correlated with the side of the obstruction caused by the existing NSD.

Table 5. Statistics of tubomanometry values for Group B.

	ETD-7	NOSE	RR	RC2	LR	LC2
Std. Deviation	1.0282	5.135	1.167849634311	9.9750	1.01687805989	7.7359
Variance	1.057	26.372	1.364	99.501	1.034	59.845
Range	4.2	18	6.520	39.1	6.670	33.3
Minimum	1.1	1	0.180	0.6	0.030	1.4
Maximum	5.3	19	6.700	39.7	6.70	34.7

Finally, in Group C, 34 patients with CRS with polyps were recruited with a 41.1% male and 55.9% female ratio. The mean age of the patients was 48 with a standard deviation of 12.3 (Table 2). Clinical examination once again revealed ETD otoscopically, or tympanometry confirmed and flexible nasoendoscopy revealed nasal polyposis with polyps occurring in the middle meatus and no significant NSD. The ETDQ-7 score was 2.85 and NOSE score was 16.03, both indicating significant nasal congestion and ETD (Table 3). TMM data are represented in Table 6 and are summarised in Figures 5–7. The right-sided R score in TMM was 1.18, while the left-sided R score was 0.99. This again indicates ETD; however, the right side appears closer to normal values compared to the left.

Table 6. Statistics of tubomanometry values for Group C.

	ETD-7	NOSE	RR	RC2	LR	LC2
Std. Deviation	0.4613	2.844	0.59574	9.2261	1.08088	4.2390
Variance	0.213	8.090	0.355	85.121	1.168	17.969
Range	1.8	17	2.64	36.1	6.48	18.9
Minimum	2.1	6	0.26	0.3	0.22	16.6
Maximum	3.9	23	2.90	36.4	6.70	35.5

In terms of the PROMs used in the study, it was considered significant to correlate these to the clinical findings as well as the TMM values. Also, it was interesting to identify which nasal pathology affects more TMM values, such as R, C2-C1, and C2 values that might indicate significant ETD. PROM results among groups are presented in Figures 6–8. In Group A, it is evident that there is a statistically significant positive correlation between NOSE scores and R values (rho = 0.39, $p = 0.021$). This means that patients suffering from chronic rhinitis and higher NOSE scores come in accordance with higher R as well as increased pressure in the nasopharynx (C2) (Figure 8). In group B, ETDQ-7 and RR features show a stronger correlation compared to NOSE and TMM values (rho = 0.36, $p = 0.054$). This reflects that ETDQ-7 is more reliable in this cohort of patients to be correlated with TMM results compared to the NOSE questionnaire. NSD significantly affects the structure of the nose, and NOSE scores are higher the worse the deviation is (Figure 9). Last but not least, in Group C, the correlations of the tests are even less significant, showing that TMM confirms the presence of ETD, but TMM values are not strongly correlated with PROMs values (Figure 10). Overall PROMs scores are illustrated in Figures 7 and 8.

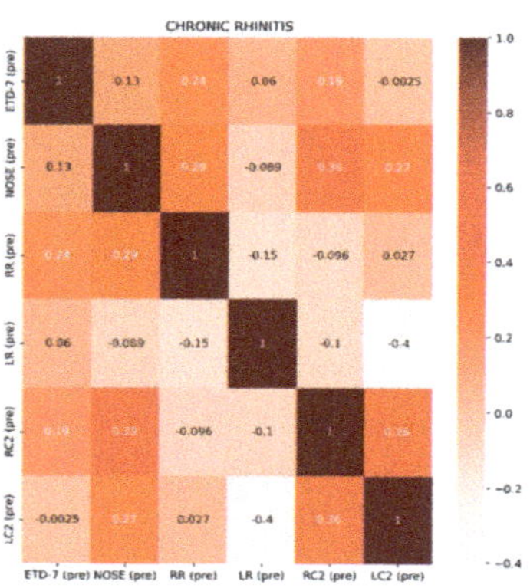

Figure 8. Spearman correlation coefficients among features ETD-7, NOSE, RR, LR, RC2, and LC2 for Group A.

To compare the two questionnaire's scores among the three groups, the analysis was conducted via the independent-samples Kruskal–Wallis test and aimed to evaluate the distribution of ETD-7 and NOSE scores across the three groups. It appears that the p value was calculated to be 0.807 for ETDQ-7, indicating uniformity in ETD among patients in the three groups. In contrast, the p value for NOSE was calculated to be 0.001, which indicates that NOSE questionnaire scores were significantly different among patients in the three different groups. After performing the independent-samples Kruskal–Wallis test among the NOSE results of each group, it was evident that NOSE was affected differently. Performing the post-hoc Dunn test showed that the most outstanding NOSE questionnaire scores belong to Group A, as these patients have milder symptoms compared to Group B and C (Table 7a,b). This is reflected in the mean NOSE questionnaire values that are 6.77, 12.48, and 16.03, respectively, for Groups A, B, and C (Table 3). Subsequently, this study confirmed the value of ETDQ-7 and NOSE questionnaires in the diagnostic pathway of ETD.

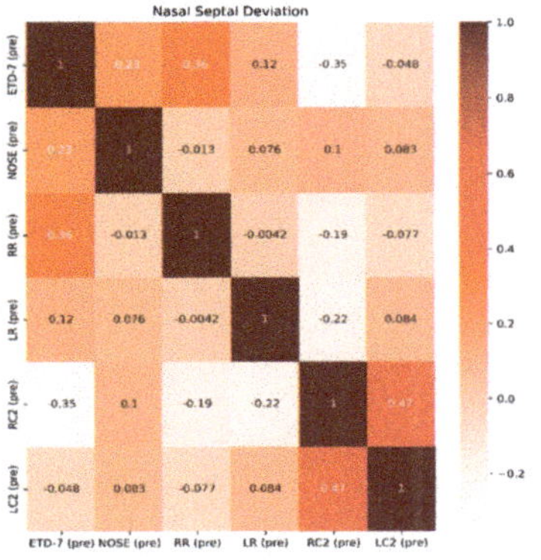

Figure 9. Spearman correlation coefficients among features ETD-7, NOSE, RR, LR, RC2, and LC2 for Group B.

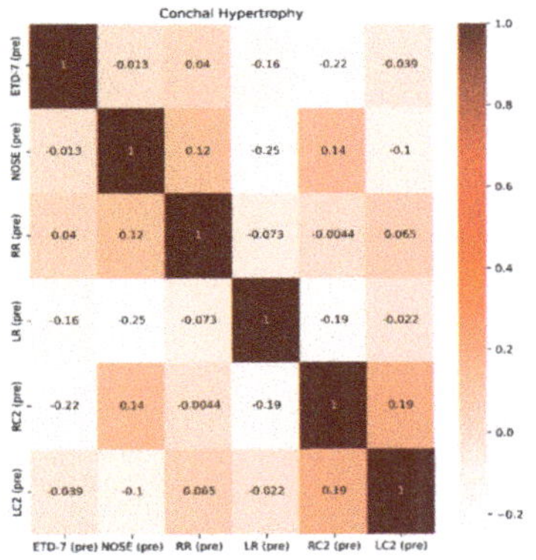

Figure 10. Spearman correlation coefficients among features ETD-7, NOSE, RR, LR, RC2, and LC2 for Group C.

Table 7. (**a**) The p-values of the Dunn post-hoc analysis with Bonferroni adjustment. (**b**) Independent-samples Kruskal–Wallis test for questionnaires.

(**a**)

Group	Chronic Rhinitis	NSD	CRS
A	1	1.95×10^{-5}	1.78×10^{-15}
B		1	0.003
C			1

(**b**)

Features	p-Value
ETD-7~Groups	0.191
NOSE-Groups	0.000

The independent-samples Kruskal–Wallis test which is a non parametric test comparing independent figures among groups, was also performed to assess the relation of TMM values, R, C2, and C2-C1 to identify possible discrepancies among the three groups. It appears that there is no statistically significant difference among the three groups in terms of TMM measurements. All patients with ETD appear to have coherent R, C2-C1, and C2 values, which might imply that nasal pathology can cause ETD irrespectively of its nature. In detail, the nasal pathology significantly affects the ET function and specifically how high the pressure can build up in the nasopharynx and how quickly this pressure rises in the area. However, there is no statistically significant difference among the three groups and their TMM values, indicating that TMM cannot discriminate among different chronic nasal pathology.

4. Discussion

The critical evaluation of TMM gains heightened significance when ETD coexists with chronic nasal diseases, including chronic rhinitis, NSD, or CRS with polyps [10–13]. The interplay between these conditions introduces additional layers of complexity and considerations that must be carefully weighed when utilising TMM in the diagnostic process.

Chronic nasal disease, characterised by persistent inflammation and anatomical variations, can exert a profound influence on Eustachian tube function. In the context of allergic rhinitis, the mucosal inflammation and increased nasal secretions may impact the patency of the Eustachian tube, contributing to the manifestation of ETD symptoms. Similarly, NSD can alter the aerodynamics of the nasal passages, influencing the pressure dynamics within the Eustachian tube [10,13]. Chronic rhinosinusitis with polyps further complicates the picture by introducing inflammatory changes and potential obstruction within the nasal and sinus cavities [11]. To our knowledge, there is no study in the current literature that correlates different nasal pathologies and compares how these affect PROMs (ETDQ-7, NOSE questionnaires) with objective TMM measurements.

4.1. *Patient-Reported Outcome Measures—PROMS*

Patient-reported outcome measures (PROMs) offer a valuable window into patient experiences, particularly when objective tests are lacking [14,15]. These questionnaire-based tools capture subjective symptoms and quality-of-life impacts, providing quantitative data that complement traditional clinical history-taking. In the context of Eustachian tube dysfunction (ETD), where a gold-standard objective test remains elusive, one specific PROM has emerged: the seven-item ETD Questionnaire (ETDQ-7) by McCoul et al. [5]. However, limitations exist. While the ETDQ-7 has gained traction in clinical and research settings, it struggles to distinguish between obstructive and patulous ETD subtypes. Additionally, its specificity drops significantly when tested against a broader population with mixed otolaryngological conditions [9,16]. This suggests that initial assessments using healthy control groups or those with unrelated pathologies may have overestimated its diagnostic accuracy. Although, while not ideal for diagnosis, this tool has been widely utilised to determine the presence and quantify the symptoms of ETD but also to monitor symptom changes and treatment response in patients with diagnosed ETD [17]. In this study, it appears that ETDQ-7 confirms the presence of ETD alongside clinical findings with otoscopy and tympanometry. It is also evident that ETDQ-7 reflects the severity of ETD, as higher scores of ETDQ-7 are correlated with pathological TMM measurements, with higher R, C2, and C2-C1 values. However, ETDQ-7 is not capable to discriminate among different nasal pathologies, as it appears to be equally affected in all three groups.

Another PROM was used in this study to identify nasal pathology and discriminate patients with severe nasal symptoms. The NOSE questionnaire was developed by Stewart et al. [18] and is used vastly in research as well as clinical practice in the field of rhinology. It can effectively quantify nasal symptoms and act as an adjunct to assess severity of the nasal condition. It has been validated in the paediatric population as well and has recently been revalidated in large groups of the population [19,20]. In this study, it was used to assess the severity of nasal symptoms, and in all three groups of patients, it showed a pathological score. After statistical analysis, it appears that NOSE scores are correlated with TMM values with higher NOSE scores to pair with abnormal R, C2, and C2-C1 scores. Even though the

NOSE questionnaire is not directly linked to ETD, there is a clear relation between the two, taking into consideration the TMM findings. It is also evident that NOSE scores are different across the three groups, with the lower scores represented in chronic rhinitis patients and statistically different to higher ones that belong to chronic rhinosinusitis patients.

4.2. Tubomanometry—TMM

Tubomanometry (TMM), as an objective diagnostic tool, must be scrutinised for its applicability in the presence of these coexisting conditions. There has already been significant discussion around the reliability and applicability of TMM to investigate ETD in an otherwise normal population [21]. The reliability and interpretability of TMM results may be affected by the altered nasal anatomy, dynamic nasal airflow patterns, and variable degrees of mucosal inflammation [10–12]. Moreover, patient discomfort and compliance during TMM may be exacerbated in individuals with chronic nasal diseases. The presence of nasal congestion, rhinorrhea, or sinonasal discomfort can influence a patient's ability to execute the required manoeuvres and may introduce confounding variables into the assessment. In this study, three different measurements were performed for every patient, in 30, 40, and 50 mbar as indicated in the literature, and the mean of all values was used for statistical analysis [2,22]. TMM was performed on all patients across all three nasal pathology groups, and the values were correlated with their ETD as well as nasal pathology. As previously mentioned, the interest of the study is focused on the R parameter, C2, and C2-C1. An R-value ≤ 1 signifies a regular and timely opening of the ET, while an R-value > 1 indicates a delayed opening. The absence of a definable R-value suggests no detectable opening of the ET. The value C2 indicates the highest-pressure measurement in the nasopharynx, and the C2-C1 indicates the speed with which the pressure rises in the nasopharynx during the measurements. A normal TMM measurement is shown in Figures 3 and 4. In this study, TMM values show statistically significant correlation with ETDQ-7 and NOSE measurements, confirming the presence of ETDQ-7 in all groups. The study also implies that TMM values are not affected in the specific population of chronic nasal disease, and it can still reflect the ETD pathology with reliably abnormal, R, C2, and C2-C1 values. This has not yet been discussed in the literature, and it is important to conduct larger studies with multiple chronic nasal pathology patients to verify our results.

4.3. Which Nasal Disease Affects the ET More?

This study aimed to shed light on the relationship between chronic nasal disease and ETD. Patients with chronic rhinitis which presents as mostly allergic have less pathological NOSE scores compared to those with NSD, and the latter group has better NOSE scores compared to the CRS with polyps. ETDQ-7 scores that reflect the severity of ETD symptoms appear similar to all three groups, implying that the nasal condition does not subjectively affect what the patients with ETD feel. TMM measurements also show high correlation with subjective measurement outcomes and also appear to be consistently pathological across all groups of patients. TMM can be used to confirm the presence of ETD in chronic nasal disease patients and is not altered based on the nature of the chronic nasal pathology. This is also confirmed in the literature; however, studies conducted to date discuss a single nasal pathology and especially nasal septal deviation and chronic nasal polyposis. Our study aims to compare multiple cohorts of patients and confirms the valid use of TMM among these groups.

However, this study shows that TMM cannot discriminate among different nasal pathologies. This is interpreted as either that chronic nasal disease influences the function of ET irrespectively of the nature of the pathology as long as the symptoms are obstructive, or that possibly TMM is not the appropriate investigation to discriminate among different nasal pathologies. There is no other study in the literature to compare our results, so TMM can reliably be used for all chronic nasal disease patients; however, TMM values do not reflect each nasal pathology. Other rhinomanometric tests might be recommended as adjuncts to correlate with ETD and its severity in various nasal pathologies.

4.4. Limitations

This study has specific limitations that need to be mentioned and presented. First, the sample size is limited, and this might affect the generalisation of the results. Second, overlapping of symptoms as well as nuances of TMM measurements and difficulties while performing the technique might have also influenced the results unintentionally. This might be the explanation for two separate extreme values of TMM, especially in Group C, that were considered inaccurate and were not included in the statistical analysis. Finally, the results should be interpreted with care and should inspire further bigger trials to be able to draw more reliable conclusions regarding chronic nasal disease and TMM measurements.

5. Conclusions

ETD in patients with chronic nasal disease are of particular interest, as these individuals often face unique challenges in ET function. In light of these considerations, a comprehensive diagnostic approach to ETD in the context of chronic nasal diseases should encompass a thorough clinical evaluation, incorporating a combination of subjective symptoms with ETDQ-7 and NOSE questionnaires. This study shows that TMM can be reliably used in this cohort of patients to diagnose ETD irrespective of their nasal pathology. Through this research, diagnostic approaches are refined to enhance clinical decision-making, and ultimately improve the management of ETD in individuals suffering with chronic nasal diseases.

Author Contributions: Conceptualization, S.A., G.P., P.K. and S.T.; methodology, S.A. and G.P.; software, P.B. and D.-E.G.; validation, S.A.; formal analysis, P.B. and D.-E.G.; investigation, S.A.; resources, writing—original draft preparation, S.A.; writing—review and editing, G.P., P.K., S.T. and J.C.; supervision, G.P., P.K., S.T. and J.C. All authors have read and agreed to the published version of the manuscript.

Funding: This research received no external funding.

Institutional Review Board Statement: The study was conducted in accordance with the Declaration of Helsinki and approved by the Ethics Committee of Aristotle University of Thessaloniki (reference number 130/2023, date of approval 10 May 2023).

Informed Consent Statement: Informed consent was obtained from all subjects involved in the study. Written informed consent was obtained from the patient(s) to publish this paper.

Data Availability Statement: All new data generated in this study are available upon request.

Conflicts of Interest: The authors declare no conflicts of interest.

References

1. Smith, M.E.; Tysome, J.R. Tests of Eustachian tube function: A review. *Clin. Otolaryngol.* **2015**, *40*, 300–311. [CrossRef] [PubMed]
2. Alper, C.M.; Teixeira, M.S.; Kim, J.H.; Swarts, J.D. Diagnostic accuracy of tubomanometry R value in detecting the Eustachian tube pressure equalizing function. *Eur. Arch. Otorhinolaryngol.* **2017**, *274*, 1865–1872. [CrossRef] [PubMed]
3. Ruan, K.; Li, J.; Tan, S.; Liu, L.; Tang, A. Comparison of sonotubometry, impedance, tubo-tympano-aerography, and tubomanometry to test eustachian tube function. *Am. J. Otolaryngol.* **2020**, *41*, 102384. [CrossRef] [PubMed]
4. Smith, M.E.; Zou, C.C.; Baker, C.; Blythe, A.J.; Hutchinson, P.J.; Tysome, J.R. The repeatability of tests of eustachian tube function in healthy ears. *Laryngoscope* **2017**, *127*, 2619–2626. [CrossRef]
5. McCoul, E.D.; Anand, V.K.; Christos, P.J. Validating the clinical assessment of eustachian tube dysfunction: The Eustachian Tube Dysfunction Questionnaire (ETDQ-7). *Laryngoscope* **2012**, *122*, 1137–1141. [CrossRef]
6. Teixeira, J.; Certal, V.; Chang, E.T.; Camacho, M. Nasal Septal Deviations: A Systematic Review of Classification Systems. *Plast. Surg. Int.* **2016**, *2016*, 7089123. [CrossRef]
7. Baumann, I.; Baumann, H. A new classification of septal deviations. *Rhinology* **2007**, *45*, 220–223.
8. Lachanas, V.A.; Tsiouvaka, S.; Tsea, M.; Hajiioannou, J.K.; Skoulakis, C.E. Validation of the nasal obstruction symptom evaluation (NOSE) scale for Greek patients. *Otolaryngol. Head Neck Surg.* **2014**, *151*, 819–823. [CrossRef]
9. Smith, M.E.; Takwoingi, Y.; Deeks, J.; Alper, C.; Bance, M.L.; Bhutta, M.F.; Donnelly, N.; Poe, D.; Tysome, J.R. Eustachian tube dysfunction: A diagnostic accuracy study and proposed diagnostic pathway. *PLoS ONE* **2018**, *13*, e0206946. [CrossRef]

10. Lima, A.F.; Moreira, F.C.; Costa, I.E.; Azevedo, C.; Mar, F.; Dias, L. Nasal septum deviation and Eustachian tube function: A prospective case-control study based on tympanometry, tubomanometry, and ETDQ-7. *Acta Otorrinolaringol. Esp.* **2021**, *73*, 34–41. (In English and Spanish) [CrossRef]
11. Vandersteen, C.; Castillo, L.; Roger, C.; Savoldelli, C.; Guevara, N. Tubomanometry: An effective and promising assessment of Eustachian tube dysfunction in chronic rhinosinusitis patients. *Eur. Ann. Otorhinolaryngol. Head Neck Dis.* **2021**, *138*, 7–12. [CrossRef] [PubMed]
12. Kaya, M.; Dağlı, E.; Kırat, S. Does Nasal Septal Deviation Affect the Eustachian Tube Function and Middle Ear Ventilation? *Turk. Arch. Otorhinolaryngol.* **2018**, *56*, 102–105. [CrossRef] [PubMed]
13. Al Karaki, V.; Hallit, S.; Nacouzi, M.; Rohayem, Z. Is there a relationship between Eustachian tube dysfunction and nasal septal deviation in a sample of the Lebanese population? *Head Face Med.* **2020**, *16*, 23. [CrossRef]
14. Roeyen, S.V.; Van de Heyning, P.; Van Rompaey, V. Responsiveness of the 7-item Eustachian Tube Dysfunction Questionnaire. *J. Int. Adv. Otol.* **2016**, *12*, 106–108. [CrossRef]
15. Roeyen, S.V.; Van de Heyning, P.; Van Rompaey, V. Value and discriminative power of the seven-item Eustachian Tube Dysfunction Questionnaire. *Laryngoscope* **2015**, *125*, 2553–2556. [CrossRef]
16. Smith, M.E.; Cochrane, I.L.; Donnelly, N.; Axon, P.R.; Tysome, J.R. The Performance of Patient-reported Outcome Measures as Diagnostic Tools for Eustachian Tube Dysfunction. *Otol. Neurotol.* **2018**, *39*, 1129–1138. [CrossRef]
17. Schröder, S.; Lehmann, M.; Sauzet, O.; Ebmeyer, J.; Sudhoff, H. A novel diagnostic tool for chronic obstructive eustachian tube dysfunction—The eustachian tube score. *Laryngoscope* **2015**, *125*, 703–708. [CrossRef]
18. Stewart, M.G.; Witsell, D.L.; Smith, T.L.; Weaver, E.M.; Yueh, B.; Hannley, M.T. Development and validation of the Nasal Obstruction Symptom Evaluation (NOSE) scale. *Otolaryngol. Head Neck Surg.* **2004**, *130*, 157–163. [CrossRef]
19. Shastri, K.; Gao, Y.; Davis, S.J.; Kimura, K.S.; Patel, P.N.; Stephan, S.J.; Yang, S.F. Normative Values of the Nasal Obstruction Symptom Evaluation Scale. *Facial Plast. Surg. Aesthet. Med.* **2023**, *25*, 35–39. [CrossRef]
20. Kawai, K.; Dombrowski, N.; AuYeung, T.; Adil, E.A. Validation of the Nasal Obstruction Symptom Evaluation Scale in Pediatric Patients. *Laryngoscope* **2021**, *131*, E2594–E2598. [CrossRef]
21. Schröder, S.; Lehmann, M.; Korbmacher, D.I.C.K.; Sauzet, O.; Sudhoff, H.; Ebmeyer, J. Evaluation of tubomanometry as a routine diagnostic tool for chronic obstructive Eustachian tube dysfunction. *Clin. Otolaryngol.* **2015**, *40*, 691–697. [CrossRef] [PubMed]
22. Zhang, J.; Zhong, Z.; Xiao, S.; Liu, Y.; Zhen, Z.; Ren, L.; Zhang, L. Tubomanometry value as an associated factor for medication outcomes in adult acute otitis media with effusion. *Eur. Arch. Otorhinolaryngol.* **2018**, *275*, 53–57. [CrossRef]

Journal of
Clinical Medicine

MDPI

Article

A Six-Year Examination of the Influence of Surgical Technique and Intraoperative Intraglandular Clostridium Botulinum Toxin Application in Salivary Gland Tumor Operations

Felix Johnson [1], Nora-Maria Burian [1,*], Matthias Santer [1], Verena Strasser [1], Teresa Steinbichler [1], Benedikt Hofauer [1], Anna Stenzl [1], Johanna Klarer [1], Robin Lochbaum [2], Haochen Lei [3], Hongyuan Cao [3], Gabriel Hillebrand [4] and Amir Bolooki [4]

1 Department of Otorhinolaryngology, Medical University of Innsbruck, Anichstraße 35, A-6020 Innsbruck, Austria
2 Department of Otorhinolaryngology, Head and Neck Surgery, Ulm University Medical Center, Frauensteige 12, 89075 Ulm, Germany
3 Department of Statistics, Florida State University, 117 N. Woodward Ave., Tallahassee, FL 32306-4330, USA
4 Department of Otorhinolaryngology, Klinikum Rechts der Isar, TUM School of Medicine and Health, Ismaninger Str. 22, 81675 Munich, Germany
* Correspondence: nora-maria.burian@tirol-kliniken.at

Abstract: Introduction: Salivary gland tumor operations are associated with complications including facial nerve dysfunction (FND) and salivary fistula. The objective of this study was to investigate the effect of extracapsular dissection (ECD) and the application of Clostridium botulinum toxin (CBT) in contrast to partial and lateral parotidectomy on complications. **Methods:** All salivary gland tumor operations performed within the last 6 years were retrospectively examined. Data were collected from electronic patient files from our otorhinolaryngology clinic. Total parotidectomies and submandibulectomies were not included in the analysis of CBT application. **Results:** In total, 418 cases were examined, including 84 (20%) malignant tumors. In total, 18 patients underwent ECD, 93 partial parotidectomy, 199 lateral parotidectomy, 76 total parotidectomy, and 32 submandibulectomy. The most common complication was transient FND (49%; $n = 205$; data available for 415 patients), which was measured at four days. Additional complications included salivary fistula ($n = 56$), infection ($n = 49$), bleeding or hematoma ($n = 21$). Preoperative facial nerve paralysis ($p < 0.0001$), pain ($p < 0.0001$), and a history of squamous cell skin carcinoma (SCC) ($p < 0.001$) were predictive of malignancy. The application of CBT did not reduce the risk of salivary fistula (p-value: 0.0182) and was associated with a higher combined complication rate (p-value: 0.0199). ECD was not associated with a lower likelihood for FND ($p = 0.350$). **Conclusions:** Preoperative pain, facial paralysis, or a history of SCC are predictors of malignancy. Use of CBT was not associated with a reduced risk of salivary fistula, but rather a higher complication rate.

Keywords: parotidectomy; extracapsular dissection; lateral parotidectomy; partial parotidectomy; clostridium botulinum toxin; intraoperative; intraglandular; pleomorphic adenoma; Warthin tumor; salivary gland tumor

1. Introduction

Salivary gland tumors account for 3–10% of all head and neck tumors [1] and represent a fair proportion of soft tissue surgery for head and neck surgeons. Removal of salivary gland tumors requires extensive surgical experience and complications are considered highly dependent on the surgeon's expertise [2]. Complications following salivary gland tumor operations include wound infections, bleeding and hematoma, chronic pain, and Frey's syndrome. Further complications include facial nerve dysfunction (FND) and salivary fistula. The surgical removal of tumors of the parotid gland is performed either via extracapsular dissection (ECD), partial parotidectomy, lateral parotidectomy (also known as superficial parotidectomy), via total parotidectomy or radical parotidectomy. Each approach has potential advantages and may be successful when appropriately performed.

A salivary fistula is a postoperative complication that may develop after a salivary gland operation. It typically presents when only part of the salivary gland has been resected. In such cases, the remaining gland tissue at the border of the resected surface continues to produce saliva. When the excreted saliva does not follow the normal anatomical drainage pathway, it may collect in the wound underneath the skin in what is known as a sialocele. In some cases, a salivary fistula may develop when the saliva drains through the sutured wound out of the skin. Frey's syndrome, also known as gustatory sweating, typically occurs after parotid surgery due to aberrant postoperative neuronal regeneration [3]. Symptomatic Frey's syndrome may be reported from patients and is confirmed through the Minor's starch–iodine test [4].

Of further interest is to determine which perioperative risk factors may be associated with sialocele or salivary fistulas, which have an estimated incidence of 9.1% [5]. The type of operation and tumor entity may influence the likelihood of developing a fistula. The intraoperative application of intraglandular Clostridium botulinum toxin may play a role in changing the chance of complications. Clostridium botulinum toxin is typically applied postoperatively in severe cases of persistent salivary fistula or sialocele. Its effect typically gradually begins about 7–10 days after application [6,7].

Currently, there are three leading types of botulinum toxin A that are produced: onabotulinum toxin A (ONA; Botox®), incobotulinum toxin A (INCO; Xeomin®), and abobotulinum toxin A (ABO; Dysport®). ONA and INCO are considered to have similar dosing units, whereas ABO is considered to have a dosing equivalent 2–3 times that of ONA or INCO [8].

Some surgeons apply approximately 200 units of Clostridium botulinum toxin type A (ABO) in order to lower the risk of postoperative fistulas, while other surgeons do not believe that it plays a role in reducing complications. To the best of our knowledge, only one clinical study has been conducted evaluating the postoperative risk of sialocele or salivary fistula when Clostridium botulinum toxin is intraoperatively applied [9]. Here, a lower rate of salivary fistulas was noted, although these results were not statistically significant.

In this study, we seek to determine if the intraoperative intraglandular application of Clostridium botulinum toxin, which some surgeons favor, is associated with a lowered risk of postoperative salivary fistula. Furthermore, the potential risk of other perioperative complications, such as bleeding, facial nerve dysfunction (FND), chronic pain, infections, hematoma, Frey's syndrome, first-bite syndrome, and emergency reoperation, will be investigated.

These perioperative factors are also to be examined in the stratification of the type of operation performed. Additionally, this study aims to describe the heterogeneous types of benign and malignant tumors that develop in salivary gland tumors in Austria, as this has rarely been investigated.

2. Methods

The study protocol is in accordance with the Declaration of Helsinki. The Institutional Ethics Board of the University Clinic of Innsbruck reviewed and approved the protocol; it was also approved by the local ethics committee (date: April 2024; protocol code EK Nmr. 1124).

2.1. Data Collection

In this monocentric retrospective study, data collection began by thoroughly inspecting the electronic patient medical database of our electronic patient file system (KIS, Klinisches Informationssystem, Oracle Health, Redwood Shores, CA, USA) at the Department of Otolaryngology and Head and Neck Surgery at the Medical University Clinic of Innsbruck to find patients who had undergone surgery for salivary gland tumors between

1 January 2018 and 1 May 2024. This included patients who had tumor operations of the parotid, submandibular, sublingual, or minor salivary glands. Patients who underwent an operation because of sialolithiasis or chronic sialadenitis were not included. Based on these criteria, 418 patients were included in the study. Following partial parotidectomy, lateral parotidectomy, or ECP, our surgeons will mix approximately 150–200 units of the Clostridium botulinum toxin type A (ABO) (Dysport®, Ipsen, München, Germany) with 2 mL of saline solution. The decision to utilize botulinum toxin is at the discretion of the individual surgeon. The decision to administer botulinum toxin is based on the extent of the resection and the amount of residual parotid tissue remaining in situ, factors that may lead to complications such as a salivary fistula or Frey's syndrome. In principle, botulinum toxin is administered in all operations where parotid tissue remains in situ. In rare cases, if the dissection of the parotid fascia, which divides the lateral from the medial part, is highly successful and the fascia remains intact, the surgeon may opt to forego the administration of botulinum toxin in our clinic. Subsequently, the CBT solution is directly injected under direct visualization into the parotid tissue that has not been removed. This is not performed in cases of total parotidectomy or submandibulectomies.

Patients who received a submandibulectomy or total parotidectomy do not typically receive CBT and therefore, were not included in the analysis of the effect of salivary fistula. However, data from these operations were still included so as to compare complication rates.

Subsequently, a review of the medical literature was conducted to identify potential factors that could affect perioperative complications. Patient records were accessed and relevant data points were identified and entered into an Excel spreadsheet. The location and histology of the primary tumor, history of squamous skin cancer or melanoma, history of smoking, age and gender were noted. Additionally, we examined the patient's history to determine if this was the first operation of a salivary gland tumor or if other operations had taken place and due to what tumor entity, if a facial paralysis or pain were preoperatively or postoperatively present. Medical records during and on the last day of stay on the ward were reviewed to determine early and late complications. Cases of post-operative bleeding or infections were noted. The intraoperative intraglandular application of Clostridium botulinum toxin was noted via surgical reports. Postoperatively, most patients presented to our clinic about 12 days to 14 days after the operation in order to have the sutures removed, to discuss histology, and to check the status of the wound. Ambulatory doctors' notes concerning wound status, facial nerve function, as well as the presence or absence of salivary fistula were consistently assessed at this point in our electronic patient database and recorded. In some cases, data points were not retrospectively able to be noted as they were not described in patient files. These cases were excluded for the specific analysis of said characteristics. In this study, patients' medical records were retrospectively examined to determine if patients reported gustatory sweating, chronic pain, or first-bite syndrome after the operation. These data were typically reported in after-treatment of patients around the 6-month mark.

2.2. Statistical Analysis

The compiled and documented data points were entered into cells of the statistical software. Prism 5 (GraphPad, Version 9.2.0, San Diego, CA, USA) and Microsoft Office Excel 2016 (Microsoft, Redmond, WA, USA) were used for data analysis. Contingency analysis was performed using one-tailed Fischer's exact test. A correlation was seen as significant if the p-value was smaller than 0.05. The predictive power of individual symptoms in relation to malignancy was also investigated. We used descriptive statistics to determine the frequency distributions (n and %) of baseline characteristics of the cohort. For continuous variables, average distributions with standard deviation (SD) or medians were utilized.

The logistic regression was performed to adjust for the potential covariates when we studied the relationship between occurrences of complications and some predictors, such as different types of operation, and the injection of CBT. The potential covariates included gender, age, diagnoses (benign or malignant tumors) and the occurrence of a re-operation. We adjusted different diagnoses by treating them as categorical variables in the logistic regression model. To decrease the number of covariates, we combined the rare diagnoses (frequency < 10) into the group "other benign" and "other malignancy".

Missing data are presented in the flowchart in Figure 1.

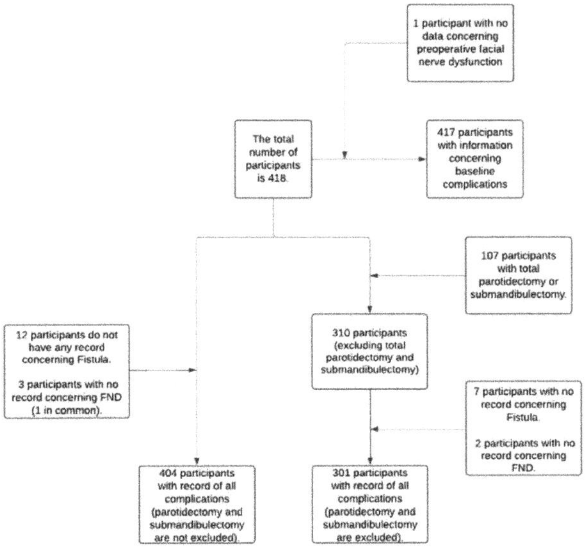

Figure 1. Flowchart illustrating the sample size and missing data points.

3. Results

A total of 418 patients were included in the study (see Table 1). The most common tumor was the pleomorphic adenoma (PA; n = 167; 39.95%) including 10 recurrent PA (RPA), which were operated on a second time with a median of 12 years (std. dev. 6.37; mean 10.11) after the first operation. The second most common tumor was the Warthin tumor (WT; n = 125; 25.90%). The salivary gland most commonly affected was the parotid gland (n = 386; 92.3% of all tumors), followed by the submandibular gland (n = 32; 7.7% of all tumors; see Table 2). No tumors were removed from the sublingual gland. The most common malignant finding was lymph node metastasis due to squamous cell carcinoma of the skin (SCC; n = 31), followed by adenocarcinoma (n = 11).

For the entire cohort noted complication rates included infection (n = 49; 12%), hematoma/bleeding (n = 21; 5%) and need for reoperation (n = 11; 3%), Frey's syndrome (n = 10; 2%), and chronic pain (n = 9; 2%). No patients were found to have first-bite syndrome.

Statistically significant correlations were observed between clinical features and malignity, which is shown in Table 3. These included preoperative facial paralysis (p-value: <0.0001), pain (p-value: <0.0001), or a history of squamous cell carcinoma ($p < 0.001$). No significant difference was noted postoperatively between the patients who had a malignant tumor vs. benign tumor and other complications (defined as bleeding, infection, Frey's syndrome, chronic pain; p-value: 0.067).

Table 1. Tumor histology and frequency.

Tumor Histology	Frequency	Percentage (%) of All Tumors
Pleomorphic adenoma	167	39.95
Warthin tumor	125	29.90
Lymph node metastasis (SCC)	31	7.42
Lymph node (benign)	14	3.35
Adenocarcinoma	11	2.63
Lymph node metastasis (malignant melanoma)	11	2.62
Lipoma	8	1.91
Cyst	8	1.91
Oncocytoma	6	1.44
Acinic cell carcinoma	6	1.44
Lymphoma	5	1.20
Mucoepidermoid carcinoma	4	0.96
Adenocystic carcinoma	4	0.96
Lymph node metastasis (Merkel cell carcinoma)	3	0.72
Myoepithelioma	2	0.48
Basal cell carcinoma	2	0.48
Basal cell adenoma	2	0.48
Carcinoma ex pleomorphic adenoma	2	0.48
Lymph node metastasis of a sarcoma	2	0.48
Secretory carcinoma	1	0.24
Schwannoma	1	0.24
Hemangioma	1	0.24
Secretory carcinoma	1	0.24
Undifferentiated carcinoma	1	0.24

Table 2. Summary of affected salivary glands and frequency of malignancy.

	Tumor Location	All Benign Tumors	All Malignant Tumors	Primary Salivary Gland Malignancy	Lymph Node Metastasis Due to SCC
Gl. parotis	386 (92.3%)	312	74	27	31
Gl. submandibularis	32 (7.7%)	22	10	10	0
Total	418	334	84	37	31

Table 3. Frequency and relationship between type of tumors and existence of complications (pain, facial paralysis and history of SCC). The number enclosed in parentheses represents the number of missing values within the specified class.

	Preoperative Pain		Preoperative Facial Paralysis (1)		History of SCC	
	Pain	No Pain	Facial Paralysis	No Facial Paralysis	History of SCC	No History of SCC
Benign	5	329	3	331	5	329
Malignant	30	54	10	73	36	48
	$p < 0.0001$		$p < 0.0001$		$p < 0.0001$	

The most common complication was facial nerve dysfunction, which occurred in 49% of patients ($n = 205$; data available for 415 patients) measured at 4 days. At 12–14 days (data available for $n = 202$ patients) there was a recorded complete improvement in 26.8% ($n = 54$) of patients, partial improvement in 107 (53%), and no improvement in 20.3% ($n = 41$). The most commonly performed surgical technique was the lateral parotidectomy ($n = 199$; 48%), followed by the partial parotidectomy ($n = 93$; 22%) (see Figure 2). The lateral parotidectomy was defined as the complete removal of the superficial parotid gland with main facial nerve exposition. A partial parotidectomy was defined as the main facial nerve exposition with the partial removal of the superficial parotid gland. Extracapsular dissection was defined as the removal of a superficial portion of the parotid gland without exposition of the main facial nerve branch (n = 18; 4%). All total parotidectomies and submandibulectomies were excluded from the analysis of the complication rates for salivary fistula.

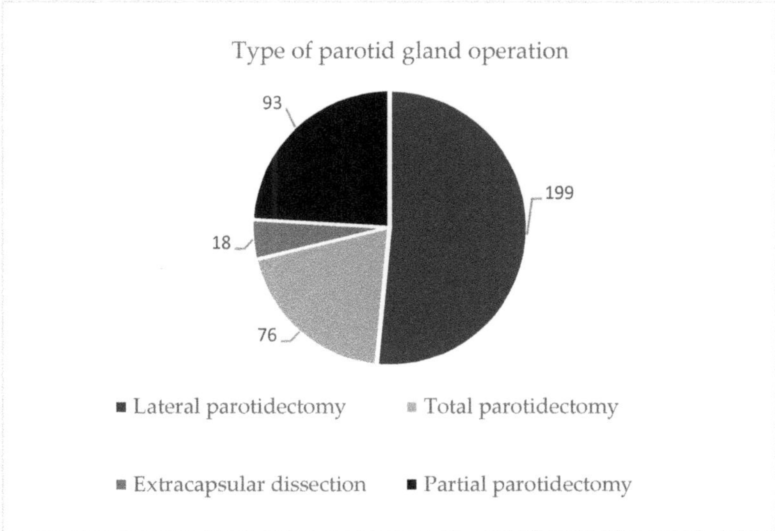

Figure 2. Type and frequency of operation performed in the parotid gland.

The logistic regression demonstrated that there was no association between the type of operation and complications (such as salivary fistula or facial nerve dysfunction, and other operation). The corresponding p-values are listed in Table 4. We also investigated the incidence of complications related to the administration of botulinum toxin and the type of surgery, excluding total parotidectomy and submandibulectomy (see Table 5 for details). As this study is retrospective, it was not possible to obtain all data. The missing data are included in parentheses.

Table 4. The number and the corresponding log odds ratio of salivary fistula and other complications stratified according to type of operation (patients with total parotidectomy or submandibulectomy were excluded). The covariates and the injection of botulinum toxin are adjusted.

	Total	Fistula	FND	Other
LP (Baseline)	199	30	83	45
PP (log odd ratio) (p-value)	93 / /	11 −0.21 p = 0.598	39 −0.04 p = 0.881	15 −0.32 p = 0.360
ECD (log odds ratio) (p-value)	18 / /	2 0.25 p = 0.767	5 −0.54 p = 0.350	3 0.11 p = 0.878

Table 5. Rate of salivary fistula and other complications stratified according to application of botulinum toxin and type of operation (patients with total parotidectomy or submandibulectomy were excluded). The number enclosed in parentheses represents the number of missing values within the specified class.

	Operation Type	Total	Fistula	Other Complications	FND
Clostridium botulinum toxin	ECD	8	2	3	3
	LP	175	29 (5)	42	74 (2)
	PP	80	11 (2)	14	34
	All	263	42 (7)	59	111 (2)
No Clostridium botulinum toxin	ECD	10	0	0	2
	LP	24	1	3	9
	PP	13	0	1	5
	All	47	1	4	16

A second operation was performed in 6% of cases. The rate of FND directly postoperatively in patients with one vs. two operations was 48.7% vs. 60.0% ($p = 0.27$). Other complications (defined as bleeding, infection, Frey's syndrome, chronic pain) were more common after the second operation (18.6% vs. 26.9%), though this was not statistically significant ($p < 0.2975$).

Additionally, we found that the injection of CBT was associated with an increased rate of the salivary fistula (2.36; $p = 0.024$) and other complications (1.25; $p = 0.030$), but did not influence the rate of postoperative facial nerve dysfunction (0.33; $p = 0.350$) when the covariates and the type of operation are adjusted. The contingency table with total parotidectomy and submandibulectomy (illustrating these both excluded and included) can be found in Tables 6 and 7.

Table 6. Contingency table of injection of botulinum toxin and type of operation (patients with total parotidectomy or submandibulectomy were excluded). The number in parentheses represents the number of missing values in that class.

	Salivary Fistula (7)		Other Complications		FND (2)	
	Salivary Fistula	No Salivary Fistula	Complications	No Complications	FND	No FND
CBT	42	214	59	204	111	150
No CBT	1	46	4	43	16	31
p-value	$p = 0.0099$		$p = 0.0289$		$p = 0.2766$	

Table 7. Contingency table of injection of botulinum toxin and type of operation (patients with total parotidectomy or submandibulectomy were not excluded). The number enclosed in parentheses represents the number of missing values within the specified class.

	Salivary Fistula (12)		Other Complications		FND (3)	
	Salivary Fistula	No Salivary Fistula	Complications	No Complications	FND	No FND
CBT	43	223	62	212	120	152
No CBT	13	127	18	126	85	58
p-value	$p = 0.0560$		$p = 0.0124$		$p = 0.003$	

4. Discussion

The cohort that received clostridium botulinum toxin consisted of 238 male and 180 female patients with a mean age of 58.29 years, who underwent a salivary gland tumor operation in Austria in the state of Tirol. Of these patients, a total of 274 patients received intraoperative intraglandular application of Clostridium botulinum toxin. While most studies examine clostridium botulinum toxin as an intervention for sialorrhea or salivary gland fistulas, the main focus of our study was to evaluate the possible prevention of such complications through intraoperative application. With 274 patients who received clostridium botulinum toxin in our cohort, our case numbers are significantly higher than in most other studies that investigated Clostridium botulinum toxin and its effect on sialorrhea or fistulas postoperatively [10–12]. Most of the literature with higher case numbers focuses mainly on neurological syndromes that lead to sialorrhea [13]. Studies focusing on primary salivary gland pathologies, such as sialadenitis or Frey's syndrome, have reported lower-case numbers [11,14–16]. Furthermore, to improve the representativeness of our study no specific patient ethnicities were excluded. Since there are also multiple publications regarding clostridium botulinum toxin for neurological pediatric disease, compared to these studies, our cohort shows a much wider age range, raising the generalizability of our findings [13]. In this cohort, the most common type of tumor was the pleomorphic adenoma (PA) followed by the Warthin tumor (WT), which conforms to the demographic data presented in other studies.

Primary salivary gland cancers are a diverse group of tumors with more than 20 different histological subtypes. These tumors can vary greatly in their appearance in histopathology. However, there is often overlap between the different subtypes in terms of their histological, immunohistochemical, molecular, and biological features [17]. The most common primary malignant tumor was the adenocarcinoma (n = 11; 2.63% of all tumors). In most demographic studies, the most common primary malignancy is described as mucoepidermoid carcinoma [18]. However, in this study, only 4 cases were reported, as compared to 11 cases of adenocarcinoma. It is notable that, when considering all malignant carcinomas, the most common malignancy in this study was lymph node metastases due to squamous cell carcinoma of the skin (n = 31; 31%).

Squamous cell carcinoma of the skin is the most common type of cancer worldwide, with 70–80% [19] estimated to develop in the head and neck area, of which 5% are estimated to metastasize [19–21]. Other studies have reported the most malignant tumor of the salivary gland to also be metastasis due to squamous cell skin cancer [22]. This reinforces the need for regular and close check-ups including ultrasound examinations in patients with a history of SCC. Patients who preoperatively clinically presented with pain, FND, or a history of SCC or malignant melanoma were significantly predictive for a malignant tumor. As such, surgeons who operate on patients who preoperatively present with said symptoms should be preoperatively prepared for a malignant outcome.

Operative methods that have been described in preventing Frey's syndrome include the use of local flaps that are interpositioned into the wound. However, this is typically primarily performed in order to improve cosmetic results or in advanced oncologic cases and is associated with further operative risks, and therefore rarely performed [23]. The use of postoperative radiotherapy in cases of refractory salivary fistula has been described [24]. However, its use is limited to its long-term adverse effects including xerostomia. The results of definitive studies concerning the association between surgical approaches and postoperative complications have been inconclusive. Some studies have indicated that ECD may be associated with a higher risk of postoperative facial nerve dysfunction (FND) and salivary fistula formation [25]. However, other studies have shown conflicting or differing results that advocate for this procedure [26,27].

In this study, the postoperative rate of FND was 49% measured at 4 days with a reported 26.8% having complete reconvalescence at 12–14 days. These results are similar to those described in other studies [28,29]. Although other studies have described lower rates of complications including FND after ECD [30], in our study, there was no association between the type of operation and FND (p-value: 0.3559) or salivary fistula (p-value: 0.6959). The rate of Frey's syndrome in our study (2%) is comparable to those described in recent studies, which also described a 2% rate following ECD and in cases of lateral or superficial parotidectomy in 1.8% of cases [25]. However, studies have presented very different rates of Frey's syndrome, some reporting symptoms in 23–43% of patients after 1 year [31]. In our study, the frequency of other complications (defined as bleeding, infection, Frey's syndrome, and chronic pain; *p*-value: 0.6706) was also not significantly lower in patients with ECD as compared to partial and lateral parotidectomy. The total rate of bleeding requiring reoperation was 3%.

The extent of surgical gland excision is the subject of discussion in various studies. Many studies show higher rates of facial palsy when higher numbers of facial nerve branches were dissected intraoperatively. This mostly correlates with the extent of parotidectomy [32]. But there are still varying study results regarding other postoperative complications. While some studies describe varying fistula rates with no significant correlation to the extent of surgery others prove a correlation to residual gland parenchyma [33–38]. In summary, the surgical trend is towards minimally invasive resections in the form of extracapsular dissection (ECD). This is due to the fact that numerous studies have shown a reduced FND risk [26]. The use of Clostridium botulinum toxin in treating salivary fistulas postoperatively is common. However, its use prophylactically via direct intraoperative intraglandular application is rarely performed. Concerning the literature there seems to be only one other study examining intraoperative application of botulinum toxin. Lee Dong-Joo et al. [9] showed that the incidence of sialoceles was significantly lower in the cohort that received botulinum toxin. The rate of salivary fistula was, however, not shown to be significantly lowered. Our study showed that the use of Clostridium botulinum toxin was associated with a higher rate of salivary fistula (*p*-value: 0.0560). The main focus of the pre-existing literature is the use of botulinum toxin only after complications, such as fistulas, have occurred. Most studies generally describe injecting between 30–100 units of Clostridium botulinum toxin, though some studies have also applied up to 225 units [39].

Furthermore, the use and potential advantages of Clostridium botulinum toxin should also be evaluated concerning the number of patients needing treatment in order to prevent a potential salivary fistula. The number of units of toxin injected was approximately 200 units, with the cost of Clostridium botulinum toxin A (ABO) at our clinic amounting to approximately EUR 238 per 500 units. In this cohort, the intraoperative application of Clostridium botulinum toxin was associated with an increased risk of complications. Studies describe rates of salivary fistula approaching 9.5% [33], suggesting that, assuming the intraglandular intraoperative application of botulinum toxin is effective, in order to potentially prevent one salivary fistula, one would need to treat 10 patients. This may be economically unfeasible for many hospitals, as the costs to hypothetically treat one patient approach EUR 1190, assuming a 100% effectivity of the botulinum toxin. Moreover, in this study, the use of botulinum toxin was associated with a higher fistula rate.

Limitations of our study include its retrospective nature, which may be associated with problems in data acquisition, as some data may not have been documented. Besides the retrospective nature of this study, other limitations should be discussed. Information concerning whether the parotid fascia was reconstructed was not recorded. Some surgeons believe that reconstruction of the parotid fascia may lower the risk of salivary fistula or Frey's syndrome [40]. Comorbidities associated with salivary gland tumor operations are difficult to quantify according to specific surgical techniques because postoperative rates of FND or salivary fistulas may be highly dependent on the type of tumor, location and size thereof, and the skill and expertise of the surgeon. Our study could be biased by the amount of surgical experience of the operating physician.

Regarding the high cost of botulinum toxin and the physician's interest in acting as minimally invasive as possible, there can still be valuable information drawn from this study. The most sensible way to use clostridium botulinum toxin would be to only use it in high-risk cases. It is likely that clostridium botulinum toxin was administered in cases in which the surgeon deemed a high risk for complications. Such cases may include instances where resection margins and the salivary gland capsule were more difficult to identify due to inflammatory processes. This could result in more extensive damage to the gland capsule, thereby raising the risk of complications. Furthermore, the tumor's location may have influenced the physician's decision-making process, as studies have shown that tumors located in the middle of the gland are associated with higher rates of sialoceles and fistulas [5,38].

Few methods are available to prevent salivary fistula. One may potentially use anticholinergic medication in the postoperative setting to reduce the production of saliva. The transdermal application of scopolamine is usually first utilized as a treatment once salivary fistulas have already become clinically apparent. One study described the prophylactic perioperative application of transdermal scopolamine and noted a significant reduction in salivary fistula with a number needed to treat of 9.17 [41]. However, this method is rarely used prophylactically over the 2- to 4-week period, in which the risk of development of salivary fistula is at its highest. Additionally, such medications can lead to unwanted side effects such as urinary retention and confusion [42]. To effectively examine the use of Clostridium botulinum toxin, prospective randomized studies should be performed, and patients should be stratified according to groups defined by tumor type and surgical approach. This is important because there could be a potential source of bias regarding the use of CBT, namely the tendency for it to be employed in challenging settings in which surgery was already deemed to be a high-risk procedure.

5. Conclusions

In this monocentric retrospective cross-sectional study, we examined 418 patients who underwent salivary gland tumor operations. The high frequency of patients with lymph node metastasis due to SCC of the skin or malignant melanoma reinforces the need for active surveillance following head and neck skin cancer. The use of Clostridium botulinum toxin did not significantly reduce the rate of salivary fistula postoperatively but was associated with a higher rate of complications and salivary fistulas. A potential bias of this study is that Clostridium botulinum toxin may have been more likely to be utilized in difficult surgical cases where resection margins and the salivary gland capsule were more difficult to identify due to inflammatory processes. This could lead to more extensive surgical trauma raising complication risks. Additionally, a potentially high number of patients needing treatment may make this unproven prophylactic treatment of salivary fistulas economically unfeasible for many surgical departments.

Author Contributions: Conceptualization, F.J. and A.B.; Investigation, F.J., N.-M.B. and R.L.; Methodology, F.J., A.B. and R.L.; Project administration, F.J. and B.H.; Validation, F.J., H.L., H.C. and R.L.; Writing—original draft, F.J., A.B., N.-M.B. and G.H.; Writing—review and editing, F.J., R.L., A.B., M.S., V.S., T.S., A.S. and J.K. All authors have read and agreed to the published version of the manuscript.

Funding: This research received no external funding.

Institutional Review Board Statement: The study was conducted in accordance with the Declaration of Helsinki and approved by the Institutional Review Board at the University Clinic of Innsbruck (protocol code 1124, date of 5 April 2024).

Informed Consent Statement: Patient consent was waived after careful consideration from the above-mentioned ethics board as no patients were identified through this study.

Data Availability Statement: The original contributions presented in the study are included in the article, further inquiries can be directed to the corresponding author.

Conflicts of Interest: The authors of this study have no conflicts of interest. Hongyuan Cao acknowledges partial support from NIH 2UL1TR001427-5. The manuscript is not under simultaneous consideration with another journal, has not been published before, and all authors concur with the submission. All authors have read and agreed to the published version of the manuscript.

Abbreviations

FND	Focal nerve dysfunction
ECD	Extracapsular dissection
SD	standard deviations
OR	Odds ratios
CI	confidence intervals
PA	Pleomorphic adenoma
RPA	Recurrent pleomorphic adenoma
WHO	World Health Organization
WT	Warthin's tumor
CBT	Clostridium botulinum toxin
ONA	Onabotulinum toxin A
INCO	Incobotulinum toxin A
ABO	Abobotulinum toxin A
SCC	Squamous cell carcinoma

References

1. Tian, Z.; Li, L.; Wang, L.; Hu, Y.; Li, J. Salivary Gland Neoplasms in Oral and Maxillofacial Regions: A 23-Year Retrospective Study of 6982 Cases in an Eastern Chinese Population. *Int. J. Oral Maxillofac. Surg.* **2010**, *39*, 235–242. [CrossRef] [PubMed]
2. Deschler, D.G.; Kozin, E.D.; Kanumuri, V.; Devore, E.; Shapiro, C.; Koen, N.; Sethi, R.K.V. Single-Surgeon Parotidectomy Outcomes in an Academic Center Experience during a 15-Year Period. *Laryngoscope Investig. Otolaryngol.* **2020**, *5*, 1096–1103. [CrossRef] [PubMed]
3. Marchese-Ragona, R.; De Filippis, C.; Marioni, G.; Staffieri, A. Treatment of Complications of Parotid Gland Surgery. *Acta Otorhinolaryngol. Ital.* **2005**, *25*, 174. [PubMed]
4. Motz, K.M.; Kim, Y.J. Auriculotemporal Syndrome (Frey Syndrome). *Otolaryngol. Clin. N. Am.* **2016**, *49*, 501–509. [CrossRef] [PubMed]
5. Britt, C.J.; Stein, A.P.; Gessert, T.; Pflum, Z.; Saha, S.; Hartig, G.K. Factors Influencing Sialocele or Salivary Fistula Formation Postparotidectomy. *Head Neck* **2017**, *39*, 387–391. [CrossRef]
6. Jeung, I.S.; Lee, S.; Kim, H.S.; Yeo, C.K. Effect of Botulinum Toxin a Injection into the Salivary Glands for Sialorrhea in Children with Neurologic Disorders. *Ann. Rehabil. Med.* **2012**, *36*, 340. [CrossRef]
7. Ledda, C.; Artusi, C.A.; Tribolo, A.; Rinaldi, D.; Imbalzano, G.; Lopiano, L.; Zibetti, M. Time to Onset and Duration of Botulinum Toxin Efficacy in Movement Disorders. *J. Neurol.* **2022**, *269*, 3706–3712. [CrossRef]
8. Scaglione, F. Conversion Ratio between Botox®, Dysport®, and Xeomin® in Clinical Practice. *Toxins* **2016**, *8*, 65. [CrossRef]
9. Lee, D.J.; Lee, Y.M.; Park, H.J.; Lee, J.W.; Cha, W. Intraoperative Botulinum Toxin Injection for Superficial Partial Parotidectomy: A Prospective Pilot Study. *Clin. Otolaryngol.* **2021**, *46*, 998–1004. [CrossRef]
10. Sławek, J.; Madaliński, M. Botulinum Toxin Therapy for Nonmotor Aspects of Parkinson's Disease. *Int. Rev. Neurobiol.* **2017**, *134*, 1111–1142. [CrossRef]
11. Graillon, N.; Le Roux, M.K.; Chossegros, C.; Haen, P.; Lutz, J.C.; Foletti, J.M. Botulinum Toxin for Ductal Stenosis and Fistulas of the Main Salivary Glands. *Int. J. Oral Maxillofac. Surg.* **2019**, *48*, 1411–1414. [CrossRef] [PubMed]
12. Lungren, M.P.; Halula, S.; Coyne, S.; Sidell, D.; Racadio, J.M.; Patel, M.N. Ultrasound-Guided Botulinum Toxin Type a Salivary Gland Injection in Children for Refractory Sialorrhea: 10-Year Experience at a Large Tertiary Children's Hospital. *Pediatr. Neurol.* **2016**, *54*, 70–75. [CrossRef]
13. Heikel, T.; Patel, S.; Ziai, K.; Shah, S.J.; Lighthall, J.G. Botulinum Toxin A in the Management of Pediatric Sialorrhea: A Systematic Review. *Ann. Otol. Rhinol. Laryngol.* **2023**, *132*, 200–206. [CrossRef] [PubMed]
14. Schwalje, A.T.; Hoffman, H.T. Intraductal Salivary Gland Infusion with Botulinum Toxin. *Laryngoscope Investig. Otolaryngol.* **2019**, *4*, 520–525. [CrossRef]
15. Golding, C.N.; Larsen, D.G. The Incidence of Frey Syndrome and Treatment with Botulinum Toxin in the Central Denmark Region. *Laryngoscope Investig. Otolaryngol.* **2022**, *7*, 1814. [CrossRef]
16. Strohl, M.P.; Chang, C.F.; Ryan, W.R.; Chang, J.L. Botulinum Toxin for Chronic Parotid Sialadenitis: A Case Series and Systematic Review. *Laryngoscope Investig. Otolaryngol.* **2021**, *6*, 404–413. [CrossRef] [PubMed]
17. Bradley, P.J. Frequency and Histopathology by Site, Major Pathologies, Symptoms and Signs of Salivary Gland Neoplasms. *Adv. Otorhinolaryngol.* **2016**, *78*, 9–16. [CrossRef] [PubMed]
18. Karia, P.S.; Jambusaria-Pahlajani, A.; Harrington, D.P.; Murphy, G.F.; Qureshi, A.A.; Schmults, C.D. Evaluation of American Joint Committee on Cancer, International Union Against Cancer, and Brigham and Women's Hospital Tumor Staging for Cutaneous Squamous Cell Carcinoma. *J. Clin. Oncol.* **2014**, *32*, 327–334. [CrossRef]
19. Veness, M.J.; Porceddu, S.; Palme, C.E.; Morgan, G.J. Cutaneous Head and Neck Squamous Cell Carcinoma Metastatic to Parotid and Cervical Lymph Nodes. *Head Neck* **2007**, *29*, 621–631. [CrossRef]

20. Mourouzis, C.; Boynton, A.; Grant, J.; Umar, T.; Wilson, A.; Macpheson, D.; Pratt, C. Cutaneous Head and Neck SCCs and Risk of Nodal Metastasis—UK Experience. *J. Craniomaxillofac. Surg.* **2009**, *37*, 443–447. [CrossRef]
21. O'Brien, C.J.; Malka, V.B.; Mijailovic, M. Evaluation of 242 Consecutive Parotidectomies Performed for Benign and Malignant Disease. *ANZ J. Surg.* **1993**, *63*, 870–877. [CrossRef] [PubMed]
22. Kato, M.G.; Erkul, E.; Nguyen, S.A.; Day, T.A.; Hornig, J.D.; Lentsch, E.J.; Gillespie, M.B. Extracapsular Dissection vs Superficial Parotidectomy of Benign Parotid Lesions: Surgical Outcomes and Cost-Effectiveness Analysis. *JAMA Otolaryngol. Head Neck Surg.* **2017**, *143*, 1092. [CrossRef] [PubMed]
23. Pellitteri, P.K. Prevention of Frey Syndrome. *Oper. Tech. Otolaryngol. Neck Surg.* **2018**, *29*, 177–184. [CrossRef]
24. Rao, J.K.D.; Gehlot, N.; Laxmy, V.; Siwach, V. Management of Parotid Fistula Using Hypertonic Saline. *Natl. J. Maxillofac. Surg.* **2011**, *2*, 177. [CrossRef]
25. Kadletz, L.; Grasl, S.; Grasl, M.C.; Perisanidis, C.; Erovic, B.M. Extracapsular Dissection versus Superficial Parotidectomy in Benign Parotid Gland Tumors: The Vienna Medical School Experience. *Head Neck* **2017**, *39*, 356–360. [CrossRef]
26. Thölken, R.; Jering, M.; Mayer, M.; Schiele, S.; Müller, G.; Zenk, J. Prospective Study on Complications Using Different Techniques for Parotidectomy for Benign Tumors. *Laryngoscope Investig. Otolaryngol.* **2021**, *6*, 1367. [CrossRef] [PubMed]
27. Psychogios, G.; Bohr, C.; Constantinidis, J.; Canis, M.; Vander Poorten, V.; Plzak, J.; Knopf, A.; Betz, C.; Guntinas-Lichius, O.; Zenk, J. Review of Surgical Techniques and Guide for Decision Making in the Treatment of Benign Parotid Tumors. *Eur. Arch. Otorhinolaryngol.* **2021**, *278*, 15–29. [CrossRef]
28. Molinari, G.; Calvaruso, F.; Barbazza, A.; Vanelli, E.; Nizzoli, F.; Reggiani, E.; Guidotti, M.; Borghi, A.; Marchioni, D.; Presutti, L.; et al. Patterns and Timing of Recovery from Facial Nerve Palsy after Nerve-Sparing Parotid Surgery: The Role of Neuromuscular Retraining. *Eur. Arch. Otorhinolaryngol.* **2024**, *281*, 5465–5472. [CrossRef]
29. Otanez, E.S.; Trokhimtchouk, T.F.; Semanate, F.; Palacios, C. Incidence of Facial Nerve Paralysis After Parotidectomy: Our Experience. *Cureus* **2024**, *16*, e55045. [CrossRef]
30. Neumann, A.; Rosenberger, D.; Vorsprach, O.; Dazert, S. The Incidence of Frey Syndrome Following Parotidectomy: Results of a Survey and Follow-Up. *HNO* **2011**, *59*, 173–178. [CrossRef]
31. Grosheva, M.; Pick, C.; Granitzka, T.; Sommer, B.; Wittekindt, C.; Klussmann, J.P.; Guntinas-Lichius, O.; Beutner, D. Impact of Extent of Parotidectomy on Early and Long-Term Complications: A Prospective Multicenter Cohort Trial. *Head Neck* **2019**, *41*, 1943–1951. [CrossRef] [PubMed]
32. Koch, M.; Zenk, J.; Iro, H. Long-Term Results of Morbidity after Parotid Gland Surgery in Benign Disease. *Laryngoscope* **2010**, *120*, 724–730. [CrossRef]
33. Guntinas-Lichius, O.; Klussmann, J.P.; Wittekindt, C.; Stennert, E. Parotidectomy for Benign Parotid Disease at a University Teaching Hospital: Outcome of 963 Operations. *Laryngoscope* **2006**, *116*, 534–540. [CrossRef]
34. Dulguerov, P.; Marchai, F.; Lehmann, W. Postparotidectomy Facial Nerve Paralysis: Possible Etiologic Factors and Results with Routine Facial Nerve Monitoring. *Laryngoscope* **1999**, *109*, 754–762. [CrossRef]
35. Tuckett, J.; Glynn, R.; Sheahan, P. Impact of Extent of Parotid Resection on Postoperative Wound Complications: A Prospective Study. *Head Neck* **2015**, *37*, 64–68. [CrossRef]
36. Witt, R.L. The Incidence and Management of Siaolocele after Parotidectomy. *Otolaryngol. Head Neck Surg.* **2009**, *140*, 871–874. [CrossRef]
37. Roh, J.L.; Kim, H.S.; Park, C.I. Randomized Clinical Trial Comparing Partial Parotidectomy versus Superficial or Total Parotidectomy. *Br. J. Surg.* **2007**, *94*, 1081–1087. [CrossRef]
38. Liu, Y.; Yuan, W.; Sun, H.; Su, M.; Kong, X.; Huang, X. Predictors of Sialocele or Salivary Fistula After Partial Superficial Parotidectomy for Benign Parotid Tumor: A Retrospective Study. *J. Oral Maxillofac. Surg.* **2022**, *80*, 327–332. [CrossRef]
39. Maharaj MBBCH, S.; Mungul, S.; Laher, A.; Shivesh Maharaj, C.; Maxeke, C. Botulinum Toxin a Is an Effective Therapeutic Tool for the Management of Parotid Sialocele and Fistula: A Systematic Review. *Laryngoscope Investig. Otolaryngol.* **2020**, *5*, 37. [CrossRef]
40. Ogino, A.; Onishi, K.; Nakamichi, M.; Okaneya, T. Use of Parotid Gland Fascia in the Prevention of Frey Syndrome After Parotidectomy. *J. Craniofac. Surg.* **2019**, *30*, 1009–1011. [CrossRef]
41. Mantsopoulos, K.; Goncalves, M.; Iro, H. Transdermal Scopolamine for the Prevention of a Salivary Fistula after Parotidectomy. *Br. J. Oral Maxillofac. Surg.* **2018**, *56*, 212–215. [CrossRef] [PubMed]
42. Antor, M.A.; Uribe, A.A.; Erminy-Falcon, N.; Werner, J.G.; Candiotti, K.A.; Pergolizzi, J.V.; Bergese, S.D. The Effect of Transdermal Scopolamine for the Prevention of Postoperative Nausea and Vomiting. *Front. Pharmacol.* **2014**, *5*, 55. [CrossRef] [PubMed]

Journal of
Clinical Medicine

MDPI

Article

Ten-Year Trends in Otolaryngological Surgery Volumes and the Impact of Infection Prevention During the COVID-19 Pandemic—A National Study

Ville-Emil Valajärvi [1,*], Satu Lamminmäki [2], Marie Lundberg [2] and Lena Hafrén [2]

1 Faculty of Medicine, University of Helsinki, 00014 Helsinki, Finland
2 Department of Otorhinolaryngology–Head and Neck Surgery, Helsinki University Hospital, University of Helsinki, 00029 Helsinki, Finland; satu.lamminmaki@hus.fi (S.L.); marie.lundberg@hus.fi (M.L.); lena.hafren@hus.fi (L.H.)
* Correspondence: ville.valajarvi@helsinki.fi

Abstract: Background/Objectives: This register study elucidates the national trends in the otolaryngologic surgery volume in Finland over a ten-year period. In particular, we investigated whether the pandemic, which had a marked effect on communicable diseases, had an impact on infection-related ear, nose, and throat (ENT) procedures. For reference, we used noninfectious ENT procedures. **Methods:** The data of this study consisted of the volumes of different otolaryngological surgical procedures in Finland from 2012 to 2022. A linear regression model was applied to calculate long-term trends in surgery volumes. The annual predicted and observed surgical volumes of each procedure were compared. In addition, different procedures were compared based on whether they were mostly infection-related, non-infection-related, or both. **Results:** The results revealed that the pandemic altered the trends of many ENT procedures, and during the pandemic, infection-related surgeries declined more than non-infection-related surgeries did. The decline in infection-related surgery volumes seems to have lasted longer than the coronavirus disease 2019 (COVID-19) pandemic itself, as only tympanostomies and mastoidectomies of all the infection-related procedures included in this study have returned to the pre-pandemic trend. Some non-infection-related procedures and procedures with mixed indications also declined during the pandemic and sustained their reduction even in 2022. **Conclusions:** This study provides a nationwide insight into ENT surgery volumes in Finland over a ten-year period. Although causative reasoning cannot be conducted based on this study, it still provides a good indication of how the absence of respiratory viruses and multifactorial societal restriction measures could have a long-lasting effect on the epidemiology and management of many ENT diseases.

Keywords: otolaryngology; ENT; COVID-19; surgery rate

1. Introduction

The coronavirus disease 2019 (COVID-19) pandemic has had wide-ranging and far-reaching effects on health care systems worldwide. One of the most affected medical specialties has been otolaryngology. In the US at the onset of the pandemic, otolaryngological surgery volumes decreased by more than 80% in outpatient settings and by more than 40% in inpatient settings [1]. In many clinics, postponing elective surgery during the early pandemic caused prompt reductions in ear, nose, and throat (ENT) surgery volumes [1–3]. However, later studies suggested that some of the reduction may not have been related to surgery cancelation policies themselves but rather to other restrictive measures, particularly the implementation of nonpharmaceutical interventions (NPIs), such as social distancing, mask wearing, and improved hygiene practices [4–7]. Especially in ENT, a significant proportion of surgical procedures are related to respiratory infections.

In the US, influenza and human metapneumovirus (hMPV) viruses circulated at historically low levels in 2020 and 2021 [8]. Respiratory syncytial virus (RSV) circulation was also historically low in 2020 but increased atypically during the summer of 2021. The incidence of parainfluenza viruses (PIVs) decreased early in the pandemic and returned to normal in spring 2021 [8]. Non-enveloped viruses such as rhinoviruses (RVs) and respiratory adenoviruses initially decreased in number during the early pandemic but quickly returned to their normal seasonal levels [8,9]. In Canada, the detection rates of influenza A and B, RSVs, PIVs, hMPVs, and adenoviruses decreased substantially amid the early pandemic, whereas enteroviruses and rhinoviruses remained in circulation [10].

In Finland, where this study was conducted, the implementation of pandemic NPIs reduced the most common respiratory viral infections. National lockdown led to shorter influenza and RSV seasons and reduced the number of emergency room visits caused by respiratory virus infections in children [11,12]. The RSV and influenza A and B seasonality also diminished among children from 2020 to 2021, when travel restrictions and mask mandates for adults were in place [13]. When these preventive measures were lifted in September 2021, both influenza and RSV cases returned. However, the peak of the RSV epidemic occurred atypically early [13]. On the other hand, NPIs caused only minimal changes in the spread of rhinovirus in Finland [14].

In France, the total number of ENT cancer surgeries decreased between 2010 and 2021 and more rapidly during the COVID-19 pandemic [15]. However, detailed data on the surgical rates of different ENT procedures are lacking. Here, we aim to assess the long-term trends in separate ENT procedures and evaluate the effects of the altered epidemiology of seasonal viruses during the COVID-19 pandemic.

2. Materials and Methods

The data of this study consisted of the volumes of different otolaryngological surgical procedures in Finland from 2012 to 2022. The data were collected from an open-access register of the Finnish Institute for Health and Welfare (THL). In this register, all the procedures performed in Finland are classified according to the Nordic Classification of Surgical Procedures (NCSP) codes. The register contains the annual volumes of 57 different otolaryngological procedures, of which 27 large-volume procedures were included in this study. Based on the judgments of three ENT specialists, the procedures were divided into three categories: infection-related, non-infection-related, or uncategorizable (Table 1). Procedures related to the treatment of otitis media and sinusitis, such as myringotomies, tympanostomy tubes, and sinus lavages, were classified as infection-related, whereas procedures related to the treatment of malignancies, such as laryngectomies and the insertion of cochlear implants, were categorized as noninfectious. Tonsillectomies were classified as infection-related since they are performed mainly because of chronic, recurrent, or complications of tonsillitis, whereas the main indication for a partial tonsillectomy is airway obstruction, and hence it was classified as noninfectious. Some procedures, such as adenotonsillectomies, adenoidectomies, tracheostomies, and middle meatal antrostomies (MMAs), are performed both for infectious and noninfectious diseases and were thus excluded from this binary grouping (Table 1).

Information about the Finnish government's policy responses to the COVID-19 pandemic was obtained from the Finnish Institute for Health and Welfare and the Ministry of Social Affairs and Health.

Table 1. Volumes of otolaryngologic procedures performed in Finland from 2012 to 2022. The procedures are classified by the Nordic Classification of Surgical Procedures (NCSP) codes. The surgeries were categorized into those related to infections, those not related, and those that were performed in both situations and thus excluded from the comparisons.

NCSP Code	Procedure	Infection-Related	2012	2013	2014	2015	2016	2017	2018	2019	2020	2021	2022	Total
UJC01	Hypopharyngoscopy	No	161	164	149	198	231	350	501	513	397	409	457	3530
EMB00	Excision of lesion of tonsil or adenoids	No	14	17	18	20	24	22	7	24	15	5	10	176
PJD41, PJD51, PJD91, PJD71	Cervical lymph node biopsy and neck dissection	No	1185	1191	1186	1253	1230	1254	1288	1381	1298	1279	1024	13,569
DQB20, DQB30, DQB40, DQB50	Partial or total laryngectomy	No	35	43	28	31	38	37	43	30	18	33	23	359
DQE00	Placement of tracheoesophageal voice prosthesis	No	170	168	184	221	223	242	256	226	206	260	179	2335
DFE00	Cochlear implantation	No	158	136	153	221	173	195	196	228	232	223	231	2146
EMB15	Partial tonsillectomy	No	382	490	825	1147	1151	1238	1364	1697	1195	811	792	11,092
EMB10	Tonsillectomy	Yes	6283	5955	5495	5686	5504	5090	5348	5538	3730	3465	3047	55,141
DCA20	Tympanostomy	Yes	14,872	12,356	12,419	13,161	11,272	9512	9041	9838	4559	2420	3963	103,413
DEB00, DEB10, DEB20, DEB25	Mastoidectomy	Yes	207	215	223	199	228	204	232	216	148	178	181	2231
TDM10	Puncture or lavage of maxillary sinus	Yes	6859	6175	5803	6591	6452	6212	6152	5936	3278	2860	2039	58,357
DCA10	Myringotomy	Yes	1659	1536	1681	1860	1866	1643	1780	1768	1138	856	1036	16,823
ENA32	Incision of deep cervical abscess	Yes	160	186	164	143	180	213	237	270	223	249	328	2353
ENA00	Incision of peritonsillar abscess	Yes	241	319	420	613	655	647	706	789	685	692	620	6387
EMB30	Adenoidectomy	Excluded	5612	4636	4929	5203	4657	4416	4418	5210	2777	1860	2300	46,018
DMB20	Middle meatal antrostomy	Excluded	3368	3373	3650	3585	3717	3682	3717	3794	2776	2357	2067	36,083
EMB20	Adenotonsillectomy	Excluded	2850	2206	1852	1984	1708	1471	1444	1482	894	494	385	16,770
GBB00	Tracheostomy	Excluded	-	912	796	838	816	847	842	796	685	811	697	8040

Statistical analysis was performed via SPSS (version 28.0; IBM, Armonk, NY, USA). A linear regression model was applied to calculate trends in surgery volumes between 2012 and 2019. This trend was extrapolated to the pandemic years 2020–2022 via 95% prediction intervals. The annual predicted and observed surgical volumes of each procedure were compared, and the percentage change between these two procedures was calculated. The observed values outside of the prediction interval indicated a significant change. To compare infection-related and non-infection-related procedures, a residual for each procedure was calculated by subtracting the predicted value from the observed value. The residuals of procedures in the infection-related and non-infection-related groups were summed. The nonparametric Mann–Whitney U test was used to test whether the summed residuals differed significantly between the groups in 2020, 2021, and 2022. Further, a 2 × 2 contingency table was formed of infection-related and non-infection-related procedures for each year, observed surgery numbers, and the residuals. A Chi-Squared test was used to study whether there was a difference between infection-related and non-infection-related groups.

Figure 1 illustrates the course of the COVID-19 pandemic in Finland. Five major hospitalization waves can be distinguished, which somewhat aligns with laboratory-confirmed positive tests. At the onset of the pandemic, social restriction measures were announced at the national level, and restrictions were subsequently made more regionally. Regional restrictions of varying severity were lifted by February 2022. Appendix A contains a more detailed description of the restrictions and vaccinations in Finland during the pandemic [16–21].

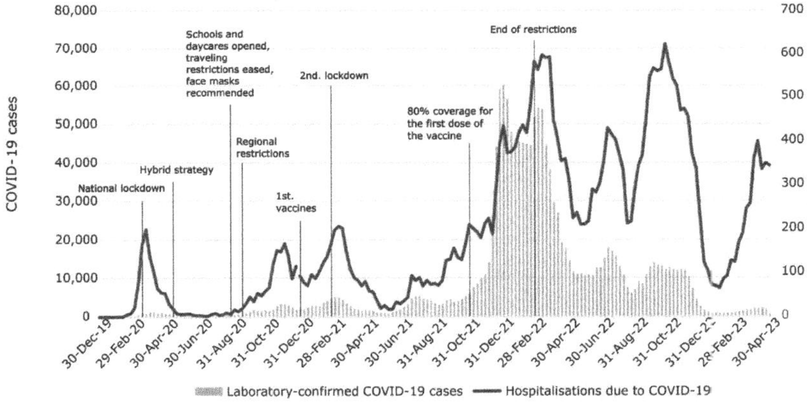

Figure 1. Social restriction measures in Finland during the pandemic, laboratory-confirmed positive COVID-19 tests, and hospitalizations due to COVID-19.

3. Results

Altogether, 384,823 ENT procedures of the selected categories were performed in Finland between 2012 and 2022. Table 1 shows the annual volumes of the 27 types of procedures. Tympanostomies were the most common infection-related surgeries (n = 103,413) during the decade, followed by maxillary lavages (n = 58,357) and tonsillectomies (n = 55,141). Among noninfectious cases, the most common were cervical lymph node biopsies or neck dissections (n = 13,569) and partial tonsillectomies (n = 11,092).

3.1. Infection-Related Procedure Volumes

The trends in the volume of infection-related procedures in Finland between 2012 and 2022 are illustrated in Figure 2. Before the COVID-19 pandemic, the annual surgical volumes of tympanostomies (Figure 2A) and tonsillectomies (Figure 2B) declined, whereas the volumes of peritonsillar abscess incisions (Figure 2C) and incisions of deep cervical abscesses (Figure 2D) demonstrated increasing trends. The annual volumes of myringotomies, mastoidectomies, and punctures/lavages of maxillary sinuses remained rather stable between 2012 and 2019 (Figure 2E–G).

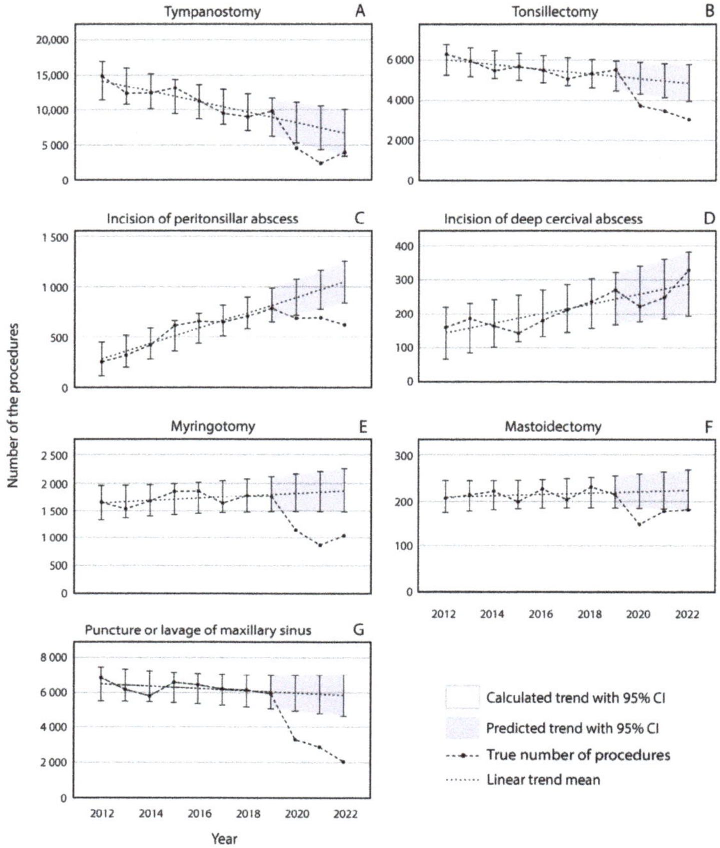

Figure 2. The annual number of infection-related otolaryngologic procedures performed in Finland from 2012 to 2022. The black dots depict the true number of procedures, and the gray and blue areas represent the 95% prediction intervals.

Compared with the predicted trend, the pandemic affected all other infection-related procedure volumes negatively except incisions of deep cervical abscesses (Figure 2D), which remained statistically significant for the predicted volumes. Compared with the predicted pre-pandemic trend, the tympanostomy volume decreased by 44.5% in 2020 and further decreased by 67.6% in 2021. However, in 2022, the volumes had recovered to the prediction (Figure 2A). For mastoidectomies (Figure 2F), recovery occurred sooner, with a reduction of 33.3% in 2020 and a smaller but still significant reduction of 20.3% compared with the predicted mean in 2021. In 2022, the surgical volume returned to the predicted trend. For myringotomies (Figure 2E), the recovery during 2022 was very slight, with only 44.6% of the procedures performed compared with the prediction. This figure was lower than that in 2020 during the pandemic (a reduction of 37.6%) but greater than that in 2021 (53.7% of the prediction).

For maxillary punctures, the decline continued throughout the pandemic, with 45.2% fewer procedures than predicted in 2020, 51.6% in 2021, and 65.1% in 2022 (Figure 2E). Compared with the predicted values, the tonsillectomy (Figure 2B) and peritonsillar abscess incision (Figure 2C) volumes were reduced by 26.8% and 23.4%, respectively, in 2020. The decline continued in 2021 and 2022, with 30.0% and 37.4% fewer tonsillectomies and 28.8% and 40.8% fewer peritonsillar abscess incisions, respectively, than expected.

3.2. Noninfectious Procedure Volumes

The annual volumes of most non-infection-related procedures, such as partial tonsillectomies, cochlear implantations, hypopharyngoscopies, cervical lymph node biopsies, and the placements of tracheoesophageal voice prostheses, slowly increased in Finland before the COVID-19 pandemic, as shown in Figure 3. The only exceptions were laryngectomies and excisions of adenoid or tonsillar lesions, which remained relatively stable.

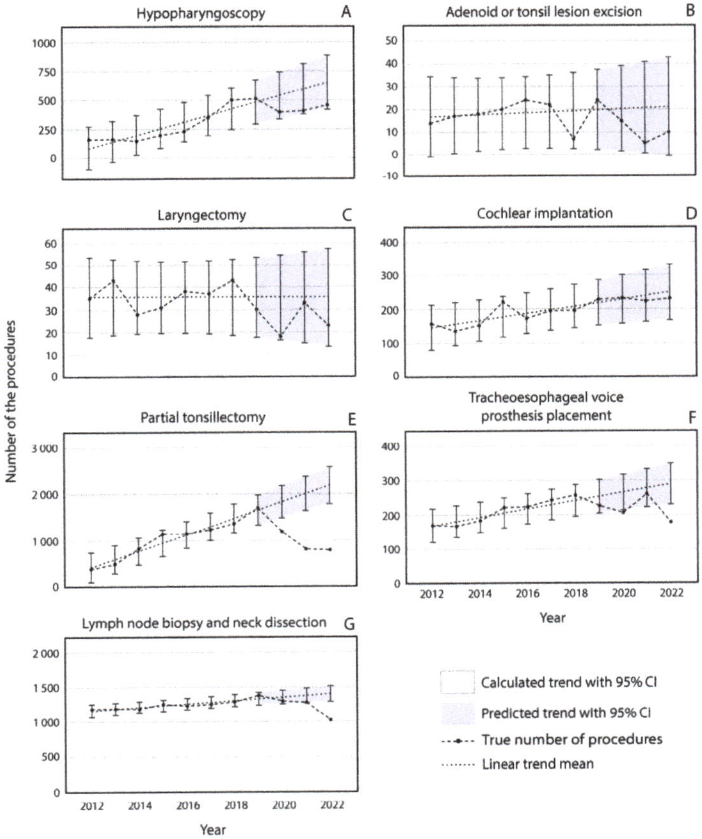

Figure 3. The annual number of non-infection-related otolaryngologic procedures performed in Finland from 2012 to 2022.

During the pandemic years, no significant change was observed compared with the pre-pandemic trend in the number of hypopharyngoscopies, adenoid or tonsil lesion excisions, laryngectomies, or cochlear implantations (Figure 3A–D). Partial tonsillectomies and, to a lesser degree, placements of tracheoesophageal voice prostheses and cervical lymph node biopsies diverged from the predicted trend during the pandemic years (Figure 3E–G). A lesser, non-significant decrease was observed in every noninfectious procedure during the pandemic, except cochlear implantations, which stayed on an increasing trend throughout the pandemic (Figure 3). Cervical lymph node excision volumes were stable in 2020 and 2021, but in 2022, a 27% reduction was observed. The partial tonsillectomy procedure volume decreased by 34.7% in 2020, by 59.6% in 2021, and by 63.7% in 2022 (Figure 3E). Compared with the predicted trend, the prevalence of placements of tracheoesophageal voice prostheses was barely significantly lower (21.1%) during 2020 but rose back to the prediction in 2021, with a decrease in 2022 to 38.1% of the predicted trend (Figure 3F).

3.3. Procedures with Infectious and Noninfectious Indications

Figure 4 illustrates the trends of uncategorized procedures in Finland from 2012 to 2022. Adenoidectomies, adenotonsillectomies, maxillary antrostomies, and tracheostomies were labeled uncategorized since their indications could not be exclusively categorized as either infection-related or nonrelated. Before the COVID-19 pandemic, the number of MMAs increased (Figure 4A), whereas adenotonsillectomies demonstrated a decreasing trend (Figure 4B). Adenoidectomies and tracheostomies were rather stable (Figure 4C,D). Compared with the predicted trend, significantly fewer endoscopic maxillary antrostomies were performed during the pandemic, with reduced volumes of 28.3% in 2020, 40.0% in 2021, and 48.2% in 2022 (Figure 4A). A similar trend was observed for adenoidectomies, with rates of 39.2%, 59.0%, and 48.0% from 2020 to 2022, respectively (Figure 4C). Adenotonsillectomies and tracheostomy procedure volumes were associated with the predicted trend during the pandemic (Figure 4B–D).

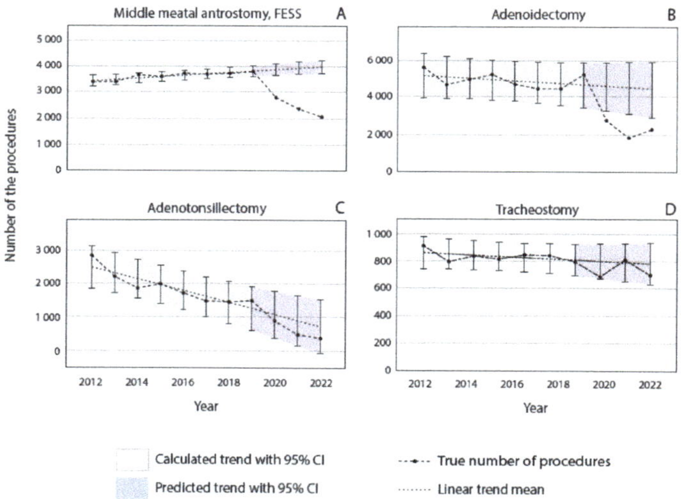

Figure 4. The annual number of otolaryngologic procedures performed for both infectious and noninfectious indications in Finland from 2012 to 2022.

3.4. Comparison of Infection-Related Procedures to Non-Infection-Related Procedures

To study whether the pandemic time affected procedure volumes differently in procedures related to infections vs. non-infection-related, we calculated a residual, i.e., the difference between the observed and predicted procedure rates. The difference between the two groups indicates that the trend in surgical volumes was different between the infectious and noninfectious procedures. The number of infection-related procedures decreased significantly more than the number of non-infection-related otolaryngologic procedures in 2020 (Mann–Whitney U test, $p = 0.026$). The difference between these two categories was sustained through 2021 ($p = 0.038$). In 2022, no statistically significant difference was detected between the groups. Using the Chi-Squared test, a statistically significant difference between the two groups was observed in 2020 ($p < 0.001$), 2021 ($p < 0.001$), and 2022 ($p = 0.002$).

4. Discussion

This study analyzed Finnish national health care records before (2012–2019), during (2020–2021), and after (2022) the COVID-19 pandemic to understand how the pandemic and preventive infection control measures affected long-term trends in ENT surgery volumes. The results revealed that the pandemic altered the trends of many ENT procedures, and during the pandemic, the number of infection-related surgeries declined more than non-infection-related surgeries did. The decline in infection-related surgery volumes seems to have lasted longer than the COVID-19 pandemic itself, as only tympanostomies and mastoidectomies of all the infection-related procedures included in this study have returned to the pre-pandemic trend. Some non-infection-related procedures and procedures with mixed indications also declined during the pandemic and sustained their reduction even in 2022.

This study revealed that the number of infection-related surgeries declined more than non-infection-related surgeries did. The findings imply that the decline in circulating respiratory viruses during the pandemic reduced the need for infection-related procedures. Demonstrative examples include tympanostomies and myringotomies, which are performed due to recurrent acute otitis media or chronic otitis media with effusion [22]. The annual number of tympanostomies has been decreasing steadily annually in Finland, but the pandemic has induced an extra decrease, which differs statistically significantly from the pre-pandemic trend. The long-term downward trend is probably at least partially related to the steady decrease in the number of births and thus the number of small children in Finland [23]. In addition, pneumococcal vaccination, which has been part of the national vaccination program since 2007, has decreased the incidence of otitis media (OM) [24], as *Streptococcus pneumoniae* is one of the most important pathogens of middle ear infections. Furthermore, smoking, a well-known risk factor for middle ear infections [25], has decreased throughout this time period in Finland [26]. A decline in tympanostomies was reported in the US between 2005 and 2019, in a study examining otolaryngology residents' caseloads [27]. A similar long-term downward trend was not observed in the number of myringotomies, probably since they were performed mainly on adults. The decrease in the number of tympanostomies related to the pandemic is in line with several previous studies demonstrating similar changes [5,7,28,29]. Additionally, a growing body of evidence demonstrates the impact of social isolation on middle ear infections. In particular, quarantine periods have been associated with the resolution of OM, especially its acute and chronic forms [28,30,31]. Additionally, the volumes of all other infection-related ENT surgeries included in this study, except incisions for deep cervical abscesses, decreased during the pandemic. The number of peritonsillar abscess incisions has steadily increased over the long term. A similar long-term increase was observed in the UK over a ten-year period, which could be related to fewer tonsillectomy operations and reduced antibiotic prescribing in primary care [32]. However, they decreased steeply toward the end of the pandemic, probably due to a lower circulation of *Streoptococcus pyogenes*, as it has been identified as a key etiological factor in peritonsillar abscess formation [33]. This result is in line with data from the whole Korean population, which revealed decreases in the numbers of peritonsillar, retropharyngeal, and parapharyngeal abscess diagnoses during the first year of the pandemic compared with those before the pandemic [34]. On the other hand, a study from the US reported no difference in the number of peritonsillar abscesses from the beginning of the pandemic through the end of 2021 compared with 2019 [35]. Maxillary punctures have also been substantially affected by the pandemic. They are performed to help with diagnosis and to relieve symptoms in acute maxillary sinus infections. The evidence that maxillary punctures relieve sinusitis symptoms is not well established; hence, maxillary punctures are rarely used in other countries. The lack of evidence for their benefits could be an explanatory factor for the long-term decline.

In addition to reduced infections during the pandemic leading to a further decrease in maxillary punctures, the decrease could be potentiated by reluctance to perform procedures with controversial efficacy during the pandemic. Another reason is that aerosol-producing procedures, such as maxillary punctures, were restricted during the pandemic. The rather stable long-term trend in the increase in mastoidectomies was momentarily interrupted during the pandemic.

As an exception to other infection-related procedures, the number of incisions for deep cervical abscesses tended to increase during the pandemic. This could be related to the fact that a large proportion of deep neck infections have an odontogenic etiology, and during the pandemic, access to dental care was very limited. The reason for the long-term increasing trend of deep neck infections is unclear but might be related to the aging of the population and an increase in the number of comorbidities [36]. In the future, it will be interesting to determine whether the number of deep neck infections will show a delayed increase from the trendline because of poor dental care during the pandemic.

While the idea that reduced infectious disease is the reason for the decline in surgical volume is persuasive, it does not completely explain these results. For example, in the category of non-infection-related procedures, partial tonsillectomies declined both during and after the pandemic. Tonsillectomies are performed due to infections, whereas partial tonsillectomies are mostly related to obstructive disorders [37]. Adenoidectomies and adenotonsillectomies are performed because of both indications. Considering our hypothesis of a reduced need for infection-related surgeries, it would have been expected that tonsillectomies would reduce and that partial tonsillectomies would remain rather stable. In Germany, the first lockdown resulted in an abrupt decrease in the national levels of tonsillectomies, adenotonsillectomies, and partial tonsillectomies. The levels remained lower after the lockdown, compared to 2019 [6]. A noticeable decrease in the number of adenotonsillectomies during the beginning of the COVID-19 pandemic was also detected in 51 children's hospitals in the US. Adenotonsillectomies sustained their reduction throughout 2020 and 2021, without signs of recovery [35]. One reason for the reduction in tonsillar surgery during the pandemic might be the capacity of health care, which prioritizes more urgent procedures. Some of the reduction in adenoidectomies could be explained by a decrease in infection-caused adenoid hypertrophy [38]. Additionally, the long-term trend in the use of tonsillectomies, adenotonsillectomies, and adenoidectomies has been declining. The only exceptions are partial tonsillectomies, which have been increasing in the long term. Partial tonsillectomies are currently preferred over a tonsillectomy for the surgical management of children with sleep apnea and snoring, which could explain this trend. Additionally, the criteria for tonsillar surgery were tightened during this period.

In addition to reduced infections contributing to a decrease in surgery volume, other explanatory factors, such as health care prioritization and differences in health-seeking behavior, could be influential. More chronic conditions, such as chronic sinusitis, which is the main indication for an MMA [39], might not have been an equal concern during the pandemic. This could be one reason why the long-term upward trend in MMAs shifted into a steeply declining trend during these three years. The pandemic has increased waiting times for surgery in Finland [40]. Additionally, a reduction in the number of referrals to ENT doctors was also observed early in the pandemic [29]. This could imply altered access to primary care or changes in health-seeking behavior. This still does not reflect the number of elective surgeries, such as cochlear implantation, laryngectomies, and adenoid or tonsil lesion excision. In our study, of the noninfectious procedures, cochlear implantations were the only surgeries that were not affected by the pandemic in 2020. Especially in children, implantation could not be postponed by months since children with congenital, severe-to-profound hearing loss can only develop near-normal language skills if they are implanted early. Further, cochlear implantation surgeries have been shown to be safe and effective even during the pandemic, given that proper precautionary measures are taken [41]. In other countries, delays in these surgeries have been reported. According to one study analyzing manufacturing data, cochlear implantation in adults decreased in the US by 10.1% between 2019 and 2020. The decrease was less pronounced among children. A total of 2.2% of those aged <3 years and 3.8% of those aged 4–17 years were included [42]. Significant delays between cochlear implant evaluation and surgery were reported in a single tertiary center in the US among patients with prelingual deafness [43] as well as in lower esophageal cancer diagnosis and in endoscopic diagnostics between March 2020 and December 2020 compared to 2019 [44]. Cancer diagnoses have been delayed in Finland because head and neck cancer symptoms have been interpreted as symptoms of COVID-19 infection [45]. This type of diagnostic delay during the pandemic could have influenced cancer-related surgeries with a delay, which was reflected by the number of neck dissections and lymph node biopsies, which decreased from the trend only in 2022. The same explanation could be applied to tracheoesophageal voice prosthesis surgeries for laryngeal cancer patients, which slightly decreased from the long-term trend in 2020 and more clearly in 2022. Contrary to ENT cancer, which may have similar symptoms to respiratory infections, a study reported an increase in diagnosed basal cell carcinoma in the skin of the head and neck region and no reduction in the diagnoses of all other non-melanoma skin cancers during the pandemic. These findings were attributed to the noticeable lesions in the head and neck area that encouraged patients to seek medical care [46]. In the future, it will be interesting to see whether there will be a delayed increase in the cancer-related surgeries that have now decreased in Finland, such as neck dissections, lymph node biopsies, and tracheoesophageal voice prosthesis surgeries.

In the US, otolaryngological surgery volumes quickly rebounded in September 2020 to 99.7% of the 2019 levels of inpatient volumes and 96.5% of outpatient volumes nationwide, after the initial decrease in the early pandemic [47]. However, significant differences among the subspeciality surgery volumes have been reported. A study conducted in the US found out that two years from the onset of the pandemic, the only subspecialities that did not exhibit a rebound in surgery volumes were pediatric otolaryngology and otology [48]. Others such as general surgery, endoscopy, rhinology, laryngology, facial plastics and reconstructive surgery, and head and neck surgery have returned to the pre-pandemic levels. This is in line with our findings that common pediatric otolaryngological procedures such as tympanostomies, adenoidectomies, and tonsillectomies have not returned to the pre-pandemic trend. The researchers reported non-significant increases only in emergency endotracheal intubations and incision procedures of the trachea during the post-pandemic period among otolaryngological procedures [48]. However, the volumes of some procedures have even surpassed the pre-pandemic trend. A register study in the US reported an increase in laryngological procedures and a shift to office-based procedures after the onset of the pandemic that was sustained throughout 2022 [49]. Also, the volumes of head and neck microvascular free flap surgery have increased and surpassed the pre-pandemic volumes [50].

In our study, surgery volumes did not fully recover even after the pandemic time was over. In June 2023, COVID-19 was removed from the list of generally hazardous communicable diseases in Finland [51], but respiratory viruses returned to the circulation earlier. The influenza season from 2021 to 2022 began normally, although the epidemic peak was delayed to May 2022 due to restrictions imposed by the Omicron variant [52]. RSV experienced a substantial epidemic in the winter between 2020 and 2021, and a second epidemic began around October 2022 [53]. There are multiple possible reasons for the continuing decline in surgical volumes. A delay in the resumption of infection-related surgical volumes would be expected, since the indications require a certain number of consecutive infections, which the pandemic interrupted. However, this does not explain why tympanostomies and mastoidectomies are the only infection-related procedures that have returned to pre-pandemic trends. Age could be another explanatory factor, since the highest incidence of OM is among young children of the age of 6–24 months [54], whose social restrictive measures were loose compared with those of older children and adults. Primary care centers were closed in Finland only during the first wave of the pandemic (Figure 1). In addition, compliance with NPIs is presumably higher for kindergarten-aged children. Another age-related explanatory factor could be related to the time delay between diagnosis and operative management. As children typically undergo surgery more swiftly, it is intuitive that tympanostomies have recovered more quickly since the pandemic. Third, the pandemic might have had a longer lasting effect on surgery indications, i.e., a more conservative approach in some ENT diseases, such as punctures of the maxillary sinuses, although it is worth mentioning that the management guidelines have remained unchanged. This could also explain the prolonged decline in some of the non-infection-related surgery volumes, such as those of partial tonsillectomies and surgeries with mixed indications, such as MMAs and adenoidectomies.

We acknowledge some limitations of the study. In the statistical analysis, we assume a linear trend for the number of procedures but can, of course, not be certain that it would have been linear without the COVID-19 pandemic. Another potential limitation is the accuracy of the reporting of the procedures, even though health care providers in Finland are legally obliged to report procedures.

5. Conclusions

In conclusion, this study provides a nationwide insight into ENT surgery volumes in Finland over a ten-year period and shows that the COVID-19 pandemic caused a significant decline in ENT surgical volumes, with varying rates of recovery across subspecialties. While some areas have recovered to or exceeded pre-pandemic levels, others continue to experience reduced volumes, highlighting the lasting impact of the pandemic on ENT surgical practice. Although causative reasoning cannot be conducted based on this study, it still provides a good indication of how the absence of respiratory viruses and multifactorial societal restriction measures could have a long-lasting effect on the epidemiology and management of many ENT diseases.

Author Contributions: Conceptualization, L.H., M.L. and S.L.; formal analysis, V.-E.V.; investigation, L.H. and V.-E.V.; writing—original draft preparation, V.-E.V.; writing—review and editing, V.-E.V., L.H., M.L. and S.L.; visualization, V.-E.V. and S.L. All authors have read and agreed to the published version of the manuscript.

Funding: This research received no external funding. Open access funding provided by University of Helsinki.

Institutional Review Board Statement: Ethical review and approval were waived for this study due to data being openly accessible.

Informed Consent Statement: Patient consent was waived due to the retrospective nature of the study.

Data Availability Statement: The data are freely available from the Finnish Institute for Health and Welfare (THL), https://sampo.thl.fi/pivot/prod/fi/thil/perus01/fact_thil_perus01 (accessed on 22 March 2023).

Acknowledgments: We would like to thank the Biostatistics Unit of the University of Helsinki for their valuable assistance in the design and execution of the statistical analysis for this study.

Conflicts of Interest: The authors declare no conflicts of interest.

Appendix A

On 16 March 2020, a state of emergency was declared, leading to a national lockdown. Public premises, schools, and universities were closed, and gatherings of more than 10 people were prohibited. Finland's borders were closed from noncitizens, and traveling abroad was prohibited. Social distancing, hand washing, and proper sneezing techniques were recommended. The use of a face mask in public places was not encouraged at that time [16]. Two months later, on the 14 May, Finland moved to a "hybrid strategy", which meant milder restrictions, effective testing, and the isolation of those exposed to COVID-19. A gathering of 50 people was allowed. In July, the limit was increased to 500, and at the end of August 2020, limitations were lifted, travel restrictions were loosened, and schools and daycares were reopened [17]. Instead, using face masks if social distancing was impossible was recommended for those over 15 years of age [18]. With the increase in hospitalizations, restrictions were implemented more regionally starting on 16 September 2020 and were based on three categories of COVID-19 epidemiological activity (the base level, acceleration stage, and spreading stage) [19].

In December 2020, the first COVID-19 vaccines were dispensed in Finland [20]. By November 2021, the coverage was over 80% for the first vaccine. In February 2021, a state of emergency was again declared. Districts that were in the acceleration stage went under a lockdown similar to that during 2020 [21]. Regional restrictions of varying severity were continued until February 2022, after which restriction measures were lifted.

References

1. Saraswathula, A.; Shippey, E.; Sprankle, L.A.; Kachalia, A.; Miller, R.G.; Gourin, C.G.; Stewart, C.M. Comparison of subspecialty major surgical volume in the United States during the COVID-19 pandemic. *Laryngoscope* **2022**, *132*, 2139–2141. [CrossRef] [PubMed]
2. Hervochon, R.; Atallah, S.; Levivien, S.; Teissier, N.; Baujat, B.; Tankere, F. Impact of the COVID-19 epidemic on ENT surgical volume. *Eur. Ann. Otorhinolaryngol. Head Neck Dis.* **2020**, *137*, 269–271. [CrossRef]
3. Mattingly, A.S.; Rose, L.; Eddington, H.S.; Trickey, A.W.; Cullen, M.R.; Morris, A.M.; Wren, S.M. Trends in US Surgical Procedures and Health Care System Response to Policies Curtailing Elective Surgical Operations during the COVID-19 Pandemic. *JAMA Netw. Open* **2021**, *4*, e2138038. [CrossRef]
4. Kourelis, K.; Angelopoulou, M.; Goulioumis, A.; Fouzas, S.; Kourelis, T. Surgery for adenotonsillar hypertrophy and otitis media in children is less demanded in quarantine times. *Int. J. Pediatr. Otorhinolaryngol.* **2022**, *158*, 111159. [CrossRef]
5. Allen, D.Z.; Challapalli, S.; McKee, S.; Lee, K.H.; Bell, C.S.; Roy, S.; Bowe, S.; Balakrishnan, K.; Chang, C.W.D.; Huang, Z. Impact of COVID-19 on nationwide pediatric otolaryngology: Otitis media and myringotomy tube trends. *Am. J. Otolaryngol.* **2022**, *43*, 103369. [CrossRef] [PubMed]
6. Windfuhr, J.P.; Günster, C. Impact of the COVID-pandemic on the incidence of tonsil surgery and sore throat in Germany. *Eur. Arch. Oto-Rhino-Laryngol.* **2022**, *279*, 4157–4166. [CrossRef] [PubMed]
7. Diercks, G.R.; Cohen, M.S. The Effect of the COVID-19 Pandemic on Pediatric Tympanostomy Tube Placement. *Otolaryngol. Neck Surg.* **2022**, *166*, 167–170. [CrossRef] [PubMed]
8. Olsen, S.J.; Winn, A.K.; Budd, A.P.; Prill, M.M.; Steel, J.; Midgley, C.M.; Kniss, K.; Burns, E.; Rowe, T.; Foust, A.; et al. Changes in influenza and other respiratory virus activity during the COVID-19 pandemic—United States, 2020–2021. *Am. J. Transplant.* **2021**, *21*, 3481–3486. [CrossRef]
9. Rankin, D.A.; Spieker, A.J.; Perez, A.; Stahl, A.L.; Rahman, H.K.; Stewart, L.S.; Schuster, J.E.; Lively, J.Y.; Haddadin, Z.; Probst, V.; et al. Circulation of Rhinoviruses and/or Enteroviruses in Pediatric Patients with Acute Respiratory Illness Before and during the COVID-19 Pandemic in the US. *JAMA Netw. Open* **2023**, *6*, e2254909. [CrossRef]
10. Groves, H.E.; Piché-Renaud, P.-P.; Peci, A.; Farrar, D.S.; Buckrell, S.; Bancej, C.; Sevenhuysen, C.; Campigotto, A.; Gubbay, J.B.; Morris, S.K. The impact of the COVID-19 pandemic on influenza, respiratory syncytial virus, and other seasonal respiratory virus circulation in Canada: A population-based study. *Lancet Reg. Health–Am.* **2021**, *1*, 100015. [CrossRef]
11. Kuitunen, I.; Artama, M.; Mäkelä, L.; Backman, K.; Heiskanen-Kosma, T.; Renko, M. Effect of Social Distancing Due to the COVID-19 Pandemic on the Incidence of Viral Respiratory Tract Infections in Children in Finland during Early 2020. *Pediatr. Infect. Dis. J.* **2020**, *39*, e423–e427. [CrossRef] [PubMed]
12. Kelloniemi, S.; Heikkilä, P.; Palmu, S. COVID-19 restrictions probably brought the 2019–2020 Finnish influenza season to an early end and led to fewer respiratory viruses among infants. *Acta Paediatr.* **2021**, *110*, 3327–3328. [CrossRef] [PubMed]
13. Kuitunen, I.; Artama, M.; Haapanen, M.; Renko, M. Respiratory virus circulation in children after relaxation of COVID-19 restrictions in fall 2021—A nationwide register study in Finland. *J. Med. Virol.* **2022**, *94*, 4528–4532. [CrossRef] [PubMed]
14. Kuitunen, I.; Artama, M.; Haapanen, M.; Renko, M. Rhinovirus spread in children during the COVID-19 pandemic despite social restrictions—A nationwide register study in Finland. *J. Med. Virol.* **2021**, *93*, 6063–6067. [CrossRef]
15. Le Bihan-Benjamin, C.; Rocchi, M.; Putton, M.; Méric, J.-B.; Bousquet, P.J. Estimation of Oncologic Surgery Case Volume Before and After the COVID-19 Pandemic in France. *JAMA Netw. Open* **2023**, *6*, e2253204. [CrossRef]
16. Government Communications Department, Ministry of Education and Culture, Ministry of Social Affairs and Health. Available online: https://valtioneuvosto.fi/en/-/10616/hallitus-totesi-suomen-olevan-poikkeusoloissa-koronavirustilanteen-vuoksi?languageId=en_US (accessed on 29 October 2023).
17. Finnish Government. Available online: https://valtioneuvosto.fi/paatokset/paatos?decisionId=0900908f806a9de2 (accessed on 29 October 2023).
18. Finnish Institute for Health and Welfare. Available online: https://thl.fi/fi/-/thl-suosittaa-kasvomaskin-kayttoa-toisten-suojaamiseksi-kasienpesu-ja-turvavalit-ovat-tarkeimmat-keinot-ehkaista-koronatartuntoja (accessed on 29 October 2023).

19. Government Communications Department. Ministry of Social Affairs and Health. Available online: https://valtioneuvosto.fi/en/-//10616/government-discusses-action-plan-to-manage-covid-19 (accessed on 29 October 2023).
20. Hartonen, T.; Jermy, B.; Sõnajalg, H.; Vartiainen, P.; Krebs, K.; Vabalas, A.; Metspalu, A.; Esko, T.; Nelis, M.; Hudjashov, G.; et al. Nationwide health, socio-economic and genetic predictors of COVID-19 vaccination status in Finland. *Nat. Hum. Behav.* **2023**, *7*, 1069–1083. [CrossRef]
21. Government Communications Department. Available online: https://valtioneuvosto.fi/en/-//10616/government-decides-on-immediate-transition-to-tier-2-of-covid-19-prevention-and-is-prepared-to-declare-a-state-of-emergency (accessed on 29 October 2023).
22. Rosenfeld, R.M.; Schwartz, S.R.; Pynnonen, M.A.; Tunkel, D.E.; Hussey, H.M.; Fichera, J.S.; Grimes, A.M.; Hackell, J.M.; Harrison, M.F.; Haskell, H.; et al. Clinical Practice Guideline: Tympanostomy Tubes in Children. *Otolaryngol. Neck Surg.* **2013**, *149*, S1–S35. [CrossRef]
23. Vastasyntyneet Alueittain—THL Kuutio-ja Tiivistekäyttöliittymä. Available online: https://sampo.thl.fi/pivot/prod/fi/synre/vastasyalue/fact_synre_vastasyalue (accessed on 6 July 2024).
24. Prymula, R.; Peeters, P.; Chrobok, V.; Kriz, P.; Novakova, E.; Kaliskova, E.; Kohl, I.; Lommel, P.; Poolman, J.; Prieels, J.-P.; et al. Pneumococcal capsular polysaccharides conjugated to protein D for prevention of acute otitis media caused by both Streptococcus pneumoniae and non-typable Haemophilus influenzae: A randomised double-blind efficacy study. *Lancet* **2006**, *367*, 740–748. [CrossRef]
25. DiFranza, J.R.; Lew, R.A. Morbidity and Mortality in Children Associated with the Use of Tobacco Products by Other People. *Pediatrics* **1996**, *97*, 560–568. [CrossRef]
26. Finnish Institute for Health and Welfare. Tobacco Statistics 2022. Available online: https://thl.fi/en/statistics-and-data/statistics-by-topic/alcohol-drugs-and-addiction/tobaccostatistics (accessed on 21 April 2024).
27. Welschmeyer, A.; Coerdt, K.; Crossley, J.; Malekzadeh, S. Critical Evaluation of Trends in Otolaryngology Resident Caseload by Subspecialty from 2005 to 2019. *Ann. Otol. Rhinol. Laryngol.* **2021**, *130*, 915–922. [CrossRef]
28. Pereira, N.M.; Maresh, A.M.; Modi, V.K.; Rosenblatt, S.D. Tympanostomy tubes in the age of quarantine. *Int. J. Pediatr. Otorhinolaryngol.* **2022**, *154*, 111047. [CrossRef] [PubMed]
29. Haapanen, M.; Renko, M.; Artama, M.; Manninen, I.; Mattila, V.M.; Uimonen, M.; Ponkilainen, V.; Kuitunen, I. Tympanostomies and tonsillar surgery in children during the COVID-19 pandemic in Finland. *Laryngoscope Investig. Otolaryngol.* **2021**, *6*, 878–884. [CrossRef]
30. Aldè, M.; Di Berardino, F.; Marchisio, P.; Cantarella, G.; Ambrosetti, U.; Consonni, D.; Zanetti, D. Effects of COVID-19 Lockdown on Otitis Media with Effusion in Children: Future Therapeutic Implications. *Otolaryngol. Neck Surg.* **2021**, *165*, 710–715. [CrossRef] [PubMed]
31. Torretta, S.; Capaccio, P.; Coro, I.; Bosis, S.; Pace, M.E.; Bosi, P.; Pignataro, L.; Marchisio, P. Incidental lowering of otitis-media complaints in otitis-prone children during COVID-19 pandemic: Not all evil comes to hurt. *Eur. J. Pediatr.* **2021**, *180*, 649–652. [CrossRef] [PubMed]
32. Powell, J.; Wilson, J.A. An evidence-based review of peritonsillar abscess. *Clin. Otolaryngol.* **2012**, *37*, 136–145. [CrossRef]
33. Saar, M.; Vaikjärv, R.; Parm, Ü.; Kasenõmm, P.; Kõljalg, S.; Sepp, E.; Jaagura, M.; Salumets, A.; Štšepetova, J.; Mändar, R. Unveiling the etiology of peritonsillar abscess using next generation sequencing. *Ann. Clin. Microbiol. Antimicrob.* **2023**, *22*, 98. [CrossRef]
34. Kim, S.Y.; Yoo, D.M.; Kim, J.H.; Kwon, M.J.; Kim, J.H.; Chung, J.; Choi, H.G. Changes in Otorhinolaryngologic Disease Incidences before and during the COVID-19 Pandemic in Korea. *Int. J. Environ. Res. Public Health* **2022**, *19*, 13083. [CrossRef]
35. Allen, D.Z.; Challapalli, S.; Lee, K.H.; Bell, C.S.; Roy, S.; Bowe, S.; Balakrishnan, K.; Chang, C.W.D.; Huang, Z. Impact of COVID-19 on nationwide pediatric otolaryngology practice: Adenotonsillectomies (TA) and tonsil-related diagnoses trends. *Am. J. Otolaryngol.* **2022**, *43*, 103526. [CrossRef]
36. Velhonoja, J.; Lääveri, M.; Soukka, T.; Irjala, H.; Kinnunen, I. Deep neck space infections: An upward trend and changing characteristics. *Eur. Arch. Oto-Rhino-Laryngol.* **2020**, *277*, 863–872. [CrossRef]
37. Blackshaw, H.; Springford, L.R.; Zhang, L.-Y.; Wang, B.; Venekamp, R.P.; Schilder, A.G.M. Tonsillectomy versus tonsillotomy for obstructive sleep-disordered breathing in children. *Cochrane Database Syst. Rev.* **2020**, *2020*, CD011365. [CrossRef]
38. Niedzielski, A.; Chmielik, L.P.; Mielnik-Niedzielska, G.; Kasprzyk, A.; Bogusławska, J. Adenoid hypertrophy in children: A narrative review of pathogenesis and clinical relevance. *BMJ Paediatr. Open* **2023**, *7*, e001710. [CrossRef]
39. Fokkens, W.J.; Lund, V.J.; Hopkins, C.; Hellings, P.W.; Kern, R.; Reitsma, S.; Toppila-Salmi, S.; Bernal-Sprekelsen, M.; Mullol, J.; Alobid, I.; et al. European Position Paper on Rhinosinusitis and Nasal Polyps 2020. *Rhinol. J.* **2020**, *58* (Suppl. S29), 1–464. [CrossRef]
40. Uimonen, M.; Kuitunen, I.; Ponkilainen, V.; Mattila, V.M. Prioritizing Elective Surgery during the COVID-19 Pandemic Has Caused Age-Related Inequality: A Multicenter Study. *SN Compr. Clin. Med.* **2022**, *4*, 25. [CrossRef]
41. Skarzynski, H.; Lorens, A.; Dziendziel, B.; Wlodarczyk, E.; Obrycka, A.; Walkowiak, A.; Skarzynski, P.H. Resumption of Cochlear Implant Surgery under COVID-19 Pandemic Conditions. *Life* **2021**, *11*, 929. [CrossRef] [PubMed]
42. Marinelli, J.P.; Nassiri, A.M.; Lohse, C.M.; Driscoll, C.L.W.; Neff, B.A.; Carlson, M.L. Effect of a Global Pandemic on Adult and Pediatric Cochlear Implantation across the United States. *Otol. Neurotol.* **2023**, *44*, 148–152. [CrossRef]
43. Noij, K.S.; Huang, E.Y.; Walsh, J.; Creighton, F.X.; Galaiya, D.; Bowditch, S.P.; Stewart, C.M.; Jenks, C.M. Trends in Timing and Provision of Pediatric Cochlear Implant Care during COVID-19. *OTO Open* **2023**, *7*, 37. [CrossRef]

44. Khan, H.; Johnson, C.; Malwankar, J.; Battafarano, R.; Yang, S.; Broderick, S.; Huang, P.; Lam, V.; Ha, J. The COVID-19 Era Is Associated with Delays in Esophageal Cancer Diagnosis and Treatment. *J. Surg. Res.* **2023**, *285*, 100–106. [CrossRef]
45. Paajanen, J.; Mäkinen, L.K.; Suikkila, A.; Rehell, M.; Javanainen, M.; Lindahl, A.; Kekäläinen, E.; Kurkela, S.; Halmesmäki, K.; Anttila, V.-J.; et al. Isolation precautions cause minor delays in diagnostics and treatment of non-COVID patients. *Infect. Prev. Pract.* **2021**, *3*, 100178. [CrossRef]
46. Benedetti, S.; Frosolini, A.; Catarzi, L.; Marsiglio, A.; Gennaro, P.; Gabriele, G. Impact of the COVID-19 Pandemic on the Diagnosis and Management of Non-Melanoma Skin Cancer in the Head and Neck Region: A Retrospective Cohort Study. *Healthcare* **2024**, *12*, 501. [CrossRef]
47. Saraswathula, A.; Gourin, C.G.; Stewart, C.M. National Trends in US Otolaryngology Surgical Volume during the Early COVID-19 Pandemic. *JAMA Otolaryngol. Head Neck Surg.* **2021**, *147*, 397. [CrossRef]
48. Qatanani, A.M.; Kshirsagar, R.S.; Douglas, N.O.; Andrade, C.; Adappa, N.D.; Eide, J.G. Trends in otolaryngology-head and neck surgery procedural volumes during the COVID-19 pandemic. *Int. J. Otorhinolaryngol. Head Neck Surg.* **2022**, *9*, 12. [CrossRef]
49. Gray, R.; Ryan, M.A.; Mehta, V. Volume and Practice-Setting Shift of Laryngology Procedures during the COVID-19 Pandemic: A Reg-ENT Database Analysis. *OTO Open* **2024**, *8*, e128. [CrossRef] [PubMed]
50. Wu, S.; Shirley, R.B.; Genther, D.; Ciolek, P.; Prendes, B.; Hopkins, B.; Ku, J. Trends in Surgical Volume and Postoperative Outcomes of Head and Neck Free Flap Reconstruction Using the Finance-Electronic Medical Record Digital Dashboard. *J. Clin. Otorhinolaryngol.* **2023**, *5*, 1–5. [CrossRef]
51. Ministry of Social Affairs and Health. Available online: https://valtioneuvosto.fi/en/-//1271139/covid-19-no-longer-classified-as-generally-hazardous-communicable-disease (accessed on 29 October 2023).
52. Kuitunen, I.; Renko, M.; Tapiainen, T. Unusual late epidemic peak during influenza season 2021–2022: A nationwide register-based analysis in Finland. *Influenza Other Respi. Viruses* **2022**, *16*, 1199–1201. [CrossRef] [PubMed]
53. Finnish Institute for Health and Welfare. Available online: https://thl.fi/fi/web/infektiotaudit-ja-rokotukset/taudit-ja-torjunta/taudit-ja-taudinaiheuttajat-a-o/rsv/rsv-esiintyvyys-suomessa (accessed on 29 October 2023).
54. Acute Otitis Media (Children). Current Care Guidelines. Working Group Set Up by the Finnish Medical Society Duodecim, Finnish Association of Otorhinolaryngology—Head and Neck Surgery, Finnish Paediatric Society, Finnish General Medicine Society. Helsinki. Available online: https://www.kaypahoito.fi/hoi31050#K1 (accessed on 29 October 2023).

Journal of
Clinical Medicine

MDPI

Article

Evolving Trends and Future Demands in ENT Procedures: A Nationwide 10-Year Analysis

Akash Jangan [1,*], Satvir Minhas [1], Emmanuel Diakos [1], Mark Simmons [1] and Zahir Mughal [2]

[1] Department of ENT, Walsall Healthcare NHS Trust, Moat Rd., Walsall WS2 9PS, UK
[2] Department of ENT, Oxford University Hospitals NHS Foundation Trust, Headley Way, Oxford OX3 9DU, UK
* Correspondence: a.jangan@nhs.net; Tel.: +44-01922-721172

Abstract: Objective: This study aims to investigate the trends in otology, rhinology, and head and neck (H&N) operations over the past decade in England. These trends will allow for predictive modelling to forecast the demand over the coming years to aid workforce and resource planning in ENT. **Methods**: Hospital Episode Statistics data were extracted between April 2012 and April 2023. A total of 121 otology, 114 rhinology, and 122 H&N procedure codes were included. Correlation and linear regression analyses were conducted to examine trends and produce a forecast model for the volume of operations. **Results**: A gradual upward trend in the volume of operations was observed in rhinology, with a positive correlation coefficient (R = 0.74). In contrast, otology (R = −0.67) and H&N (R= −0.75) showed negative trends, indicating a moderate decline in operational volumes over time. The COVID-19 pandemic significantly disrupted operating activity in rhinology and otology. To address the backlog and reach the pre-pandemic forecasted levels within the next five years, surgical capacity must increase by an additional 33,807 rhinology 25,486 otology, and 10,300 head procedures per year in England. **Conclusions**: This analysis highlights a need for prioritization and expansion of the ENT workforce and resources to manage the current backlog and anticipated increase in demand over the next five years.

Keywords: Hospital Episodes Statistics (HES); workforce planning; otolaryngology; otology; rhinology; head and neck

1. Introduction

Ear, Nose, and Throat (ENT) surgery encompasses a diverse range of conditions, including those affecting hearing, balance, breathing, swallowing, voice, and head and neck (H&N) cancers. Over time, the landscape of ENT procedures has undergone significant changes, influenced by rapid technological advancements, shifting patient demographics, evolving patterns of disease burden, and the impact of healthcare policies. These dynamic factors present considerable challenges for the National Health Service (NHS) in the United Kingdom, which is already under significant strain due to increasing demands and stretched resources.

Technological advancements, such as endoscopic sinus surgery, cochlear implants, laser techniques, robotic surgery, and the use of artificial intelligence, are constantly changing the field of otolaryngology, enhancing the precision and scope of surgical procedures [1–5]. However, these innovations have also introduced a level of unpredictability to the demand for specific procedures, requiring flexible and forward-thinking approaches to resource planning. Additionally, demographic shifts, such as the aging population in the UK, are contributing to changes in the prevalence of ENT conditions. For instance, the number of people aged over 85 is projected to grow by 55% by 2037 [6]. This is expected to lead to an increased prevalence of chronic conditions such as hearing loss, H&N cancers, and chronic rhinosinusitis. Therefore, it is likely to intensify the demand for otology, rhinology, and H&N surgical services, necessitating strategic planning to meet future healthcare needs.

The Coronavirus Disease 2019 (COVID-19) pandemic has further compounded the challenges faced by the NHS, profoundly disrupting healthcare delivery worldwide. In the UK, elective surgical waiting lists grew from 4.4 million before the pandemic to 6 million in 2022, with an estimated 10 million patients delaying or forgoing treatment altogether [7]. This unprecedented backlog has placed additional pressure on an already-overstretched healthcare system. Although the NHS Constitution mandates that 92% of patients should wait no longer than 18 weeks from referral to treatment, this standard has not been achieved since 2015 [8]. The 2022 delivery plan for tackling the elective care backlog highlighted the difficulty in predicting how quickly services could recover, reinforcing the urgent need for improved resource allocation and workforce optimization.

Effective workforce planning is essential for ensuring the sustainability of ENT services and optimizing healthcare delivery. The UK surgical workforce census published in 2023 emphasized that the current workload is unsustainable for the existing workforce, underscoring the importance of understanding trends in procedural demand to anticipate and address future challenges [9]. The NHS believes that workforce planning requires aligning the right people with the appropriate skills in the right locations at the right time to deliver the highest standard of patient care [6]. To achieve this, a detailed analysis of trends in procedural volumes within surgical specialties is key to guiding resource allocation and workforce development.

Despite the clinical and practical importance of procedural analyses, there remains a paucity of detailed studies examining trends in ENT procedures. Hospital Episode Statistics (HES) data provide a comprehensive dataset covering procedures performed in all NHS hospitals across England from 2000 to 2023 [10]. This publicly available resource offers a unique opportunity to analyze inpatient and outpatient activity on a national scale, providing valuable insights into trends and procedural volumes [10]. Using this dataset, this study investigates trends in otology, rhinology, and H&N procedures over the past decade to inform resource planning and workforce optimization. There is a specific focus on the impact of COVID-19 on pre-pandemic operating volumes in ENT. The goal is to ensure the NHS is equipped to meet the evolving healthcare needs of its population, to guide the pathway to recovery post-COVID-19, and to support the development of sustainable ENT services for the future.

2. Materials and Methods

2.1. Data Collection

HES data was accessed through online records on the NHS Digital website. This data included the number of patients undergoing surgical procedures in each fiscal year from April 2012 to April 2023. Procedures were entered into a Microsoft Excel spreadsheet with their specific Office of Population Censuses and Surveys (OPCS-4) codes. A total of 121 otology, 114 rhinology, and 122 H&N procedure codes were included, as listed in Supplementary File S1. The HES data from 2000–2001 to 2011–2012 was excluded from the trend analysis as there was an arbitrary shift in procedure volumes across all subspecialties between the years 2011–2012 and 2012–2013 (Supplementary File S2). This increase is not accounted for but may be related to changes in reporting practices. Therefore, in order to provide the most accurate and up-to-date analysis, only the time period beyond 2012–2013 was included in this study.

Data corresponding to the COVID-19 period (2020–2021 to 2022–2023) was excluded from trend analysis as this period was an anomaly. The fiscal year April 2020–April 2021 was selected as the beginning of the COVID-19 period because the first UK-wide lockdown was announced in March 2020 and the NHS restructured its services and workforce, severely impacting elective activity [11]. The pre-COVID-19 (2019–2020) year volumes were compared to the operative volumes in each subsequent year, and this was presented as a percentage reduction. To further assess the impact of COVID-19, we estimated the backlog created by the pandemic. First, we calculated the difference between the forecasted number of operations during the COVID-19 period and the actual number of operations during this period. This comparison enabled us to determine the annual deficit. Then, by summing these annual deficits, we estimated the cumulative backlog of operations generated by the pandemic. Finally, to propose a strategy for clearing the pandemic backlog, we calculated the additional number of operations needed for each subspeciality to clear the backlog over the next five years.

2.2. Statistical Tests

The statistical tests were performed on the total volume of ENT procedures (rhinology, otology and H&N) as well as each individual subspecialty. Correlation analysis was performed to assess the linear relationship between time and number of operations. The correlation coefficient (R) was calculated to quantify the direction and strength of the linear relationship. Linear regression analysis was conducted to evaluate the regression model and its predictive power. Coefficient of determination (R^2) was reported to evaluate the goodness of fit of the regression model. Our analysis was based on the data from 2012–2013 to 2019–2020. All analyses were performed using Python 3.11. This study involved secondary analysis of anonymized HES data, and, therefore, no ethical approval was required according to the NHS Health Research Authority online tool.

3. Results

3.1. Trend Analysis

The trend for the total ENT procedure volumes across all subspecialties showed that pre-pandemic (2012–2013 to 2019–2020) volumes were generally stable, with no significant fluctuations (Figure 1). The correlation coefficient was −0.08, indicating a very weak correlation. The trend of ENT procedures across the three subspecialties over time is shown in Figure 2. Rhinology showed a positive correlation coefficient (R = 0.74), indicating a strong upward trend in the number of operations. However, H&N (R = −0.75) and otology (R = −0.67) showed negative trends, reflecting moderate declines in operating numbers during the analyzed period.

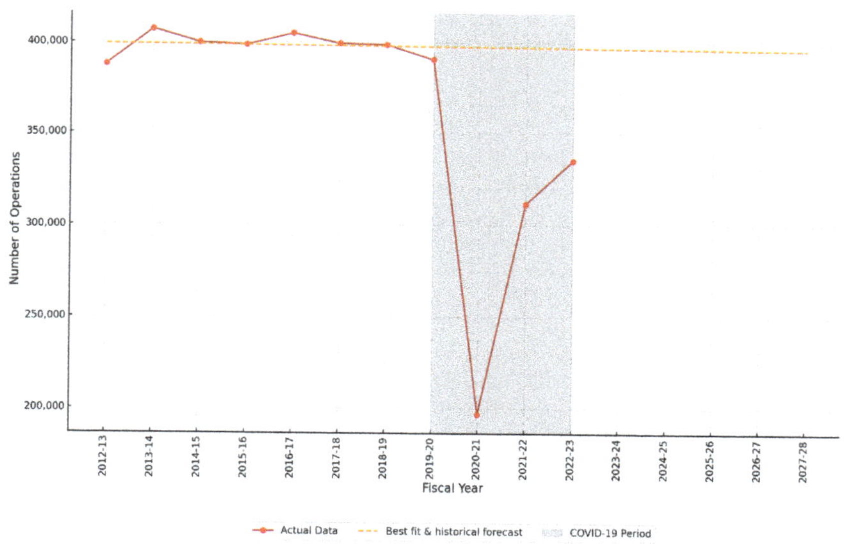

Figure 1. Trend analysis of cumulative ENT procedures. The line of best fit represents the linear regression trend based on pre-pandemic (2012–2013 to 2019–2020) volumes with a five-year forecast regression line. Grey area = COVID-19 period. Fiscal year = April to April.

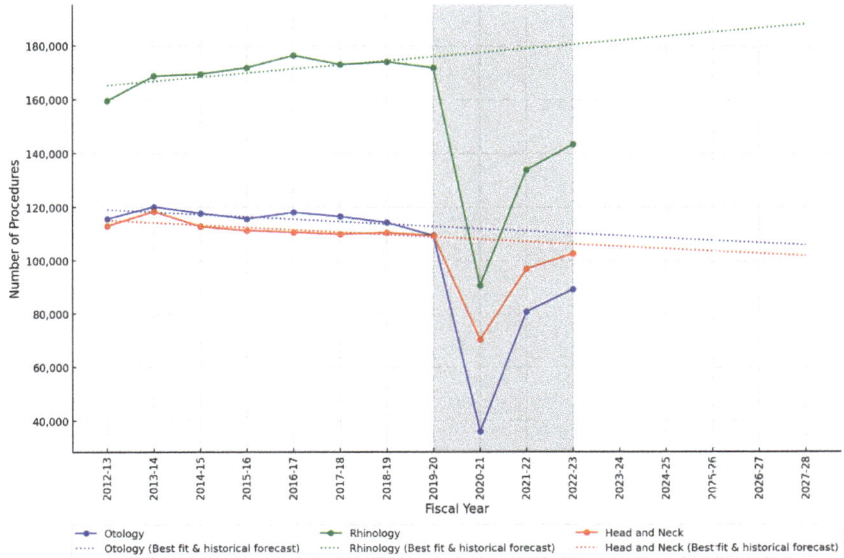

Figure 2. Trend analysis of ENT subspecialties with five-year forecast regression lines for each subspecialty based on pre-COVID-19 data. Grey area = COVID-19 period. Fiscal year = April to April.

3.2. Forecast Analysis

The coefficient of determination (R^2) values quantified the proportion of variance in procedure volumes that could be explained by the linear regression model. The R^2 was 0.007 for the cumulative number of ENT procedure volumes, suggesting that time alone explained only a very small portion of the variation in procedure volumes, likely due to other influencing factors. The R^2 values were rhinology 0.54, H&N 0.56, and otology 0.45. These values indicated a moderate linear trend over time, implying the model captured the trend reasonably well.

3.3. Impact of COVID-19

The pandemic caused significant disruption to operating activity, as depicted by a sharp deviation from the predicted trends, highlighted in grey shade in both Figures 1 and 2. Compared to pre-pandemic levels, in 2020–2021, there was an overall 50.7% decrease in the total number of ENT procedures performed (Figure 1). This improved to a 22.0% decrease in 2021–2022 and 16.1% decrease in 2022–2023 (Figure 1).

The volume of operations in the most recent recorded year, 2022–2023, showed near-complete recovery in H&N, but procedure volumes in otology and especially rhinology remained below the predicted pre-pandemic forecasted levels for 2022–2023 (Figure 2).

The estimated cumulative backlog of operations created by the pandemic was significant, with approximately 169,034 operations in rhinology, 127,431 in otology, and 51,499 operations in H&N (Table 1).

Table 1. Year-by-year COVID-19 backlog breakdown. Derived by calculating the difference between the forecasted levels and the actual volume of procedures.

Year	Otology	Rhinology	Head & Neck
2020–2021	76,034	86,750	37,664
2021–2022	30,330	45,111	10,282
2022–2023	21, 067	37,173	3553
Cumulative backlog	127,431	169,034	51,449

3.4. Strategy for the Next Five Years

To address the backlog created by the pandemic within the next five years, by 2027–2028, 33,807 procedures in rhinology, 25,486 in otology, and 10,300 in H&N are needed in addition to new cases.

4. Discussion

4.1. Main Findings

The findings show that, nationally, across England, the overall ENT procedure volumes remained stable between April 2012 and April 2020, suggesting that demand for ENT services was relatively constant during this pre-pandemic period. Interestingly, however, whilst overall trends were stable, amongst the subspecialities, an upward trend was observed in rhinology and downward trends in otology and H&N procedures. A scoping review of the literature suggests that this study is the most comprehensive analysis of the nationwide ENT subspecialty procedure volumes during the pre-pandemic and pandemic period. The total number of ENT procedures in this study was stable over a decade; in contrast, globally, multiple single-center studies report an increase in ENT operating, but this may be more reflective of local practices as opposed to national demand [12,13]. Institutional practices and local expertise often influence the choice and adoption of medical procedures. For instance, a recent single-center study advocates incorporating sliding epiglottoplasty as an additional step for pharyngeal reconstruction following laryngectomy, rather than relying solely on primary closure. This approach not only affects procedural volumes but also underscores the role of institutional preferences in shaping clinical practices [14]. Similarly, the National Institute for Health and Care Excellence (NICE) issued guidance on the use of Hypoglossal Nerve Stimulation for moderate to severe obstructive sleep apnea (OSA) in 2017 [15]. Despite this, the first UK center to perform this procedure was Guy's and St Thomas' Hospital in London in 2023 [16]. This demonstrates how geographical location, and local expertise can significantly influence the availability and adoption of new procedures, leading to disparities in procedural volumes.

The upward trend in rhinology is likely multifactorial and influenced by changes in technology, adoption of new techniques, and evolving management guidelines and policies. For instance, an increase in endoscopic sinus surgery has been observed in multiple previous studies [1,17,18]. This may be attributable to advancements in technologies and increasing popularity and application of endoscopic techniques, which are minimally invasive. Similarly, there has been a significant development in the usage of laser technologies in rhinology [19]. Additionally, the positive trend in rhinology may be inflated by the coding of multiple procedures performed during a single session. For example, endoscopic sinus surgeries often encompass multiple individual procedures, such as septoplasty or turbinate surgery. Therefore, a single operative encounter may be coded under multiple procedures, which could account for the relatively increased number of rhinology procedures over H&N and otology. Furthermore, in recent years, there has been a change in the management guidelines of certain conditions, such as chronic rhinosinusitis (CRS), with a push for early surgical intervention [20]. This shift in patient management may be contributing to the increasing demand for rhinology procedures. Similarly, a recent randomized controlled trial recommended septoplasty as a more effective intervention than medical management for nasal obstruction associated with a deviated nasal septum [21]. This recommendation is likely to drive future demand for these procedures for functional indications. Patient expectations and behavior may have evolved with time and patients may increasingly seek surgical options for chronic conditions affecting quality of life, such as obstructive nasal airflow and snoring.

A downwards trend was observed in otology and H&N procedures. This may be attributable to changes in the clinical management of chronic conditions. Additionally, the downwards trend in H&N can be explained by advances in non-surgical alternatives to managing malignancies, such as radiotherapy, chemotherapy and biological therapies. Comparably, in France, the overall number of ENT cancer surgeries declined between

2010 and 2021, with a sharper decrease observed during the COVID-19 pandemic [22]. There have been limited studies which looked at nationwide data on otological or H&N procedure volumes. However, trends in specific procedures within each subspecialty have been reported. A national study in Scotland reported a decline in ventilation tube insertion in children between 2001 and 2018 [23]. Finland and the US report similar declines in tympanostomies [24,25]. Similarly, a nationwide South Korean study shows a reduction in cholesteatoma surgery between 2012 and 2018 [26]. These individual studies are comparable to our findings for otology. In contrast, several studies report that total thyroidectomies, a common H&N procedure, appears to have increased in the United States of America (US) over a similar period [27,28].

4.2. Impact of COVID-19

The findings suggest that, compared to 2019–2020, there was an approximately 50.7% reduction in elective ENT procedures in the year 2020–2021 and this has gradually improved but has not reached pre-pandemic levels yet. These findings are comparable to other studies in the literature. In the US, similar trends have been seen in ENT as well as other specialties, including cardiology, orthopedics, and ophthalmology [29–32]. A single-center UK study conducted in 2021 showed a 31.2% reduction in ENT surgical procedures post-COVID-19, and despite low volumes of COVID-19 infection, the operating levels have not returned to baseline [33]. Similarly, our study shows that operating volumes in 2022–2023 are only 84% of the levels in 2019–2020. This may be secondary to changes in elective practices as new safety protocols have reduced the efficiency and speed at which elective surgery is administered, suggesting that, nationally, we are yet to return to pre-pandemic operating levels, let alone clear the backlog generated by the pandemic.

Considering the subspeciality data, a relatively small difference in pre- and post-COVID-19 forecasts was observed in H&N procedures. The data show that rhinology and otology were more severely impacted by COVID-19 compared to H&N. This difference might be due to the nature of these procedures, many of which are urgent or oncological and, thus, less susceptible to deferral or cancellation compared to more elective or non-urgent procedures in rhinology and otology.

There is an urgent need for strategic expansion and optimization of operational capacity to manage the anticipated increase in demand for new cases and address the backlog of deferred treatments. Our analysis indicates that, to clear the backlog within the next five years, the volume of operations per year must increase by an additional 10,300 in H&N, 25,468 in otology, and 33,807 in rhinology. This significant upscaling in surgical capacity is essential to address the current backlog while meeting the ongoing demand for ENT surgery.

4.3. Application of Findings and Recommendations

This study can be used to provide several recommendations for workforce planning. ENT departments should prioritize addressing the significant variations in backlog and demand across the specialties. Based on these data, rhinology has the largest backlog as well as the strongest upward trend in demand. This suggests that a significant investment in additional workforce, training, and theatre allocation is needed in this subspecialty. The five-year timeline for recovery suggested by our forecast analysis is an example of how our study can be used to set a clearance target nationally. These data may be used to advocate for national policy changes to prioritize specialties like rhinology, which are facing high demand and backlogs. Furthermore, they can be used to advocate for targeted funding programs to accelerate recovery.

Our study highlights the need for integrating predictive models into national healthcare strategies to proactively allocate resources appropriately, to plan for future demands. It is apparent that although a linear regression model does give a foundational idea of basic trends, it does not fully account for the multiple cofounding variables that have been discussed. Furthermore, we recommend the integration of real-time analytics into hospital systems to provide more accurate forecasting for future procedural demands. Transparency and availability of these data to the general population can aid in public awareness about the backlog and its impact in order to help manage patient expectations for delayed procedures.

Training and workforce development are key areas for translating the findings of this study. This study highlights the need for targeted workforce training programs in rhinology. For instance, additional fellowship programs may address the high demand for procedures by upskilling surgeons in emerging techniques and recruiting additional specialists in departments. Alternatively, H&N and otology, whilst experiencing a moderate backlog, should focus on sustaining procedure volumes and address challenges related to the declining pre-pandemic trend. This may suggest that more focus and attention are needed in the outpatient workload management of these subspecialties, as this may help to identify patients who may benefit from surgery. Insights into the trends in outpatient workload will be extremely valuable.

In addition, these data can help provide a framework for scheduling activity within departments. For instance, the data show that the volume ratio of otology/rhinology/H&N in the year 2022–2023 was approximately equal to 1:2:1. These proportions can be utilized to dictate how theatre time is divided between subspecialities. Similarly, they can influence the proportion of subspecialists that are recruited into a department. These data can also aid in prioritizing cases for waiting list initiatives such as additional operating theatre sessions scheduled outside of regular contractual hours. A potential partnership with the private healthcare providers that can perform low-risk, high-volume procedures may aid in freeing up NHS resources for more complex cases.

4.4. Limitations

This study relied on retrospective HES data, using an administrative dataset, and, therefore, may not fully capture the breadth of clinical practice. The reporting and coding of procedures are likely to evolve with technologies, practice, and computer software within the NHS. For example, the Royal College of Physicians, in collaboration with the Department of Health, aimed to improve the quality and accuracy of clinical coding through the iLab project [34]. While these improvements are beneficial, they can introduce arbitrary shifts in data over extended periods of time, leading to measurement bias and complicating trend analysis. We observed a notable unexplained shift in reporting trends between the first and second decade of the 20-year span of HES data, as illustrated in Supplementary File S2. Consequently, we used the latter segment of data to ensure the most up-to-date and accurate data analysis.

The predictive modelling provided an estimate of the anticipated volume of operations. However, it was based on pre-COVID-19 activity levels and, therefore, assumes that in the post-COVID-19 period, the rate of trend will be the same. With only a few years of post-COVID-19 data available, these data were volatile and had to be excluded from the trend analysis. The R^2 values for the three subspecialties were moderate, suggesting that a linear model does not fully account for unexamined factors influencing the observed trends. For instance, a report by the Financial Times highlighted a record surge in private healthcare demand in 2023 [35]. This trend is largely attributed to public dissatisfaction with NHS waiting times and resource constraints. As a result, our forecast model may overestimate the pandemic-induced backlog, as a portion of these cases may have already been addressed by the private sector.

A key limitation of predictive modelling is its inability to account for unforeseen changes in future healthcare delivery innovations, or policy shifts that could impact on future clinical activity. For example, while not currently funded by the NHS, biologic therapy has the potential to reduce the need for repeated endoscopic sinus surgery for CRS with nasal polyps in the future [36]. Conversely, in otology, the expanding criterion for cochlear implantation is likely to increase the demand for this procedure [37]. Such advancements could alter the demand for certain surgical procedures.

4.5. Future Research

Trend analysis of national data provides valuable insights into overall service demand but may not be generalizable to individual ENT departments. Resource availability, patient demographics, and clinical practices may vary significantly across regions. Therefore, local audits of activity and assessment of local needs are critical in addressing specific local demands and will complement these national data. We are still in the early stages of recovery post-COVID-19. Future work should also be directed at seeing how the dynamic rate of recovery evolves, and predictive modelling should be repeated and resource allocation periodically adjusted in response to new trends.

Another avenue for future research is the analysis of emergency ENT services. Emergency procedures constitute a significant component of hospital workload and often influence the availability of resources for elective surgeries. Understanding trends in emergency ENT services and comparing these to elective services will be useful in evaluating their impact on elective care as well as aid in workforce allocation and infrastructure planning.

5. Conclusions

This nationwide study shows that, in the UK, the demand for ENT procedures has remained stable over the last decade. However, rhinology procedures demonstrated the most significant upward trend and greatest deficit from COVID-19. The impact of COVID-19 highlighted the vulnerabilities in the current system, with a prolonged recovery period expected. Our findings advocate that ongoing monitoring and strategic planning are essential to ensure the NHS remains responsive to evolving clinical needs.

Supplementary Materials: The following supporting information can be downloaded at: https://www.mdpi.com/article/10.3390/jcm13247850/s1, Supplementary File S1: Table S1: Otology procedures and the OPCS-4 codes included from hospital episode statistics (HES) data; Table S2: Rhinology procedures and OPCS4 codes included from hospital episode statistics (HES) data; Table S3: Head and neck procedures and OPCS4 codes included from hospital episode statistics (HES) data; Supplementary File S2: Trends in the annual volume of otology, rhinology, and head and neck (H&N) procedures in England from 2000–2001 to 2022–2023.

Author Contributions: Conceptualization, A.J. and Z.M.; methodology, A.J., Z.M. and S.M.; software and validation, A.J. and Z.M.; formal analysis, A.J. and Z.M.; data curation, A.J.; supervision, S.M., M.S. and E.D.; writing—original draft preparation, A.J.; writing—review and editing, all authors; project administration, Z.M., M.S. and E.D. All authors have read and agreed to the published version of the manuscript.

Funding: This research received no external funding.

Institutional Review Board Statement: This study involved secondary analysis of anonymized HES data, and, therefore, no ethical approval was required according to the NHS Health Research Authority online tool.

Informed Consent Statement: Not applicable.

Data Availability Statement: The data used in this study was obtained from the Hospital Episode Statistics (HES) database, which is openly available through NHS Digital. This is accessible on the following website: https://digital.nhs.uk/data-and-information/data-tools-and-services/data-services/hospital-episode-statistics.

Conflicts of Interest: The authors declare no conflicts of interest.

References

1. Gupta, K.; Jolly, K.; Bhamra, N.; Osborne, M.S.; Ahmed, S.K. The evolution of sinus surgery in England in the last decade—An observational study. *World J. Otorhinolaryngol. Head Neck Surg.* **2020**, *7*, 240–246. [CrossRef]
2. Mackay, S.G.; Every, J.D. Advances in pharyngeal surgery over the past 10 years: New techniques and technology. *Otolaryngol. Clin. N. Am.* **2024**, *57*, 501–510. [CrossRef]
3. Byrd, J.K.; Duvvuri, U. Current trends in robotic surgery for otolaryngology. *Curr. Otorhinolaryngol. Rep.* **2013**, *1*, 153–157. [CrossRef]

4. Tama, B.A.; Kim, D.H.; Kim, G.; Kim, S.W.; Lee, S. Recent advances in the application of artificial intelligence in otorhinolaryngology-head and neck surgery. *Clin. Exp. Otorhinolaryngol.* **2020**, *13*, 326–339. [CrossRef] [PubMed]
5. Ciorba, A.; Skarżyński, P.H.; Gocmenler, H.; Hatzopoulos, S. Advances in pediatric and adult cochlear implant and middle ear prostheses. *J. Clin. Med.* **2021**, *10*, 3152. [CrossRef] [PubMed]
6. NHS England. NHS Long-Term Workforce Plan. Available online: https://www.england.nhs.uk/long-read/nhs-long-term-workforce-plan-2/#5-next-steps (accessed on 3 December 2024).
7. NHS England. Delivery Plan for Tackling the COVID-19 Backlog of Elective Care. Available online: https://www.england.nhs.uk/coronavirus/wp-content/uploads/sites/52/2022/02/C1466-delivery-plan-for-tackling-the-covid-19-backlog-of-elective-care.pdf (accessed on 3 December 2024).
8. The King's Fund. Waiting Times for Non-Urgent Treatment. Available online: https://www.kingsfund.org.uk/insight-and-analysis/data-and-charts/waiting-times-non-urgent-treatment (accessed on 3 December 2024).
9. The Royal College of Surgeons of England. UK Surgical Workforce Census Report. Available online: https://www.rcseng.ac.uk/standards-and-research/surgical-workforce-census/ (accessed on 3 December 2024).
10. NHS Digital. Hospital Episode Statistics (HES). Available online: https://digital.nhs.uk/data-and-information/data-tools-and-services/data-services/hospital-episode-statistics (accessed on 3 December 2024).
11. NHS COVID-19 Framework. Operating Framework for Urgent and Planned Services. Available online: https://www.covidlawlab.org/wp-content/uploads/2020/06/Operating-framework-for-urgent-and-planned-services-within-hospitals.pdf (accessed on 3 December 2024).
12. Muhammed Afsal, E.; Suma, R. Retrospective analysis of otorhinolaryngology-related elective surgeries performed in a tertiary care centre, North Kerala, India. *J. Clin. Diagn. Res.* **2023**, *17*, MC01–MC03. [CrossRef]
13. Choi, K.J.; Kahmke, R.R.; Crowson, M.G.; Puscas, L.; Scher, R.L.; Cohen, S.M. Trends in otolaryngology consultation patterns at an academic quaternary care center. *JAMA Otolaryngol. Head Neck Surg.* **2017**, *143*, 472–477. [CrossRef]
14. Grošelj, A.; Tancer, I.; Jerman, A.; Paučič, J.; Pušnik, L. Pharyngeal reconstruction after total laryngectomy with sliding epiglottis: Technical aspects with retrospective review. *Front. Oncol.* **2024**, *13*, 1284266. [CrossRef]
15. National Institute for Health and Care Excellence. Interventional Procedures Guidance—Hypoglossal Nerve Stimulation for Moderate to Severe Obstructive Sleep Apnoea. 2017. Available online: https://www.nice.org.uk/guidance/ipg598/resources/hypoglossal-nerve-stimulationfor-moderate-to-severe-obstructive-sleep-apnoea-pdf1899872235842245 (accessed on 15 December 2024).
16. Yakubu, K. ENT & Audiology News. First UK Hypoglossal Nerve Stimulation Implant in the Treatment for Moderate to Severe OSA. 2023. Available online: https://www.entandaudiologynews.com/development/spotlight-on-innovation/post/first-uk-hypoglossal-nerve-stimulation-implant-in-the-treatment-for-moderate-to-severe-osa (accessed on 15 December 2024).
17. Venkatraman, G.; Likosky, D.; Zhou, W.; Finlayson, S.R.G.; Goodman, D.C. Trends in endoscopic sinus surgery rates in the Medicare population. *Arch. Otolaryngol. Head Neck Surg.* **2010**, *136*, 426–430. [CrossRef]
18. Pynnonen, M.A.; Davis, M.M. Extent of sinus surgery, 2000 to 2009: A population-based study. *Laryngoscope* **2014**, *124*, 820–825. [CrossRef] [PubMed]
19. Lau, K.; Stavrakas, M.; Ray, J. Lasers in rhinology—An update. *Ear Nose Throat J.* **2021**, *100*, 77S–82S. [CrossRef] [PubMed]
20. Guideline Development Group for Rhinosinusitis. Commissioning Guide: Chronic Rhinosinusitis. Royal College of Surgeons of England. Available online: https://www.rcseng.ac.uk/-/media/files/rcs/standards-and-research/commissioning/rhinosinusitis-commissioning-guide-for-republication.pdf (accessed on 21 July 2024).
21. Carrie, S.; O'Hara, J.; Fouweather, T.; Homer, T.; Rousseau, N.; Rooshenas, L.; Bray, A.; Stocken, D.D.; Ternent, L.; Rennie, K.; et al. Clinical effectiveness of septoplasty versus medical management for nasal airway obstruction: Multicentre, open-label, randomised controlled trial. *BMJ* **2023**, *18*, 383. [CrossRef]
22. Le Bihan-Benjamin, C.; Rocchi, M.; Putton, M.; Méric, J.-B.; Bousquet, P.J. Estimation of oncologic surgery case volume before and after the COVID-19 pandemic in France. *JAMA Netw. Open* **2023**, *6*, e2253204. [CrossRef]
23. Wescott, R.A.; Downie, L.S.; Kubba, H. Retrospective observational study analysing the trends in ventilation tube insertion in children in Scotland between 2001 and 2018. *Clin. Otolaryngol.* **2024**, *49*, 199–206. [CrossRef] [PubMed]
24. Valajärvi, V.-E.; Lamminmäki, S.; Lundberg, M.; Hafrén, L. Ten-year trends in otolaryngological surgery volumes and the impact of infection prevention during the COVID-19 pandemic—A national study. *J. Clin. Med.* **2024**, *13*, 7190. [CrossRef] [PubMed]
25. Welschmeyer, A.; Coerdt, K.; Crossley, J.; Malekzadeh, S. Critical evaluation of trends in otolaryngology resident caseload by subspecialty from 2005 to 2019. *Ann. Otol. Rhinol. Laryngol.* **2021**, *130*, 915–922. [CrossRef] [PubMed]
26. Im, G.J.; Han, K.D.; Park, K.H.; Cho, C.H.; Jang, H.; Lee, J.H.; Lee, S.H. Rate of chronic otitis media operations and cholesteatoma surgeries in South Korea: A nationwide population-based study (2006–2018). *Sci. Rep.* **2020**, *10*, 11356. [CrossRef]
27. Al-Qurayshi, Z.; Robins, R.; Hauch, A.; Randolph, G.W.; Kandil, E. Association of surgeon volume with outcomes and cost savings following thyroidectomy: A national forecast. *JAMA Otolaryngol. Head Neck Surg.* **2016**, *142*, 32–39. [CrossRef]
28. Nouraei, S.A.; Virk, J.S.; Middleton, S.E.; Aylin, P.; Mace, A.; Vaz, F.; Kaddour, H.; Darzi, A.; Tolley, N.S. A national analysis of trends, outcomes, and volume–outcome relationships in thyroid surgery. *Clin. Otolaryngol.* **2017**, *42*, 354–365. [CrossRef] [PubMed]
29. Saraswathula, A.; Gourin, C.G.; Stewart, C.M. National trends in U.S. otolaryngology surgical volume during the early COVID-19 pandemic. *JAMA Otolaryngol. Head Neck Surg.* **2021**, *147*, 397–399. [CrossRef]

30. Ad, N.; Luc, J.G.Y.; Nguyen, T.C.; COVID-19 North American Cardiac Surgery Survey Working Group. Cardiac surgery in North America and coronavirus disease 2019 (COVID-19): Regional variability in burden and impact. *J. Thorac. Cardiovasc. Surg.* **2021**, *162*, 893–903. [CrossRef] [PubMed]
31. Bedard, N.A.; Elkins, J.M.; Brown, T.S. Effect of COVID-19 on hip and knee arthroplasty surgical volume in the United States. *J. Arthroplast.* **2020**, *35*, S45–S48. [CrossRef]
32. Breazzano, M.P.; Nair, A.A.; Arevalo, J.F.; Barakat, M.R.; Berrocal, A.M.; Chang, J.S.; Chen, A.; Eliott, D.; Garg, S.J.; Ghadiali, Q.; et al. Frequency of urgent or emergent vitreoretinal surgical procedures in the United States during the COVID-19 pandemic. *JAMA Ophthalmol.* **2021**, *139*, 456–463. [CrossRef] [PubMed]
33. Arman, S.; Hopkins, M.; McKean, S. The impact of COVID-19 on elective otolaryngology surgery in a rural hospital in the United Kingdom. *Clin. Otolaryngol.* **2021**, *46*, 1282–1285. [CrossRef] [PubMed]
34. Croft, G.P.; Williams, J.G. The RCP Information Laboratory (iLab): Breaking the cycle of poor data quality. *Clin. Med.* **2005**, *5*, 47–49. [CrossRef]
35. Financial Times. Demand for Private Healthcare Hits Record High in UK. 2024. Available online: https://www.ft.com/content/a4f07a08-b7e9-4330-9915-c2640edf7866 (accessed on 22 November 2024).
36. Xian, M.; Zhang, L. Potential of biologics to alter the need for repeated surgery in patients with chronic rhinosinusitis with nasal polyps. *Allergy* **2023**, *78*, 623–625. [CrossRef] [PubMed]
37. Varadarajan, V.V.; Sydlowski, S.A.; Li, M.M.; Anne, S.; Adunka, O.F. Evolving criteria for adult and pediatric cochlear implantation. *Ear Nose Throat J.* **2021**, *100*, 31–37. [CrossRef]

Journal of
Clinical Medicine

MDPI

Review

Contemporary Management of Cerebrospinal Fluid Rhinorrhoea: A Review of the Literature

Zahir Mughal [1,*], Pablo Martinez-Devesa [1], Alexandros Boukas [2], Sanjeeva Jeyaretna [2,3] and Ali Qureishi [1]

[1] Department of ENT, John Radcliffe Hospital, Headley Way, Headington, Oxford OX3 9DU, UK; pablo.martinez-devesa@ouh.nhs.uk (P.M.-D.); ali.qureishi@ouh.nhs.uk (A.Q.)
[2] Department of Neurosurgery, John Radcliffe Hospital, Headley Way, Headington, Oxford OX3 9DU, UK; alex.boukas@ouh.nhs.uk (A.B.); sanjeeva.jeyaretna@ouh.nhs.uk (S.J.)
[3] Nuffield Department of Clinical Neurosciences, University of Oxford, John Radcliffe Hospital, Headley Way, Headington, Oxford OX3 9DU, UK
* Correspondence: zahir.mughal@ouh.nhs.uk

Abstract: Background/Objectives: Cerebrospinal fluid (CSF) rhinorrhoea carries a significant risk of life-threatening intracranial complications. This review provides a contemporary overview of current management strategies for CSF rhinorrhoea. **Methods:** We conducted a literature review, examining studies from Medline, Embase, and Google Scholar published within the last 20 years. This narrative synthesis summarises the current and future trends in the management of CSF rhinorrhoea. **Results:** The management of CSF leaks requires a multidisciplinary approach, encompassing a thorough clinical assessment, targeted diagnostic testing, and a spectrum of surgical and non-surgical interventions. Endoscopic techniques, particularly the use of vascularised flaps such as the nasoseptal flap, has become central to anterior skull base reconstruction. Numerous graft and flap choices provide tailored solutions based on defect size and CSF flow characteristics, with reported success rates exceeding 90%. **Conclusions:** Endoscopic repair of CSF rhinorrhoea continues to evolve, with modern techniques significantly enhancing success rates and reducing morbidity. Further understanding of underlying aetiologies, advances in technology, and refinement in surgical technique are areas for future innovation in CSF rhinorrhoea management.

Keywords: anterior skull base; cerebrospinal fluid; endoscopic; idiopathic intracranial hypertension; rhinorrhoea

1. Introduction

Cerebrospinal fluid (CSF) is primarily produced by the choroid plexus within the ventricles at an approximate rate of 0.35 mL/min, equating to 350–500 mL/day [1]. It circulates through the ventricular system and subarachnoid space, where it serves a role in cushioning the brain, regulating intracranial pressure, and clearing metabolic waste. Reabsorption occurs into the venous system via arachnoid villi. In adults, the total CSF volume averages 140 mL, with the total volume being turned over approximately three times per day [1]. CSF rhinorrhoea is characterised by abnormal communication between the subarachnoid space and the nasal cavity. This occurs due to a defect in the dura mater, skull base bone, and nasal mucosa, creating a fistulous connection.

The aetiology of CSF rhinorrhoea can be broadly classified into traumatic or non-traumatic (Figure 1), with craniofacial trauma being the most common cause [1]. Anterior skull base fractures account for nearly 25% of all skull fractures, emphasising their clinical

https://doi.org/10.3390/jcm14030995

relevance [2]. A systematic review identified the most common sites of injury as the ethmoid/cribriform plate (46%), frontal sinus (44%), orbital roof (15%), and sphenoid sinus (11%) [2]. The incidence of spontaneous CSF leaks is rising, particularly amongst females in regions with high obesity rates [3]. Traditionally, spontaneous CSF leaks have been defined as occurring without an identifiable inciting factor. However, growing evidence suggests that a substantial proportion of these cases are attributable to underlying idiopathic intracranial hypertension (IIH) [4]. IIH predominantly affects middle-aged obese females and is characterised by symptoms and signs of raised intracranial pressure (ICP) in the absence of hydrocephalus or mass lesions, a normal CSF composition, and no underlying cause for the elevated ICP [5]. Epidemiological data indicate a correlation between the rising levels of obesity and the increasing incidence of spontaneous CSF leaks [6]. Since obesity is a known risk factor for IIH, this association reinforces the hypothesis that many spontaneous leaks are secondary to IIH. The proposed mechanism for CSF leakage in IIH involves elevated ICP and associated dural pulsations, which can exert direct pressure on the skull base, leading to bone thinning, resorption, and formation of meningoceles or meningoencephaloceles [7]. These defects are most commonly observed in the sphenoid sinus (30%), ethmoid sinus (17%), and cribriform plate (16%) [8].

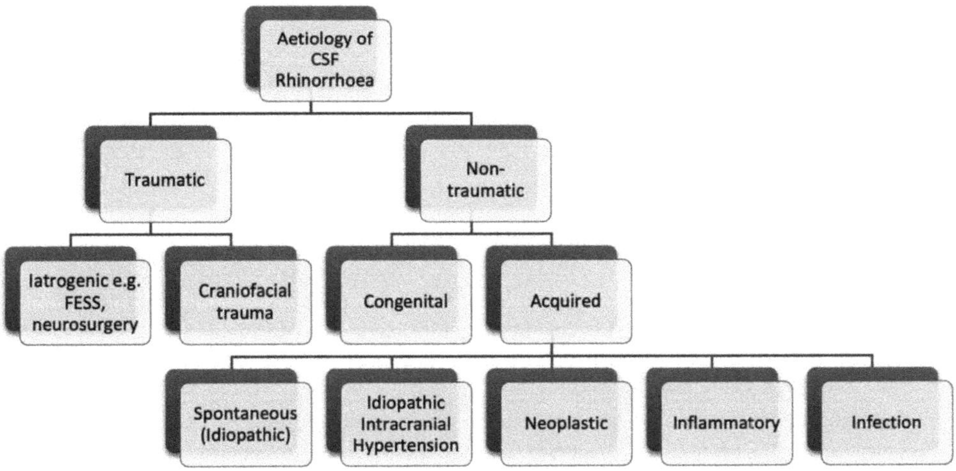

Figure 1. Classification of the aetiology of CSF rhinorrhoea. FESS = Functional Endoscopic Sinus Surgery.

CSF rhinorrhoea carries a significant risk of life-threatening intracranial complications, including meningitis, seizure, pneumocephalus, epidural abscess, and hydrocephalus [9]. Prompt diagnosis and treatment are therefore essential to prevent these complications. The advent of endonasal endoscopic techniques has greatly expanded the armamentarium of reconstructive methods for anterior skull base defects. This review aims to provide an updated overview of the contemporary assessment and management of CSF leaks originating from the anterior skull base. We highlight current innovations in treatments and future potential directions.

2. Materials and Methods

A literature review was conducted by searching the Medline, Embase, and Google Scholar databases using the following key terms: CSF, cerebrospinal fluid, leak, rhinorrh*, fistula, defect, endoscop*, repair, closure, reconstruction, management, treatment, approach, and seal*. Additional studies were identified through forward citation tracking and manually reviewing reference lists. Articles published in the last 20 years, focusing on diagnosis, management, and surgical techniques for anterior skull base defects, were included. We excluded studies focusing on indirect CSF rhinorrhoea from the middle or posterior fossae via the eustachian tube. Articles were selected based on their relevance, with the aim of identifying key themes and discussing recent advancements in the field of CSF rhinorrhoea. The analysis was narrative in nature, synthesising findings qualitatively.

3. Results

3.1. Clinical Assessment

The clinical presentation of CSF rhinorrhoea is typically unilateral, clear, watery nasal discharge [10]. The clinical history should focus on the consistency of the nasal discharge, laterality, duration, onset, timing, aggravating factors, such as straining or posture, and any episodes of meningitis. Symptoms of raised intracranial pressure, such as headaches associated with visual disturbance, should be elicited. However, patients with an active CSF leak may paradoxically present with symptoms of reduced ICP, including orthostatic headache and neck stiffness [10]. The history should also explore potential underlying causes, such as intracranial pathology, prior head trauma, or sinonasal surgery. Particular attention should be paid to identifying IIH, a condition that can result in significant morbidity, including permanent visual loss and disabling headache [11]. IIH is typically seen in females of childbearing age and is associated with obesity, obstructive sleep apnea, and hypertension [3]. Symptoms include headache, visual obscuration, blurry vision, diplopia, pulsatile tinnitus, dizziness, and neck pain [12]. These symptoms may be masked by the presence of a CSF leak, which can act as a 'pressure release valve' [13]. Consequently, symptoms of IIH may only manifest after the leak is repaired, complicating the preoperative diagnosis of this condition.

A comprehensive ENT examination is essential, with particular emphasis on nasendoscopy for direct visualisation of the leak. This evaluation should also include the inspection of the Eustachian tubes and an otologic examination to identify otologic sources of CSF rhinorrhoea [10]. The 'halo sign' [8], characterised by an internal blood ring and an external lighter fluid ring on filter paper, may indicate the presence of CSF in traumatic cases. Subtle CSF leaks may be provoked by having the patient sit up, lean forward, and flex the neck after lying supine—known as the 'reservoir sign' [14]. The remainder of the examination focuses on neuro-ophthalmology signs.

3.2. Investigations

Confirmation of CSF rhinorrhoea requires laboratory analysis of nasal fluid for beta-2 transferrin or beta-trace protein [8,15]. Once CSF has been confirmed, imaging studies are essential to localise the defect. High-resolution computed tomography (HRCT) of the skull base and paranasal sinuses is the initial imaging of choice, providing detailed bony anatomy [15]. If the osseous defect is not visualised on CT, magnetic resonance imaging (MRI) with heavily T2-weighted sequences and fat suppression is recommended for detecting CSF fistula [16]. The MRI protocol should utilise fast imaging employing steady-state acquisition cycled phases (FIESTA-C) or constructive interference steady state (CISS), combined with fluid attenuation inversion recovery (FLAIR) sequences, or their equivalents [10]. At our institution, we prefer a dual imaging approach incorporating both CT and MRI, leveraging their complementary strengths to improve the localisation of CSF leak(s) and facilitate precise surgical planning. This approach is particularly beneficial for patients with spontaneous CSF rhinorrhoea or IIH, who often present with multiple skull base defects [10].

For cases with active leaks that remain undetected by non-invasive imaging, CT cisternography with intrathecal dye injection may be more definitive [15]. Additionally, intrathecal fluorescein (ITF) administration may aid in intraoperative identification of the fistula [17]. However, this off-label use of fluorescein carries rare but potentially serious neurological complications [17]. The use of intraoperative neuronavigation with CT (with or without MRI fusion) is recommended in complex cases and can assist in localising the area of bony defect and associated CSF leak [10].

The diagnostic workup for suspected IIH follows recommendations of recent international consensus guidelines [10,12]. It begins with an ophthalmology evaluation to assess for papilledema and visual function. If papilledema is detected, the first step is to measure blood pressure to exclude malignant hypertension, followed by an urgent MRI venogram. Radiological indicators of IIH include an empty sella, posterior globe flattening, tortuosity of the optic nerve, optic nerve sheath distention, and widening of the foramen ovale [18]. Transverse sinus stenosis is considered to be the most sensitive and reliable imaging indicator marker for IIH [19]. After ruling out hydrocephalus, mass, structural, vascular lesion, and abnormal meningeal enhancement on imaging, all patients should have a lumbar puncture. This test is used to ensure that the composition is normal and to measure opening pressures, with >25 cm of CSF consistent with a diagnosis of IIH [10]. This diagnostic approach aligns with the modified Friedman criteria [20].

3.3. Management

Management of CSF leaks is multidisciplinary, typically including skull base surgeons (ENT and neurosurgery), ophthalmologists, neurologists, and radiologists, coordinated through a skull base multidisciplinary team meeting.

Once the diagnosis has been established, vaccination should be administered against common pathogens (*Streptococcus pneumoniae*, *Haemophilus influenzae* type b, and *Neisseria meningitidis*) to prevent ascending bacterial meningitis [21]. The approach to management depends on whether the leak is acute or chronic [1]. The management algorithm is summarised in Figure 2.

In acute traumatic CSF leaks, management varies based on the cause. Iatrogenic surgical trauma is unlikely to resolve spontaneously and therefore requires prompt surgical treatment [15]. In contrast, leaks from accidental craniofacial trauma are likely to resolve spontaneously and can often be initially managed conservatively with bed rest, head elevation by 30 degrees, avoidance of straining, and laxatives [1]. Lumbar drains may reduce the duration of leakage during conservative management [15]. A step-wise escalation has been proposed, with a three-day trial of conservative treatment, followed by three days of CSF diversion [22], and surgical repair is considered if the leak persists beyond seven days despite these measures [15]. Prophylactic antibiotics are generally not recommended for this group, as they do not significantly reduce infection risk [23].

For delayed presentations of traumatic CSF rhinorrhoea, and all non-traumatic cases, the mainstay of management is surgical repair. Since the introduction of rigid endoscopes for transnasal skull base repair in 1981 [24], the endoscopic approach has become the standard of care, achieving success rates exceeding 90% [25]. This minimally invasive technique has largely replaced traditional open craniotomy approaches due to reduced morbidity and mortality [26].

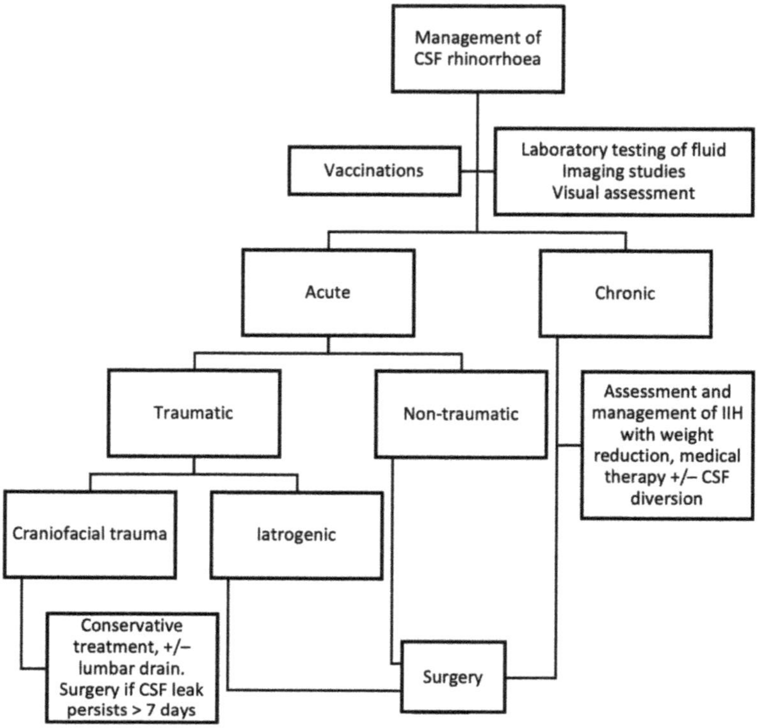

Figure 2. Algorithm for the management of cerebrospinal fluid (CSF) rhinorrhoea. IIH—Idiopathic intracranial hypertension.

3.4. Surgical Technique

The surgical technique for endoscopic repair involves several key steps [10,22]: the mucosa surrounding the defect is meticulously removed circumferentially to expose the underlying bone. If a meningocele or meningoencephalocele is present, it is reduced using bipolar diathermy and resected to the level of the skull base. Careful inspection is necessary to identify and protect any herniated cerebral vessels, which must be placed back into the intracranial space to avoid a distal infarct. The defect is reconstructed using a variety of grafts and flaps, as outlined in Figure 3. Autologous materials are commonly used but require a donor site, introducing additional risks, such as infection, hematoma, or seroma formation, and a longer operation time [27]. Since the description of the vascularised nasoseptal flap in 2006 [28], this flap has become the workhorse for anterior skull base reconstruction. While allografts and xenografts present an alternative, mitigating donor site morbidity, they carry risks of foreign body reaction and aseptic meningitis [14]. Alloplastic materials provide another option, but they remain susceptible to complications such as infection and extrusion [14,27]. Currently, there is no definite evidence favoring one type of material over another, and material selection is typically based on the surgeon's preference [29].

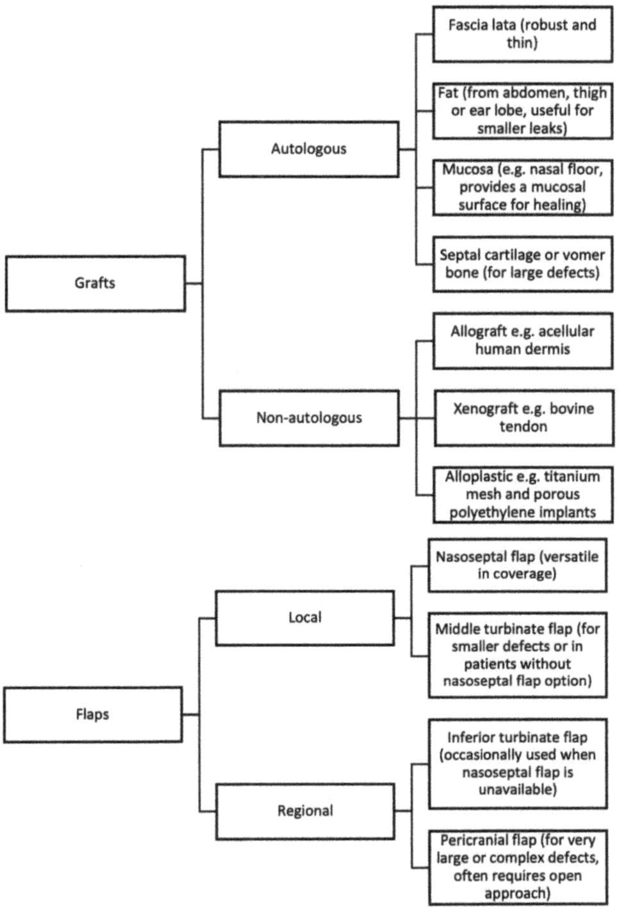

Figure 3. Common materials used in anterior skull base reconstruction.

Grafts can be placed as under-lay, on-lay, or in combination. Techniques such as 'bath-plug' [30] or 'parachute' [31] involve intradural placement of grafts to achieve a secure seal. For small defects, a single-layer closure with a graft may be sufficient, while multi-layered reconstruction with grafts and vascularised flaps is preferred for large or high-flow leaks [22,29]. For larger osseous defects or high-flow leaks, the gasket-seal technique [32] can be employed, incorporating a rigid buttress of bone or cartilage or Medpor (alternative synthetic material) between the layers to enhance structural support. Some authors advocate for over-correction, even in smaller defects, to accommodate for an expected 20% shrinkage in mucosal tissue postoperatively [8,33]. Stabilisation of the reconstruction is achieved with various adjunctive materials, including glues, sealants, and nasal packing. While these adjuncts are commonly used, evidence supporting their effectiveness is limited [29]. Our usual practice involves a multi-layered reconstruction with autologous grafts and nasoseptal flap, and lumbar drainage is generally avoided unless strongly indicated, such as in cases of high-flow leaks or revision surgeries.

3.5. Postoperative Care

Postoperative management includes maintaining head elevation at 30 degrees, bed rest, laxatives, and avoidance of straining for six weeks [22]. Patients should be admitted overnight and undergo monitoring of vital and neurological signs [10]. A temporary lumbar drain may be beneficial in cases of raised intracranial pressure (ICP) [29]. An early postoperative CT scan is performed to check graft position and exclude postoperative intracranial complications such as pneumocephalus, which may predict repair failure [34]. If the scan is satisfactory, patients are typically allowed to mobilise after 48 h, although evidence supporting the optimal duration of bed rest remains limited. Upon discharge, patients are instructed to use a saline nasal spray for six weeks [22]. As dissection occurs through a clean–contaminated operative field, most surgeons elect to use perioperative antibiotics with anti-staphylococcal coverage [14]. At ENT follow-up review, the nasal cavity is assessed for mucosal healing and identification of postoperative problems such as sinonasal infection, CSF leak recurrence, and intracranial complications.

Patients with spontaneous CSF leaks require close neurology and ophthalmological follow-up to monitor for papilledema and to formally assess intracranial pressure, which may develop after closure of the skull base defect if they have underlying IIH [10,13].

3.6. Idiopathic Intracranial Hypertension

The management of IIH involves collaboration between ENT surgeons, neurologists, ophthalmologists, and neurosurgeons. The three primary goals of IIH treatment are to reduce body weight, aid vision protection, and headache control [35]. The management of IIH is summarised in Figure 4. Weight reduction is the only disease-modifying therapy currently available for IIH and is recommended for all patients with a body mass index (BMI) greater than 30 kg/m^2 [11]. A systematic review of weight loss strategies demonstrated that lifestyle interventions achieved modest weight reductions ranging from 1.4 to 15.7 kg, while bariatric surgery yielded significantly greater weight loss, with an average reduction of 27.2–27.8 kg at 24 months [36]. Weight loss has been shown to correlate with a decrease in ICP, with bariatric surgery producing the most pronounced reduction, averaging 11.9 cm H_2O at 24 months [36]. This highlights the importance of weight management in contributing to IIH disease remission. In view of this, expert consensus recommends considering bariatric surgery referral for patients with a BMI $\geq$ 35 kg/m^2 [36].

Acetazolamide, a carbonic anhydrase inhibitor that interferes with CSF production, is considered the mainstay of pharmacological treatment of IIH [11], although evidence supporting its efficacy is not strong [37]. Additionally, due to its side-effect profile, it is not routinely prescribed in the UK [12]. Alternative medications that have been used in the management of IIH include furosemide, topiramate, and octreotide [38]. If medical therapy fails, is poorly tolerated, or if vision is threatened, surgical intervention such as CSF diversion procedures or optic nerve sheath fenestration (ONSF) may be necessary, with the choice of procedure depending on local expertise [11,12]. In urgent sight-threatening cases, a temporising lumbar drain may serve as a bridge to surgery, providing protection for vision [12].

Promising upcoming medical therapies include 11β-HSD1 inhibitors, glucagon-like peptide-1 receptor agonists (GLP-1RAs), anti-calcitonin gene-related peptide (CGRP), and receptor monoclonal antibodies [11,35,38]. Cerebral venous sinus stenting (VSS) has also gained attention as an emerging surgical intervention, demonstrating significant improvements in papilledema, headache, and pulsatile tinnitus rates, with a superior safety profile compared to CSF shunting and ONSF [38]. These novel approaches hold promise for improving outcomes and expanding future treatment options in IIH management.

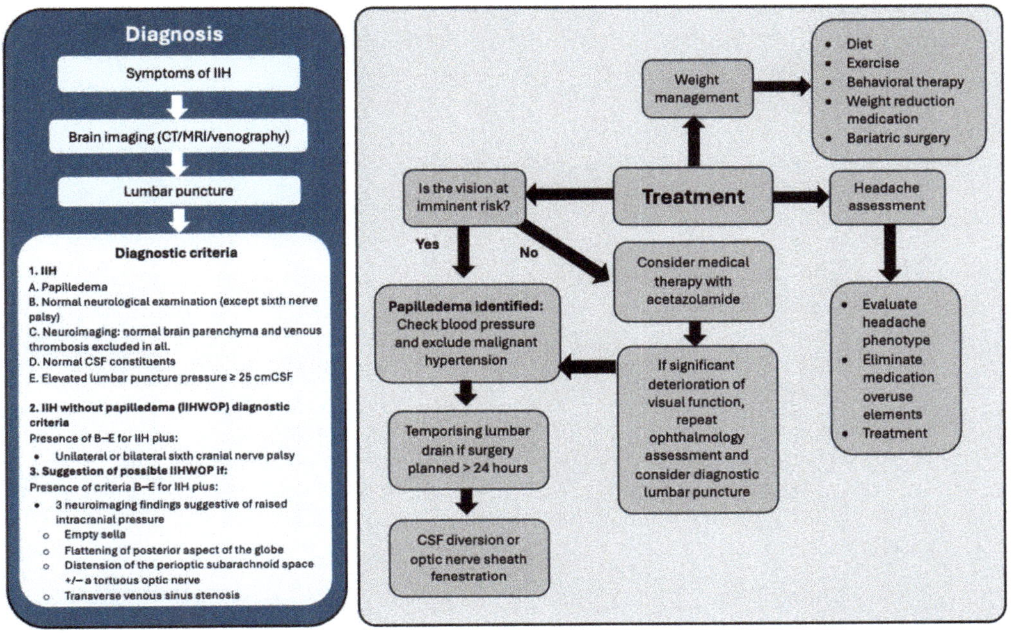

Figure 4. Algorithm for the management of idiopathic intracranial hypertension. Adapted from Mollan et al. [12].

4. Discussion

4.1. Summary of Main Findings

CSF rhinorrhoea presents significant challenges in both diagnosis and management due to its diverse clinical presentations, aetiologies, and treatment approaches. This review highlights the importance of a systematic and multidisciplinary approach to clinical assessment, advanced imaging, pharmacological therapies, and tailored treatments. IIH adds further complexity to the diagnostic process during an active CSF leak, as elevated opening pressures may not be demonstrable, necessitating a high index of clinical suspicion. Beyond repairing the CSF leak, effective management of IIH requires a comprehensive strategy involving weight reduction, pharmacotherapy, and surgical interventions. This holistic approach is essential to address the underlying condition and prevent recurrence or long-term complications.

This review highlights the significant advancements in imaging and surgical techniques for the management of CSF rhinorrhoea, which have evolved considerably over the past two decades. Endoscopic repair has become the standard of care, offering a minimally invasive approach with excellent outcomes. Among these advancements, the use of the vascularised nasoseptal flap has shown remarkable effectiveness in achieving durable closure, especially for high-flow or complex skull base defects. While conservative management remains a viable option for acute, non-iatrogenic traumatic leaks, often with good outcomes, non-resolving or chronic leaks typically require surgical intervention.

4.2. Implications of Findings

The findings carry key implications for clinical practice. First, the importance of a multidisciplinary approach, as effective management requires collaboration among ENT surgeons, neurosurgeons, ophthalmologists, radiologists, and neurologists. Ideally, this collaboration should occur within a dedicated skull base MDT to ensure coordinated care. Second, the results highlight the need for early and accurate diagnosis of CSF rhinorrhoea with laboratory testing and precise localisation with advanced skull base imaging techniques. Third, while the adoption of endoscopic techniques has transformed surgical management, the need for individualised treatment based on aetiology, defect size, and CSF leak flow characteristics is central to effective management. Lastly, the recognition and management of underlying IIH in spontaneous cases of CSF rhinorrhoea is essential to prevent recurrence and associated morbidity.

4.3. Limitations

This review is limited by challenges within the existing body of literature. Many recommendations are derived from retrospective, observational studies and expert consensus, which may limit their generalisability and strength of evidence. There is a paucity of randomised controlled trials evaluating optimal surgical repair strategies. The evidence supporting pharmacological strategies for ICP control and headache management in IIH remains insufficient, highlighting the need for more robust, high-quality studies in these areas.

As a narrative review, this study did not include the systematic data extraction or analytic techniques characteristic of systematic reviews. However, it provided a broad and comprehensive exploration of the available evidence, identifying trends and highlighting areas for future research.

4.4. Future Research

Future research should focus on high-quality, prospective studies and randomised controlled trials to address the current gaps in evidence for the diagnosis and management of CSF leaks. Habenbacher et al. [39] proposed a diagnostic protocol combining beta trace protein testing, HRCT, and ITF for reliably confirming and localising CSF leaks. ITF was instrumental in identifying multiple defects and ensuring watertight closure during surgical repair. However, their study highlighted limitations, such as the potential for false negatives with ITF and cases where leaks were not confirmed intraoperatively despite positive beta trace and HRCT findings. These observations underscore the need for further refinement of diagnostic protocols. Advancements in technology, including MRI sequences, angled scopes, navigation systems, and high-definition cameras [40], could potentially improve the localisation of small or complex leaks and potentially reduce the need for invasive procedures like ITF. Additionally, these advances may facilitate further innovation in endoscopic techniques and reconstructive options.

A diagnosis of IIH is often made retrospectively, as it can be challenging to meet the diagnostic criterion of elevated opening lumbar pressures during an active leak. Future research should aim to develop and validate diagnostic approaches, including the use of characteristic radiological findings, to identify these patients more reliably.

5. Conclusions

CSF rhinorrhoea from anterior skull base defects poses a significant clinical challenge. The advent of endoscopic techniques and vascularised flaps, such as the nasoseptal flap, have revolutionised the management of these leaks, offering effective and less invasive solutions with high success rates. A multidisciplinary approach is essential, with tailored interventions based on the nature of the defect and underlying aetiology. Continued innovation in diagnostic approaches, technology, and surgical technique will be key to advancing the field and enhancing patient outcomes with CSF rhinorrhoea.

Author Contributions: Conceptualisation, Z.M. and A.Q.; methodology, Z.M. and P.M.-D.; data curation, Z.M.; formal analysis, Z.M., A.B. and S.J.; writing—original draft preparation, Z.M. and

P.M.-D.; writing—review and editing, all authors; supervision, A.Q. All authors have read and agreed to the published version of the manuscript.

Funding: This research received no external funding.

Institutional Review Board Statement: Not applicable.

Informed Consent Statement: Not applicable.

Data Availability Statement: No new data were created or analysed in this study. Data sharing is not applicable to this article.

Conflicts of Interest: The authors declare no conflict of interest.

References

1. Le, C.; Strong, E.B.; Luu, Q. Management of anterior skull base cerebrospinal fluid leaks. *J. Neurol. Surg. B Skull Base* **2016**, *77*, 404–411. [CrossRef]
2. Umana, G.E.; Pucci, R.; Palmisciano, P.; Cassoni, A.; Ricciardi, L.; Tomasi, S.O.; Strigari, L.; Scalia, G.; Velentini, V. Cerebrospinal fluid leaks after anterior skull base trauma: A systematic review of the literature. *World Neurosurg.* **2022**, *157*, 193–206.e2. [CrossRef]
3. Nelson, R.F.; Gantz, B.J.; Hansen, M.R. The rising incidence of spontaneous cerebrospinal fluid leaks in the United States and the association with obesity and obstructive sleep apnea. *Otol. Neurotol.* **2015**, *36*, 476–480. [CrossRef]
4. Bidot, S.; Levy, J.M.; Saindane, A.M.; Oyesiku, N.M.; Newman, N.J.; Biousse, V. Do most patients with a spontaneous cerebrospinal fluid leak have idiopathic intracranial hypertension? *J. Neuroophthalmol.* **2019**, *39*, 487–495. [CrossRef]
5. Markey, K.A.; Mollan, S.P.; Jensen, R.H.; Sinclair, A.J. Understanding idiopathic intracranial hypertension: Mechanisms, management, and future directions. *Lancet Neurol.* **2016**, *15*, 78–91. [CrossRef]
6. McCluskey, G.; Doherty-Allan, R.; McCarron, P.; Loftus, A.M.; McCarron, L.V.; Mulholland, D.; McVerry, F.; McCarron, M.O. Meta-analysis and systematic review of population-based epidemiological studies in idiopathic intracranial hypertension. *Eur. J. Neurol.* **2018**, *25*, 1218–1227. [CrossRef]
7. Alromaih, S.R. Pathophysiology of skull base defects and cerebrospinal fluid leak. *Saudi J. Otorhinolaryngol. Head Neck Surg.* **2021**, *23*, 91–94. [CrossRef]
8. Prosser, J.D.; Vender, J.R.; Solares, C.A. Traumatic cerebrospinal fluid leaks. *Otolaryngol. Clin. N Am.* **2011**, *44*, 857–873. [CrossRef]
9. Zapalac, J.S.; Marple, B.F.; Schwade, N.D. Skull base cerebrospinal fluid fistulas: A comprehensive diagnostic algorithm. *Otolaryngol. Head Neck Surg.* **2002**, *126*, 669–676. [CrossRef]
10. Georgalas, C.; Oostra, A.; Ahmed, S.; Castelnuovo, P.; Dallan, I.; van Furth, W.; Harvey, R.J.; Herman, P.; Kombogiorgas, D.; Locatelli, D.; et al. International consensus statement: Spontaneous cerebrospinal fluid rhinorrhea. *Int. Forum Allergy Rhinol.* **2021**, *11*, 794–803. [CrossRef]
11. Mollan, S.P.; Ali, F.; Hassan-Smith, G.; Botfield, H.; Friedman, D.I.; Sinclair, A.J. Evolving evidence in adult idiopathic intracranial hypertension: Pathophysiology and management. *J. Neurol. Neurosurg. Psychiatry* **2016**, *87*, 982–992. [CrossRef] [PubMed]
12. Mollan, S.P.; Davies, B.; Silver, N.C.; Shaw, S.; Mallucci, C.L.; Wakerley, B.R.; Krishnan, A.; Chavda, S.V.; Ramalingam, S.; Edwards, J.; et al. Idiopathic intracranial hypertension: Consensus guidelines on management. *J. Neurol. Neurosurg. Psychiatry* **2018**, *89*, 1088–1100. [CrossRef]
13. de Macedo Filho, L.; Machado, C.C.P.; Mendes, G.B.B.; Santana, L.M.F.; Ruella, M.E.; Grewal, S.; Chaichana, K.L.; Hinojosa, A.Q.; Fermo, O.; Almeida, J.P. Spontaneous rhinorrhea and idiopathic intracranial hypertension: A complex and challenging association. *Neurol. Neurochir. Pol.* **2024**, *58*, 31–37. [CrossRef]
14. Phang, S.Y.; Whitehouse, K.; Lee, L.; Khalil, H.; McArdle, P.; Whitfield, P.C. Management of CSF leak in base of skull fractures in adults. *Br. J. Neurosurg.* **2016**, *30*, 596–604. [CrossRef] [PubMed]
15. Wang, E.W.; Zanation, A.M.; Gardner, P.A.; Schwartz, T.H.; Eloy, J.A.; Adappa, N.D.; Bettag, M.; Bleier, B.S.; Cappabianca, P.; Carrau, R.L. ICAR: Endoscopic skull-base surgery. *Int. Forum Allergy Rhinol.* **2019**, *9*, S145–S365. [CrossRef] [PubMed]
16. Mostafa, B.E.; Khafagi, A. Combined HRCT and MRI in the detection of CSF rhinorrhea. *Skull Base* **2004**, *14*, 157–162. [CrossRef]
17. Jolly, K.; Gupta, K.K.; Banota, A.; Ahmed, S.K. The effectiveness and safety of intrathecal fluorescein in the management of cerebrospinal fluid leaks. *Am. J. Rhinol. Allergy* **2021**, *35*, 879–884. [CrossRef]
18. Butros, S.R.; Goncalves, L.F.; Thompson, D.; Agarwal, A.; Lee, H.K. Imaging features of idiopathic intracranial hypertension, including a new finding: Widening of the foramen ovale. *Acta Radiol.* **2012**, *53*, 682–688. [CrossRef]
19. Morris, P.P.; Black, D.F.; Port, J.; Campeau, N. Transverse sinus stenosis is the most sensitive MR imaging correlate of idiopathic intracranial hypertension. *Am. J. Neuroradiol.* **2017**, *38*, 471–477. [CrossRef]

20. Friedman, D.I.; Liu, G.T.; Digre, K.B. Revised diagnostic criteria for the pseudotumor cerebri syndrome in adults and children. *Neurology* **2013**, *81*, 1159–1165. [CrossRef]
21. Rimmer, J.; Belk, C.; Lund, V.J.; Swift, A.; White, P. Immunisations and antibiotics in patients with anterior skull base cerebrospinal fluid leaks. *J. Laryngol. Otol.* **2014**, *128*, 626–629. [CrossRef] [PubMed]
22. Gonen, L.; Monteiro, E.; Klironomos, G.; Alghonaim, Y.; Vescan, A.; Zadeh, G.; Gentili, F. Endoscopic endonasal repair of spontaneous and traumatic cerebrospinal fluid rhinorrhea: A review and local experience. *Neurosurg. Clin. N. Am.* **2015**, *26*, 333–348. [CrossRef] [PubMed]
23. Ratilal, B.O.; Costa, J.; Pappamikail, L.; Sampaio, C. Antibiotic prophylaxis for preventing meningitis in patients with basilar skull fractures. *Cochrane Database Syst. Rev.* **2015**, *2015*, CD004884. [CrossRef] [PubMed]
24. Wigand, M.E. Transnasal ethmoidectomy under endoscopical control. *Rhinology* **1981**, *19*, 7–15.
25. Psaltis, A.J.; Schlosser, R.J.; Banks, C.A.; Yawn, J.; Soler, Z.M. A systematic review of the endoscopic repair of cerebrospinal fluid leaks. *Otolaryngol. Head Neck Surg.* **2012**, *147*, 196–203. [CrossRef]
26. Komotar, R.J.; Starke, R.M.; Raper, D.M.S.; Anand, V.K.; Schwartz, T.H. Endoscopic endonasal versus open repair of anterior skull base CSF leak, meningocele, and encephalocele: A systematic review of outcomes. *J. Neurol. Surg. A Cent. Eur. Neurosurg.* **2013**, *74*, 239–250. [CrossRef]
27. Soneru, C.P.; Riley, C.A.; Tabaee, A.; Kacker, A.; Anand, V.K.; Schwartz, T.H. The challenge of skull base closure: Methods for reducing postoperative cerebrospinal fluid leak. *World Neurosurg.* **2019**, *124*, 502–512. [CrossRef]
28. Hadad, G.; Bassagasteguy, L.; Carrau, R.L.; Mataza, J.C.; Kassam, A.; Snyderman, C.H.; Mintz, A. A novel reconstructive technique after endoscopic expanded endonasal approaches: Vascular pedicle nasoseptal flap. *Laryngoscope* **2006**, *116*, 1882–1886. [CrossRef]
29. Oakley, G.M.; Orlandi, R.R.; Woodworth, B.A.; Batra, P.S.; Alt, J.A. Management of cerebrospinal fluid rhinorrhea: An evidence-based review with recommendations. *Int. Forum Allergy Rhinol.* **2016**, *6*, 17–24. [CrossRef]
30. Wormald, P.J.; McDonogh, M. 'Bath-plug' technique for the endoscopic management of cerebrospinal fluid leaks. *J. Laryngol. Otol.* **1997**, *111*, 1042–1046. [CrossRef]
31. Fiore, G.; Bertani, G.A.; Carrabba, G.G.; Guastella, C.; Marfia, G.; Tariciotti, L.; Gribaudi, G.L.; Mantovani, G.; Cristofori, A.D.; Locatelli, M. The "Parachute" technique for the endoscopic repair of high-flow anterior skull-base CSF leaks. *World Neurosurg.* **2021**, *151*, e880–e887. [CrossRef] [PubMed]
32. Leng, L.Z.; Brown, S.; Anand, V.K.; Schwartz, T.H. "Gasket-Seal" watertight closure in minimal-access endoscopic cranial base surgery. *Neurosurgery* **2008**, *62*, ONSE342–ONSE343. [CrossRef] [PubMed]
33. Hosemann, W.; Goede, U.; Sauer, M. Wound healing of mucosal autografts for frontal cerebrospinal fluid leaks—Clinical and experimental investigations. *Rhinology* **1999**, *37*, 108–112. [PubMed]
34. Ajlan, A.; Basindwah, S.; Hawsawi, A.; Omar, M.A.; Alsaleh, S.; Alrasheed, A.; Alroqi, A.; Alqurashi, A. Early postoperative computed tomography scan air distribution predicts postoperative CSF leak in endoscopic skull base surgery. *World Neurosurg.* **2023**, *172*, e605–e610. [CrossRef]
35. Souza, M.N.P.; Costa, B.d.A.L.; Santos, F.R.D.R.; Fortini, I. Update on idiopathic intracranial hypertension management. *Arq. Neuro-Psiquiatr.* **2022**, *80*, 227–231. [CrossRef]
36. Abbott, S.; Chan, F.; Tahrani, A.A.; Wong, S.H.; Campbell, F.E.J.; Parmar, C.; Pournaras, D.J.; Denton, A.; Sinclair, A.J.; Mollan, S.P. Weight management interventions for adults with idiopathic intracranial hypertension. *Neurology* **2023**, *101*, e2138–e2150. [CrossRef]
37. Piper, R.J.; Kalyvas, A.V.; Young, A.M.H.; Hughes, M.A.; Jamjoom, A.A.B.; Fouyas, I.P. Interventions for idiopathic intracranial hypertension. *Cochrane Database Syst. Rev.* **2015**, *2015*, CD003434. [CrossRef]
38. Zhou, C.; Zhou, Y.; Liu, L.; Jiang, H.; Wei, H.; Zhou, C.; Ji, X. Progress and recognition of idiopathic intracranial hypertension: A narrative review. *CNS Neurosci. Ther.* **2024**, *30*, e14895. [CrossRef]
39. Habenbacher, M.; Sebastnik, D.; Moser, U.; Adrianakis, A.; Kiss, P.; Alsukayt, M.; Pock, J.; Walla, K.; Maitz, E.; Tomazic, P.V. The value of beta trace protein in CSF-leakage detection confirmed by endoscopic fluorescein evaluation. *Rhinology* **2024**, *62*, 766–768. [CrossRef]
40. Riley, C.A.; Soneru, C.P.; Tabaee, A.; Kacker, A.; Anand, V.K.; Schwartz, T.H. Technological and ideological innovations in endoscopic skull base surgery. *World Neurosurg.* **2019**, *124*, 513–521. [CrossRef]

Journal of
Clinical Medicine

MDPI

Article

Impact of the COVID-19 Pandemic on the Treatment of Head and Neck Cancers

Max L. Lee [1], Andrey Finegersh [1,2] and Michelle M. Chen [1,2,3,*]

1 Department of Otolaryngology—Head and Neck Surgery, Stanford University School of Medicine, 801 Welch Road, Palo Alto, CA 94304, USA; maxlee12@stanford.edu (M.L.L.); afinegersh@stanford.edu (A.F.)
2 Department of Surgery, Palo Alto Veterans Administration, Palo Alto, CA 94304, USA
3 ValleyCare Pleasanton Cancer Center, Pleasanton, CA 94588, USA
* Correspondence: michelle.chen@stanford.edu; Tel.: +1-(650)-498-6000; Fax: +1-(650)-498-8659

Abstract: Background/Objectives: The COVID-19 pandemic led to unprecedented disruptions to cancer care, including the care of head and neck cancer. Given the necessity of timely treatment for mucosal cancers, it is important to understand how the pandemic affected the diagnosis, presentation, and treatment of mucosal head and neck cancer. **Methods**: The National Cancer Database was queried for patients with primary head and neck mucosal cancer. The number of annual diagnoses and the number of days between diagnosis and the start and end of any treatment were tracked over time from 2004 to 2020. Chi-square tests were used to compare differences in patient clinical and demographic characteristics in 2019 and 2020 to provide the most direct comparison. Multivariable linear regression and logic regression analyses were also used to compare three treatment quality measures between 2019 and 2020: number of days between diagnosis and start of treatment, number of days between surgery and start of postoperative radiation, and number of days between surgery and end of radiation. **Results**: The number of mucosal cancer diagnoses decreased (9.1%) during the early stages of the pandemic, with a larger decrease (12.4%) among patients receiving surgery. On multivariable analysis comparing 2020 to 2019, time to treatment was shorter (2.3 days; 95% CI, 1.69 to 2.85 days), and time from surgery to start of postoperative radiation was less likely to be delayed (OR, 0.91 of radiation greater than 42 days from surgery; 95% CI, 0.85 to 0.97). However, patients who were black, female, older, or uninsured were more likely to experience treatment delays. **Conclusions**: Overall, there were no treatment delays for patients with surgical head cancer and patients with neck cancer during the COVID-19 pandemic. However, vulnerable groups, such as patients who were black, female, older, and uninsured, were at higher risk of experiencing treatment delays.

Keywords: squamous cell carcinoma of head and neck; COVID-19; pandemic; outcomes; disparities; otolaryngology

1. Introduction

The impact of the early COVID-19 pandemic on in-person healthcare utilization has been well-documented [1–3], with decreases in emergency department utilization [1,4,5], inpatient hospital admissions [5,6], and cancer diagnoses [7,8]. Patients with cancer were particularly vulnerable to disruptions caused by the COVID-19 pandemic, given the importance of timely treatment [9] and increased risk of COVID-19-related complications and mortality [10,11]. Years later, research suggests patients were also at higher risk of developing longer-term complications, particularly long COVID-19, which include symptoms such as fatigue, cough, myalgias, and gastrointestinal symptoms [12].

In 2020, the pandemic led to significant delays in cancer screening, diagnosis, and treatment for many types of cancer [7,13]. Timely treatment is particularly important in patients with head and neck cancer (HNC) given there is a Commission on Cancer (CoC) quality metric associated with the time from surgery to initiation of radiation. Mucosal cancers in particular are associated with devastating complications, such as fatal bleeding, which require rigorous postoperative monitoring as well as multidisciplinary management, both of which were likely adversely affected by the COVID-19 pandemic [14]. Prior institutional studies have demonstrated that the number of patients evaluated and diagnosed with HNC in 2020 decreased, relative to 2019 [15–18]. There have been significant discrepancies in prior studies, where some did not find significant differences in patient characteristics, time to diagnosis, or time to treatment between patients diagnosed during the pandemic versus pre-pandemic [15,16], while other studies found significant delays [18]. Patients diagnosed with HNC in 2020 were also more likely to present with more advanced disease as measured by factors including tumor size, nodal disease, and staging [15,16,18–20].

Studies of the impact of the early COVID-19 pandemic on HNC treatment have primarily been conducted at individual academic centers over the span of a few months, resulting in small sample sizes with limited generalizability [15–18]. Moreover, none of these studies have evaluated the impact of the pandemic on the time from surgery to the initiation of radiation therapy. The goal of our study was to characterize differences in treatment times and clinical and demographic characteristics of patients diagnosed with HNC during the COVID-19 pandemic in the United States on a larger scale.

2. Methods

2.1. Data Source

The database used for this study was the National Cancer Database (NCDB), which captures over 70% of incident cases of cancer in the United States. This study was approved by the Institutional Review Board (IRB) of Stanford University School of Medicine, and the informed consent requirement was waived since the study was performed using a deidentified dataset.

2.2. Study Population and Covariates

2.2.1. Classification of Mucosal Head and Neck Cancer

We identified patients from the NCDB from 2004 to 2020 who were diagnosed with primary HNC based on the International Classification of Diseases for Oncology, 3rd Edition (ICD-O3) diagnosis codes, which have remained unchanged throughout the time period of the study. Mucosal cancer subsites were divided into oral cavity, oropharynx (C019, C024, C051, C052, C090, C091, C098–C109, C140, and C142), hypopharynx (C129–C132, C138, and C139), and larynx (C320–C323, C328, and C329).

2.2.2. Demographic and Clinical Variables

Patient demographic variables and clinical variables included age, sex, race, education, household income, distance from the treatment facility, insurance status, Charlson–Deyo score, tumor subsite, facility region, urban-rural classification, pathologic staging, and readmission. The percentage of adults without a high school education and median household income, by ZIP code of the patient's residence, were stratified by quartiles of the US population and based on the US Census 2000. The 2010 and 2020 US Census data were not available in the NCDB dataset. Insurance status was classified into the following groups: Medicaid, Medicare, private insurance or managed care, other government, and uninsured or unknown. Rural–urban classification was grouped into metro, urban, rural, and not available or unknown. Facility regions were based on the US Census Bureau classifications [21].

2.2.3. Cancer Staging, Treatment, and Clinical Outcomes

Clinical and pathologic TNM staging was classified according to the *8th Edition American Joint Committee on Cancer Staging Manual* (AJCC, Chicago, IL, USA) from 2018 to 2020 and according to the *Traditional AJCC Staging Manual* from 2004 to 2017 [22]. Readmission was categorized as an unplanned readmission within 30 days. Charlson–Deyo score was divided into two groups: scores of 0–1 and scores of 2–3.

Patients were also classified based on the types and combinations of treatment they received—surgery, radiation, and chemotherapy. Groups included surgery alone, surgery and adjuvant radiation, surgery and adjuvant chemoradiation, radiation alone, concurrent chemoradiation, or unknown. For example, a patient who received surgery but whose radiation and chemotherapy status was unknown was placed in the "unknown" group.

2.3. Statistical Analyses

2.3.1. Descriptive Statistics

Inclusion criteria for descriptive statistics were all adult patients diagnosed with HNC between 2004 and 2020. The average annual percentage change (AAPC) and corresponding 95% confidence interval of the trend line were calculated between the years of 2004 and 2019 to track changes in mucosal cancer diagnoses, the number of days between surgery and start of any treatment, and the number of days between surgery and start of radiation over time. Additionally, 95% confidence intervals were calculated based on the annual percent change (APC) of these variables between 2004 and 2019 to give point estimates to determine whether the changes between 2019 and 2020 were anomalous. We opted for this method of showing changes over time because the NCDB only updates their statistics annually, making a more rigorous time-series analysis difficult to perform given the small number of data points. Chi-square tests were used to compare differences in patient demographic and clinical characteristics across years. To provide the most direct year-to-year analysis, we compared patients from 2019 to 2020.

2.3.2. Regression Analyses

The regression analyses were limited to only patients diagnosed with HNC between 2019 and 2020 in order to compare 2020 directly to 2019. There were three quality metrics that we compared between 2019 and 2020 using multivariable regression analysis: number of days between diagnosis and start of treatment, number of days between surgery and start of radiation, and number of days between surgery and end of radiation. These quality measures have been shown to be associated with survival and outcomes in head and neck cancer [23–25].

To determine the relationship between the year and the number of days between diagnosis and start of treatment, we used multivariable linear regression, controlling for demographic and clinical characteristics. To determine the relationship between year and the number of days between surgery and the start of radiation, we used multivariable logistic regression, setting the cutoff for the binary variable at 42 days and controlling for demographic and clinical characteristics. This cutoff was determined using the National Comprehensive Cancer Network (NCCN) guidelines, which recommend that postoperative radiotherapy (PORT) for HNC is started within 6 weeks, or 42 days, of surgery [26,27]. To determine the relationship between year and the number of days between surgery and the end of radiation, we also used multivariable logistic regression, setting the cutoff for the binary variable at 100 days. This was determined based on evidence suggesting that the optimal treatment package time, time between surgery and completion of radiation, was less than 100 days [28]. All analysis was performed using STATA (Version 15.1, StataCorp LLC, College Station, TX, USA).

3. Results

3.1. Changes in HNC Diagnoses and Treatment over Time

Our cohort included 475,405 adult patients with HNC between 2004 and 2020. The AAPC in the number of HNC diagnosed between 2004 and 2019 was 4.2% (95% CI, 3.6% to 4.7%). However, between 2019 and 2020, the annual percent change (APC) in the number of HNC diagnoses was −9.1% (95% CI, 2.0% to 6.3%), representing a large drop in diagnoses from 37,005 to 33,652 that was significantly lower than what would be expected based on prior trends. For all of our quality metrics, we saw a similar pattern of a positive or flat trend from 2004 to 2019 followed by an abrupt negative trend between 2019 and 2020. Between 2004 and 2019, the AAPC in the number of days between diagnosis and start of treatment was 1.7% (95% CI, 0.8% to 2.6%). However, from 2019 to 2020, the APC was −4.9% (95% CI, −1.9% to 5.3%), which was lower than what would be expected based on prior trends (Figure 1A). For our time to radiation metrics, from 2004 to 2019, the AAPC in the number of days between surgery and start of radiation was flat at 0.72% (95% CI, −0.4% to 1.8%), and the APC from 2019 to 2020 was −3.3% (95% CI, −3.7% to 5.1%), which was not statistically significant (Figure 1A). Similarly, the AAPC for the number of days between surgery and completion of radiation from 2004 to 2019 was also flat at <0.1% (95% CI, −0.9% to 0.8%), and the APC between 2019 and 2020 was −2.2% (95% CI, −3.4% to 3.3%).

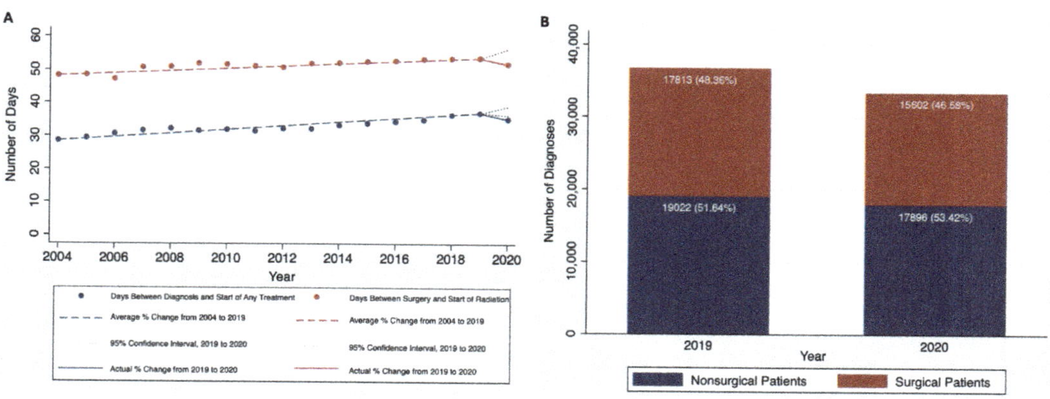

Figure 1. (**A**) Time to treatment quality metrics over time, 2004 to 2020, and (**B**) Surgical versus Nonsurgical patients (2019 and 2020).

We also divided the cohort into surgical and nonsurgical patients and compared the AAPC in the number of diagnoses from 2004 to 2020. From 2004 to 2019, the AAPC in the number of diagnoses for the surgical group was 4.14% (95% CI, 2.96% to 5.32%), which was similar to the nonsurgical group at 4.19% (95% CI, 3.69% to 4.70%). However, from 2019 to 2020, the drop in the number of diagnoses was more in the surgical group (−12.41%, 95% CI of −0.1% to 8.8%) than the nonsurgical group (−5.92%, 95% CI of 2.2% to 6.2%) (Figure 1B) and was larger in both cases than what would be expected based on prior trends.

3.2. Demographic and Clinical Characteristics of Patients with HNC in 2019 and 2020

We compared patient characteristics between these two years for our primary analysis. The total cohort size for patients with HNC in 2019 and 2020 was 70,657 patients. Chi-square tests were used to compare patient demographic and clinical characteristics between patients diagnosed with HNC in 2019 versus 2020. Since the process of clinical and pathologic staging of cancers changed in 2018 with the new AJCC staging manual, patients in 2019 and 2020 were diagnosed using the same criteria. There were no clinically significant differences in patient demographic or clinical characteristics between patients diagnosed in 2019 versus 2020, although patients in 2020 were very slightly more likely to present with higher clinical T staging (33.32% cT3 and cT4 versus 30.74% cT3 and cT4) and pathologic T staging of disease (13.96% pT3 and pT4 versus 13.17% pT3 and pT4) versus patients in 2019 (Table 1). However, compared to patients diagnosed with HNC in 2019, patients diagnosed with HNC in 2020 were slightly more likely to be node positive at diagnosis (46.75% vs. 45.27%, $p < 0.001$) but did not have a difference in the rate of metastatic disease (3.51% vs. 3.29%, $p = 0.250$). It is important to note that a number of variables, particularly surgical margins and variables related to the pathologic staging of cancer, had a high proportion of patients classified as other or unknown. The reason there are more unknowns for pathologic staging and surgical margins is due to the fact that primary treatment for head and neck cancer can be definitive chemoradiation, definitive radiation, or surgery. For non-surgical patients, there would be no pathologic staging or surgical margins. In terms of clinical staging variables, there is a moderate proportion of unknown variables (11–21%), which is not unexpected. We know that there are patients with head and neck cancer of unknown primaries who have p16+/human-papillomavirus-associated disease, and often their primary is not identified, but are classified as patients with oropharyngeal cancer. This is a real-world study, and, as such, not all patients achieved complete nodal and distant metastatic staging, and those variables may be unknown.

Table 1. Demographic and clinical characteristics, 2019 versus 2020.

	2019 N (%)	2020 N (%)	*p*-Value
Age (in years)			
≤50	3629 (9.81)	3311 (9.84)	$p = 0.059$
51–60	9799 (26.48)	8619 (25.61)	
61–70	12,853 (34.73)	11,776 (34.99)	
70+	10,724 (28.98)	9946 (29.56)	
Sex			
Male	27,413 (74.08)	24,814 (73.74)	$p = 0.233$
Female	9590 (2592)	8838 (26.26)	
Race			
White	31,748 (85.79)	28,856 (85.75)	$p = 0.068$
Black	3443 (9.30)	3035 (9.02)	
Other	1814 (4.90)	1761 (5.23)	

Table 1. *Cont.*

	2019 N (%)	2020 N (%)	*p*-Value
Proportion of adults from patient's ZIP code not graduating high school, 2000 US Census data			
29.0%	5409 (17.66)	4773 (17.22)	$p = 0.097$
20% to 28.9%	7514 (24.54)	6876 (24.80)	
14% to 19.9%	7315 (23.89)	6818 (24.60)	
Less than 14%	10,387 (33.92)	9254 (33.38)	
Median household income for patient's ZIP code, 2000 US Census data			
<USD 30,000	4421 (14.43)	3873 (13.97)	$p = 0.075$
USD 30,000–USD 34,999	5695 (18.59)	5327 (19.21)	
USD 35,000–USD 45,999	8692 (28.38)	7969 (28.74)	
USD 46,000+	11,823 (38.60)	10,555 (38.07)	
Distance from facility (miles)			
≤10	12,762 (34.66)	11,607 (34.65)	$p = 0.639$
11 to 20	6420 (17.44)	5937 (17.72)	
21 to 50	7008 (19.03)	6293 (18.78)	
51 to 100	3087 (8.38)	2872 (8.57)	
>100	7545 (20.49)	6792 (20.27)	
Insurance status			
Uninsured	1559 (4.32)	1367 (4.06)	$p = 0.302$
Private Insurance/Managed Care	12,898 (34.85)	11,656 (34.64)	
Medicaid	3951 (10.68)	3675 (10.92)	
Medicare	17,456 (47.17)	15,982 (47.49)	
Other	1101 (2.98)	972 (2.89)	
Charlson–Deyo score			
0–1	33,034 (89.27)	29,904 (88.86)	$p = 0.084$
2–3	3971 (10.73)	3748 (11.14)	
Primary site			
Oral Cavity	11,250 (30.40)	10,246 (30.45)	$p = 0.916$
Oropharynx	15,625 (42.22)	14,260 (42.37)	
Hypopharynx	1607 (4.34)	1432 (4.26)	
Larynx	8523 (23.03)	7714 (22.92)	
Readmission			
No unplanned readmission	35,990 (97.26)	32,811 (97.50)	**$p < 0.001$ ***
Unplanned readmission	628 (1.70)	583 (1.73)	
Unknown	387 (1.05)	258 (.77)	
Surgical margins			
Negative	13,569 (36.67)	11,954 (35.52)	**$p = 0.001$**
Positive	2550 (6.89)	2241 (6.66)	
Unknown	20,886 (56.44)	19,457 (57.82)	

Table 1. *Cont.*

	2019 N (%)	2020 N (%)	*p*-Value
Facility region			
East	7189 (19.43)	6208 (18.45)	**$p = 0.001$**
South	9093 (24.57)	8518 (25.31)	
Midwest	14,582 (39.41)	13,429 (39.91)	
West	5371 (14.51)	4869 (14.47)	
Unknown	770 (2.08)	628 (1.87)	
Rural–urban			
Metro	28,899 (78.09)	26,417 (78.50)	**$p < 0.001$**
Urban	6116 (16.53)	5666 (16.84)	
Rural	792 (2.14)	678 (2.01)	
Unknown	1198 (3.24)	891 (2.65)	
Treatment			
Surgery Only	9614 (25.98)	8306 (24.68)	**$p < 0.001$**
Surgery and Radiation	4147 (11.21)	3811 (11.32)	
Surgery and Chemoradiation	3490 (9.43)	2924 (8.69)	
Radiation Only	4496 (12.15)	4415 (12.23)	
Chemoradiation Only	10,594 (28.63)	9862 (29.31)	
One or More Factors Unknown	4664 (12.60)	4634 (13.77)	
Pathologic T stage			
T1	5521 (14.92)	4475 (13.30)	**$p < 0.001$**
T2	3738 (10.10)	3399 (10.10	
T3	1994 (5.39)	1867 (5.55)	
T4	2878 (7.78)	2828 (8.41)	
Other/Unknown	22,873 (61.81)	21,071 (62.64)	
Pathologic N stage			
N0	5340 (14.43)	4881 (14.50)	$p = 0.839$
N+	5923 (16.01)	5334 (15.85)	
Other/Unknown	25,742 (69.56)	23,437 (69.65)	
Pathologic M stage			
M0	16,185 (43.74)	14,203 (42.21)	**$p < 0.001$**
M+	434 (1.17)	406 (1.21)	
Other/Unknown	20,386 (55.09)	19,043 (56.59)	
Clinical T stage			
T1	7968 (23.25)	6800 (21.97)	**$p < 0.001$**
T2	8576 (25.02)	7642 (24.69)	
T3	5381 (15.70)	5262 (17.00)	
T4	5157 (15.04)	5051 (16.32)	
Other/Unknown	7196 (20.99)	6193 (20.01)	
Clinical N stage			
N0	15,108 (40.83)	13,255 (39.39)	**$p < 0.001$**
N+	16,752 (45.27)	15,733 (46.75)	
Other/Unknown	5145 (13.90)	4664 (13.86)	
Clinical M stage			
M0	31,555 (85.27)	28,662 (85.17)	$p = 0.250$
M+	1216 (3.29)	1180 (3.51)	
Other/Unknown	4234 (11.44)	3810 (11.32)	

* *p*-values < 0.05 are shown in bold font.

3.3. Changes in Treatment Time Metrics from 2019 to 2020

After adjusting for clinical and socioeconomic characteristics, patients diagnosed in 2020 were found to have a shorter interval between diagnosis and start of treatment than those diagnosed in 2019 (mean difference = −2.27 days; 95% CI, −2.85 to −1.69 days). Other covariates that had a statistically significant association included race and distance from treatment facility. Black patients had to wait longer for treatment when compared to white patients (mean difference = 3.64 days; 95% CI, 2.51 to 4.77). Additionally, patients who lived further from the treatment facility had to wait longer for treatment, with patients who lived over 100 miles from the treatment facility waiting over a week longer (mean difference = 7.75 days; 95% CI, 6.31 to 9.18) than patients who lived 10 miles or fewer from the treatment facility (Table 2).

Table 2. Multivariable linear regression analysis of time from surgery to the initiation of treatment, 2019 vs. 2020.

Independent Variable	Mean Difference (Days)	CI	p-Value
Year 2020 (ref: Year 2019)	−2.27	−2.85 to −1.69	**<0.001 ***
Age, y (ref: ≤50 y)			
51–60 y	1.99	0.80 to 3.18	**0.001**
61–70 y	1.98	0.78 to 3.18	**0.001**
71 y or older	0.31	−1.01 to 1.64	0.646
Sex (ref: Male)	1.39	0.68 to 2.11	**<0.001**
Race (ref: White)			
Black	3.64	2.51 to 4.77	**<0.001**
Other	0.84	−0.63 to 2.31	0.265
Proportion of adults from patient's ZIP code not graduating high school, 2000 US Census data (ref: 29.0%+)			
20% to 28.9%	−0.35	−1.43 to 0.72	0.518
14% to 19.9%	−0.27	−1.45 to 0.92	0.658
Less than 14%	−1.49	−2.78 to −0.21	**0.023**
Median household income for patient's ZIP code, 2000 US Census data (ref: <USD 30,000)			
USD 30,000–USD 34,999	−1.08	−2.23 to 0.61	0.064
USD 35,000–USD 45,999	−0.86	−2.05 to 0.33	0.158
USD 46,000+	−2.03	−3.35 to −0.70	**0.003**
Distance from treatment facility (ref: 0–10 miles away from treatment facility)			
11–20 miles	1.12	−0.33 to 1.91	**0.005**
21–50 miles	2.13	1.30 to 2.96	**<0.001**
51–100 miles	3.66	2.49 to 4.83	**<0.001**
>100 miles	7.75	6.31 to 9.18	**<0.001**
Insurance status (ref: uninsured or unknown)			
Private Insurance or Managed Care	−5.81	−7.57 to −4.05	**<0.001**
Medicaid	1.99	−0.02 to 4.00	0.053
Medicare	−3.47	−5.24 to −1.69	**<0.001**
Other Government	0.20	−2.25 to 2.66	0.871

Table 2. *Cont.*

Independent Variable	Mean Difference (Days)	CI	p-Value
Charlson–Deyo score of 2 or 3 (ref: score of 0 or 1)	0.31	−0.65 to 1.27	0.533
Tumor site (ref: oral)			
Oropharynx	−10.31	−11.24 to −9.37	**<0.001**
Hypopharynx	−10.05	−11.57 to −8.53	**<0.001**
Larynx	−9.46	−10.43 to −8.49	**<0.001**
Facility region (ref: east)			
South	−2.85	−3.71 to −1.99	**<0.001**
Midwest	0.02	−0.83 to 0.87	0.957
West	1.39	0.31 to 2.48	**0.012**
Unknown	−4.54	−6.73 to −2.34	**<0.001**
Rural/urban (ref: metro)			
Urban	−0.13	−1.08 to 0.83	0.793
Rural	−4.09	−5.96 to −2.22	**<0.001**
Not available/Unknown	−4.52	−6.21 to −2.83	**<0.001**
Clinical T stage (ref: T1)			
T2	4.88	4.05 to 5.72	**<0.001**
T3	7.84	6.84 to 8.84	**<0.001**
T4	9.43	8.35 to 10.52	**<0.001**
Other/Unknown	−0.82	−1.84 to 0.21	0.118
Clinical N stage (ref: N0)			
N+	−2.99	−3.82 to −2.17	**<0.001**
Other/Unknown	−2.81	−4.72 to −0.91	**0.004**
Clinical M stage (ref: M0)			
M+	−2.30	−4.21 to −0.39	**0.018**
Other/Unknown	−5.29	4.18 to 8.68	**<0.001**
Treatment (ref: surgery only)			
Surgery and Adjuvant Radiation	−3.09	−4.09 to −2.08	**<0.001**
Surgery and Adjuvant Chemoradiation	−2.75	−3.90 to −1.60	**<0.001**
Radiation only	16.86	15.70 to 18.02	**<0.001**
Definitive Chemoradiation	10.29	9.22 to 11.37	**<0.001**
Unknown	11.18	9.34 to 13.01	**<0.001**

CI: 95% confidence interval; * Significant p-values (<0.05) are shown in bold font.

Patients with HNC in 2020 were less likely than patients in 2019 to have the time between surgery and the start of radiation be greater than 42 days (OR, 0.91; 95% CI, 0.85 to 0.97) and were less likely to have the time between surgery and the end of radiation be greater than 100 days (OR, 0.88; 95% CI, 0.83 to 0.93). Older patients were more likely to have a delay between surgery and the start of radiation. Female patients were more likely to have a delay between surgery and the start of radiation (OR: 1.18; 95% CI, 1.09 to 1.28) and were more likely to have a delay between surgery and the end of radiation (OR: 1.10; 95% CI, 1.03 to 1.18) relative to male patients. Compared with white patients, black patients were more likely to have a delay between surgery and the start of radiation (OR: 1.15; 95% CI, 1.01 to 1.32). Finally, patients who had either private insurance or managed care plans were less likely to have a delay between surgery and the start of radiation (OR: 0.73; 95% CI, 0.61 to 0.87) and a delay between surgery and the end of radiation (OR = 0.77; 95% CI, 0.66 to 0.89) relative to patients who were uninsured or whose insurance status was unknown (Table 3). Only clinical staging was used in this analysis since non-surgical patients did not have pathologic staging.

Table 3. Multivariable logistic regression of time from surgery to the start and end of radiation, 2019 vs. 2020.

	Time from Surgery to Start of Radiation			Time from Surgery to End of Radiation		
Independent Variable	**Odds Ratio**	**95% Confidence Interval**	***p*-Value**	**Odds Ratio**	**95% Confidence Interval**	***p*-Value**
Year 2020 (ref: Year 2019)	0.91	0.85 to 0.97	**0.004** *	0.88	0.83 to 0.93	**<0.001** *
Age, y (ref: ≤50 y)						
51–60 y	1.16	1.03 to 1.30	**0.011**	1.23	1.11 to 1.36	**<0.001**
61–70 y	1.26	1.12 to 1.42	**0.014**	1.35	1.22 to 1.50	**<0.001**
71 y or older	1.63	1.42 to 1.87	**<0.001**	1.71	1.52 to 1.92	**<0.001**
Sex (ref: Male)	1.18	1.09 to 1.28	**<0.001**	1.10	1.03 to 1.18	**0.003**
Race (ref: White)						
Black	1.15	1.01 to 1.32	**0.039**	1.08	0.96 to 1.21	0.205
Other	0.97	0.84 to 1.12	0.689	0.96	0.85 to 1.08	0.474
Proportion of adults from patient's ZIP code not graduating high school, 2000 US Census Data (ref: 29.0%+)						
20% to 28.9%	1.02	0.91 to 1.15	0.720	1.01	0.91 to 1.11	0.904
14% to 19.9%	0.93	0.82 to 1.06	0.271	0.98	0.88 to 1.09	0.724
Less than 14%	0.90	0.79 to 1.03	0.122	0.94	0.84 to 1.05	0.269
Median household income for patient's ZIP code, 2000 US Census data (ref: <USD 30,000)						
USD 30,000–USD 34,999	0.86	0.76 to 0.98	**0.028**	0.85	0.76 to 0.95	**0.005**
USD 35,000–USD 45,999	0.87	0.76 to 0.99	**0.038**	0.81	0.72 to 0.91	**<0.001**
USD 46,000+	0.84	0.72 to 0.97	**0.019**	0.73	0.64 to 0.83	**<0.001**
Distance from treatment facility (ref: 0–10 miles)						
11–20 miles	0.98	0.90 to 1.07	0.684	1.02	0.94 to 1.10	0.627
21–50 miles	1.25	1.14 to 1.38	**<0.001**	1.23	1.14 to 1.33	**<0.001**
51–100 miles	1.35	1.19 to 1.54	**<0.001**	1.41	1.26 to 1.57	**<0.001**
>100 miles	1.11	0.96 to 1.28	0.162	1.28	1.13 to 1.45	**<0.001**

Table 3. *Cont.*

	Time from Surgery to Start of Radiation			Time from Surgery to End of Radiation		
Independent Variable	**Odds Ratio**	**95% Confidence Interval**	***p*-Value**	**Odds Ratio**	**95% Confidence Interval**	***p*-Value**
Insurance status (ref: uninsured/unknown)						
Private Insurance or Managed Care	0.73	0.61 to 0.87	**<0.001**	0.77	0.66 to 0.89	**0.001**
Medicaid	1.25	1.02 to 1.54	**0.031**	1.27	1.07 to 1.51	**0.006**
Medicare	0.88	0.73 to 1.05	0.161	0.93	0.80 to 1.09	0.365
Other Government	1.02	0.78 to 1.34	0.869	1.07	0.85 to 1.34	0.581
Charlson–Deyo score of 2–3 (ref: score of 0–1)	1.17	1.04 to 1.31	**0.011**	1.18	1.07 to 1.31	**0.001**
Tumor site (ref: Oral Cavity)						
Oropharynx	0.47	0.43 to 0.51	**<0.001**	0.58	0.53 to 0.62	**<0.001**
Hypopharynx	0.69	0.54 to 0.88	**0.002**	0.86	0.70 to 1.05	0.150
Larynx	0.42	0.38 to 0.47	**<0.001**	0.55	0.50 to 0.60	**<0.001**
Readmission (ref: no unplanned readmission)						
Unplanned Readmission	1.33	1.05 to 1.68	**0.016**	1.31	1.08 to 1.59	**0.005**
Unknown	0.73	0.53 to 0.99	**0.042**	0.73	0.55 to 0.97	**0.033**
Facility region (ref: east)						
South	0.75	0.68 to 0.83	**<0.001**	0.89	0.82 to 0.97	**0.006**
Midwest	0.89	0.80 to 0.98	**0.017**	1.13	1.04 to 1.23	**0.004**
West	0.91	0.81 to 1.02	0.108	0.99	0.90 to 1.09	0.772
Unknown	0.84	0.67 to 1.06	0.144	0.99	0.82 to 1.20	0.908
Rural/urban (ref: metro)						
Urban	0.90	0.81 to 1.01	0.062	0.86	0.78 to 0.94	**0.001**
Rural	0.86	0.67 to 1.11	0.255	0.83	0.67 to 1.03	0.087
Not available/Unknown	1.07	0.88 to 1.30	0.477	0.99	0.84 to 1.17	0.931
Pathologic T stage (ref: stage 1)						
T2	0.78	0.71 to 0.86	**<0.001**	0.63	0.58 to 0.69	**<0.001**
T3	0.61	0.54 to 0.69	**<0.001**	0.43	0.39 to 0.48	**<0.001**
T4	0.65	0.58 to 0.74	**<0.001**	0.43	0.39 to 0.48	**<0.001**
Other/Unknown	3.89	3.30 to 4.58	**<0.001**	3.83	3.33 to 4.40	**<0.001**

Table 3. *Cont.*

Independent Variable	Time from Surgery to Start of Radiation			Time from Surgery to End of Radiation		
	Odds Ratio	95% Confidence Interval	*p*-Value	Odds Ratio	95% Confidence Interval	*p*-Value
Pathologic N stage (ref: N0)						
N+	0.41	0.37 to 0.45	**<0.001**	0.37	0.34 to 0.40	**<0.001**
Other/Unknown	0.75	0.67 to 0.84	**<0.001**	1.05	0.96 to 1.15	0.305
Pathologic M stage (ref: M0)						
M+	3.39	2.35 to 4.91	**<0.001**	4.29	3.14 to 5.87	**<0.001**
Other/Unknown	1.57	1.34 to 1.85	**<0.001**	1.31	1.15 to 1.50	**<0.001**

CI: 95% confidence interval; * Significant *p*-values (<0.05) are shown in bold font.

4. Discussion

We found a gradual increase in both HNC diagnoses and treatment times from 2004 to 2019, with abrupt decreases in both diagnoses and treatment times between 2019 and 2020 corresponding with the early stages of the COVID-19 pandemic. Patients in 2020 generally had similar demographic and clinical characteristics compared to patients in 2019 and were not more likely to present with distant metastases. After controlling for social and demographic characteristics, we found that patients treated during the pandemic were more likely to have shorter times from diagnosis to treatment as well as shorter times from the start of surgery to both the start and end of radiation treatment. As a whole, these differences were small, and our results suggest that hospitals were able to effectively prioritize multidisciplinary cancer treatment for HNC and avoid delays. Despite prioritization of cancer surgery during the pandemic, there were continued disparities, with race, gender, age, and insurance status being associated with delays in care.

From 2019 to 2020, there was a larger decrease in HNC surgical cases than in non-surgical cases. This is consistent with other studies that also found a more significant decrease in patients with surgical HNC [17,29,30]. An international study assessing 15 different cancer types, including HNC, cited lockdown measures and avoidance of COVID-19-related complications as potential reasons why surgeries were postponed, with health systems in lower-middle countries experiencing more significant delays [29]. However, another study conducted at an academic hospital found that while there were fewer cases performed, this was partially compensated for through a higher proportion of oncologic surgeries being performed, suggesting prioritization of serious cases [30]. Although the stage of disease at presentation was similar across the two years, there was a slightly higher proportion of cases that underwent non-surgical treatment (Table 1). Perhaps this was due to limitations in terms of capacity for surgery or treatment locally rather than at tertiary care centers.

Our study did not show any clinically meaningful difference in stage of presentation between 2019 and 2020. A large study performed in the Netherlands reported that there were no changes in tumor stage at presentation during the pandemic [31], while other smaller studies found an increase in patients presenting with higher stage HNC [15,16,19]. Of note, many of these studies are limited by small sample sizes and shorter time frames of only a few months, suggesting that there is likely wide geographical variation in delayed presentation of HNC [15,16,19]. As a whole, the data does not suggest that there was an obvious shift during the pandemic with decreased diagnosis of early-stage disease that may be found incidentally on imaging or during routine dental exams.

We found a consistent decrease in all three treatment time metrics during the pandemic. Prior United States studies have noted no increases or even slight decreases in time from diagnosis to treatment during the COVID-19 pandemic [15,32]. One reason for this is shorter waiting lists allowed patients to be treated in a more timely manner [31,33]. That being said, some international studies did demonstrate increased time from diagnosis to cancer treatment, citing COVID-19 lockdowns and risks concerning complications as potential contributing factors [29,34,35]. Facilities had a wide degree of variation in their ability to adapt cancer care to the pandemic. One study on breast cancer surgery in New York City public hospitals found that while the pandemic was not associated with delays to treatment overall, there was wide variation between treatment centers, with some hospitals successfully prioritizing cancer surgeries, leading to faster treatment times, while treatment at other hospitals ended up with significant delays [36].

Despite evidence suggesting that cancer centers were overall able to prioritize high-risk patients and prevent treatment delays, our study also found that older patients, female patients, black patients, and patients who were uninsured were more likely to have longer treatment times. Many of these patients are part of vulnerable populations who have historically faced barriers to accessing healthcare services even prior to the pandemic [37,38]. Studies suggest that many of these pre-existing health disparities were exacerbated for patients with cancer during COVID-19, leading to cancer treatment delays and higher rates of COVID-19-related complications and mortality among vulnerable groups [37,39,40]. Further work is necessary to develop targeted interventions and practices to support vulnerable patients during cancer care when similar situations arise in the future.

One important limitation of our study is the lack of information past 2020, making it difficult to assess the long-term impact of the pandemic on HNC treatment. Additionally, since the NCDB is only updated annually, we were limited from utilizing more rigorous time trend analysis to analyze the drop in diagnoses and increase in treatment times between 2019 and 2020. Therefore, although our study found that the drop in diagnoses between 2019 and 2020 was statistically significant, there is a possibility that the decrease in patient numbers could have been due to random variation. Another limitation of our dataset was that demographic characteristics, such as income and education quartiles, were referenced to the demographic characteristics of patients' ZIP codes based on the 2000 US Census. Because demographic characteristics change significantly over time, this limits the accuracy of more recent data points. Additionally, the NCDB only contains facilities that are COC accredited, which biases the data towards cancer treatment centers that are likely better equipped to maintain high-quality cancer care during times of crisis, like the COVID-19 pandemic. This limits the generalizability of the study, considering the evidence suggesting that cancer treatment centers, particularly in lower-middle-income countries, had large variability in their ability to adapt cancer care to the pandemic, as well as our ability to calculate incidence rates [29,36]. Finally, the lack of data on disease-specific clinical outcomes such as complications and long-term survival makes it difficult to assess the impact of the COVID-19 pandemic on clinical care.

Our study demonstrated that there was no change in the clinical stage of patients who presented for care of HNC during the COVID-19 pandemic, and treatment time metrics were stable to decreased. Our findings suggest that hospitals were able to prioritize treatment of patients with HNC and avoid treatment delays. However, vulnerable groups, particularly patients who were black, female, elderly, or uninsured, were at higher risk of experiencing treatment delays. Further research is necessary to determine if there are any long-term ramifications to the COVID-19 pandemic in terms of the emergence of more advanced stage malignancies in the coming years.

Author Contributions: Conceptualization, M.L.L., A.F. and M.M.C.; methodology, M.L.L. and M.M.C.; data analysis, M.L.L. and M.M.C.; data interpretation, M.L.L., A.F. and M.M.C.; writing—original draft preparation, M.L.L. and M.M.C.; writing—review and editing, M.L.L., A.F. and M.M.C. All authors have read and agreed to the published version of the manuscript.

Funding: This research received no external funding.

Institutional Review Board Statement: Ethical review and approval were waived by the Stanford University Institutional Review Board since this study utilized a deidentified database.

Informed Consent Statement: Patient consent was waived since this study utilized a deidentified database.

Data Availability Statement: The data presented in this study are provided by the American College of Surgeons, by application.

Conflicts of Interest: The authors have no conflicts of interest to declare.

Abbreviations

The following abbreviations are used in this manuscript:

HNC	Head and Neck Cancer
NCDB	National Cancer Database
IRB	Institutional Review Board
AJCC	American Joint Committee on Cancer
APC	Average Percentage Change
CI	Confidence Intervals
NCCN	National Comprehensive Cancer Network
PORT	Postoperative Radiotherapy
AAPC	Average Annual Percentage Change

References

1. Moynihan, R.; Sanders, S.; Michaleff, Z.A.; Scott, A.M.; Clark, J.; To, E.J.; Jones, M.; Kitchener, E.; Fox, M.; Johansson, M.; et al. Impact of COVID-19 pandemic on utilisation of healthcare services: A systematic review. *BMJ Open* **2021**, *11*, e045343. [CrossRef] [PubMed]
2. Xu, S.; Glenn, S.; Sy, L.; Qian, L.; Hong, V.; Ryan, D.S.; Jacobsen, S. Impact of the COVID-19 Pandemic on Health Care Utilization in a Large Integrated Health Care System: Retrospective Cohort Study. *J. Med. Internet Res.* **2021**, *23*, e26558. [CrossRef]
3. Roy, C.M.; Bollman, E.B.; Carson, L.M.; Northrop, A.J.; Jackson, E.F.; Moresky, R.T. Assessing the indirect effects of COVID-19 on healthcare delivery, utilization and health outcomes: A scoping review. *Eur. J. Public Health* **2021**, *31*, 634–640. [CrossRef] [PubMed]
4. Hartnett, K.P.; Kite-Powell, A.; DeVies, J.; Coletta, M.A.; Boehmer, T.K.; Adjemian, J.; Gundlapalli, A.V. National Syndromic Surveillance Program Community of Practice Impact of the COVID-19 Pandemic on Emergency Department Visits—United States, 1 January 2019–30 May 2020. *MMWR Morb. Mortal. Wkly. Rep.* **2020**, *69*, 699–704. [CrossRef]
5. Rennert-May, E.; Leal, J.; Thanh, N.X.; Lang, E.; Dowling, S.; Manns, B.; Wasylak, T.; Ronksley, P.E. The impact of COVID-19 on hospital admissions and emergency department visits: A population-based study. *PLoS ONE* **2021**, *16*, e0252441. [CrossRef]
6. Kapsner, L.A.; Kampf, M.O.; Seuchter, S.A.; Gruendner, J.; Gulden, C.; Mate, S.; Mang, J.M.; Schüttler, C.; Deppenwiese, N.; Krause, L.; et al. Reduced Rate of Inpatient Hospital Admissions in 18 German University Hospitals During the COVID-19 Lockdown. *Front. Public Health* **2021**, *8*, 594117. [CrossRef]
7. Rucinska, M.; Nawrocki, S. COVID-19 Pandemic: Impact on Cancer Patients. *Int. J. Environ. Res. Public Health* **2022**, *19*, 12470. [CrossRef]
8. Boettcher, A.N.; Hammoud, D.A.; Weinberg, J.B.; Agarwal, P.; Mendiratta-Lala, M.; Luker, G.D. Cancer Imaging and Patient Care during the COVID-19 Pandemic. *Radiol. Imaging Cancer* **2020**, *2*, e200058. [CrossRef]
9. Hanna, T.P.; King, W.D.; Thibodeau, S.; Jalink, M.; Paulin, G.A.; Harvey-Jones, E.; O'Sullivan, D.E.; Booth, C.M.; Sullivan, R.; Aggarwal, A. Mortality due to cancer treatment delay: Systematic review and meta-analysis. *BMJ* **2020**, *371*, m4087. [CrossRef]
10. Chavez-MacGregor, M.; Lei, X.; Zhao, H.; Scheet, P.; Giordano, S.H. Evaluation of COVID-19 Mortality and Adverse Outcomes in US Patients With or Without Cancer. *JAMA Oncol.* **2022**, *8*, 69–78. [CrossRef]

11. Pathania, A.S.; Prathipati, P.; Abdul, B.A.; Chava, S.; Katta, S.S.; Gupta, S.C.; Gangula, P.R.; Pandey, M.K.; Durden, D.L.; Byrareddy, S.N.; et al. COVID-19 and Cancer Comorbidity: Therapeutic Opportunities and Challenges. *Theranostics* **2021**, *11*, 731–753. [CrossRef] [PubMed]
12. Conti, V.; Corbi, G.; Sabbatino, F.; De Pascale, D.; Sellitto, C.; Stefanelli, B.; Bertini, N.; De Simone, M.; Liguori, L.; Di Paola, I.; et al. Long COVID: Clinical Framing, Biomarkers, and Therapeutic Approaches. *J. Pers. Med.* **2023**, *13*, 334. [CrossRef] [PubMed]
13. Patt, D.; Gordan, L.; Diaz, M.; Okon, T.; Grady, L.; Harmison, M.; Markward, N.; Sullivan, M.; Peng, J.; Zhou, A. Impact of COVID-19 on Cancer Care: How the Pandemic Is Delaying Cancer Diagnosis and Treatment for American Seniors. *JCO Clin. Cancer Inform.* **2020**, *4*, 1059–1071. [CrossRef]
14. Consalvo, F.; De Simone, M.; Scarpa, A.; Acerra, A.; Salzano, F.A.; Fineschi, V.; Santurro, A. Challenges and Complications in the Management of Advanced Oropharyngeal Carcinoma: Role of Post-Mortem Diagnosis and Future Perspectives. *J. Clin. Med.* **2024**, *13*, 5198. [CrossRef] [PubMed]
15. Solis, R.N.; Mehrzad, M.; Faiq, S.; Frusciante, R.P.; Sekhon, H.K.; Abouyared, M.; Bewley, A.F.; Farwell, D.G.; Birkeland, A.C. The Impact of COVID-19 on Head and Neck Cancer Treatment: Before and During the Pandemic. *OTO Open* **2021**, *5*, 2473974X211068075. [CrossRef]
16. Kiong, K.L.; Diaz, E.M.; Gross, N.D.; Diaz, E.M.; Hanna, E.Y. The impact of COVID-19 on head and neck cancer diagnosis and disease extent. *Head Neck* **2021**, *43*, 1890–1897. [CrossRef]
17. Popovic, M.; Fiano, V.; Moirano, G.; Chiusa, L.; Conway, D.I.; Garzino Demo, P.; Gilardetti, M.; Iorio, G.C.; Moccia, C.; Ostellino, O.; et al. The Impact of the COVID-19 Pandemic on Head and Neck Cancer Diagnosis in the Piedmont Region, Italy: Interrupted Time-Series Analysis. *Front. Public Health* **2022**, *10*, 809283. [CrossRef]
18. Zubair, A.; Jamshaid, S.; Scholfield, D.W.; Hariri, A.A.; Ahmed, J.; Ghufoor, K.; Ali, S. Impact of COVID-19 pandemic on head-neck cancer referral and treatment pathway in North East London. *Ann. R. Coll. Surg. Engl.* **2022**, *105*, S28–S34. [CrossRef]
19. Tevetoğlu, F.; Kara, S.; Aliyeva, C.; Yıldırım, R.; Yener, H.M. Delayed presentation of head and neck cancer patients during COVID-19 pandemic. *Eur. Arch. Otorhinolaryngol.* **2021**, *278*, 5081–5085. [CrossRef]
20. Stevens, M.N.; Patro, A.; Rahman, B.; Gao, Y.; Liu, D.; Cmelak, A.; Wiggleton, J.; Kim, Y.J.; Langerman, A.; Mannion, K.; et al. Impact of COVID-19 on presentation, staging, and treatment of head and neck mucosal squamous cell carcinoma. *Am. J. Otolaryngol.* **2022**, *43*, 103263. [CrossRef]
21. Available online: https://www2.census.gov/geo/pdfs/maps-data/maps/reference/us_regdiv.pdf (accessed on 3 April 2023).
22. Amin, M.B.; Greene, F.L.; Edge, S.B.; Compton, C.C.; Gershenwald, J.E.; Brookland, R.K.; Meyer, L.; Gress, D.M.; Byrd, D.R.; Winchester, D.P. The Eighth Edition AJCC Cancer Staging Manual: Continuing to build a bridge from a population-based to a more "personalized" approach to cancer staging. *CA Cancer J. Clin.* **2017**, *67*, 93–99. [CrossRef] [PubMed]
23. Graboyes, E.M.; Garrett-Mayer, E.; Ellis, M.A.; Sharma, A.K.; Wahlquist, A.E.; Lentsch, E.J.; Nussenbaum, B.; Day, T.A. Effect of Time to Initiation of Postoperative Radiation Therapy on Survival in Surgically-Managed Head and Neck Cancer. *Cancer* **2017**, *123*, 4841–4850. [CrossRef] [PubMed]
24. Rygalski, C.J.; Zhao, S.; Eskander, A.; Zhan, K.Y.; Mroz, E.A.; Brock, G.; Silverman, D.A.; Blakaj, D.; Bonomi, M.R.; Carrau, R.L.; et al. Time to Surgery and Survival in Head and Neck Cancer. *Ann. Surg. Oncol.* **2021**, *28*, 877–885. [CrossRef]
25. Liao, D.Z.; Schlecht, N.F.; Rosenblatt, G.; Kinkhabwala, C.M.; Leonard, J.A.; Ference, R.S.; Prystowsky, M.B.; Ow, T.J.; Schiff, B.A.; Smith, R.V.; et al. Association of Delayed Time to Treatment Initiation With Overall Survival and Recurrence Among Patients with Head and Neck Squamous Cell Carcinoma in an Underserved Urban Population. *JAMA Otolaryngol. Neck Surg.* **2019**, *145*, 1001–1009. [CrossRef]
26. Pfister, D.G.; Spencer, S.; Adelstein, D.; Adkins, D.; Anzai, Y.; Brizel, D.M.; Bruce, J.Y.; Busse, P.M.; Caudell, J.J.; Cmelak, A.J.; et al. Head and Neck Cancers, Version 2.2020, NCCN Clinical Practice Guidelines in Oncology. *J. Natl. Compr. Cancer Netw. JNCCN* **2020**, *18*, 873–898. [CrossRef]
27. Ladbury, C.; Liu, J.; Nelson, R.; Amini, A.; Maghami, E.; Sampath, S. Prognostic Impact of Primary Tumor Extent and Postoperative Radiation Facility Location in Major Salivary Gland Malignancies. *Cureus* **2022**, *14*, e24038. [CrossRef]
28. Rosenthal, D.I.; Liu, L.; Lee, J.H.; Vapiwala, N.; Chalian, A.A.; Weinstein, G.S.; Chilian, I.; Weber, R.S.; Machtay, M. Importance of the treatment package time in surgery and postoperative radiation therapy for squamous carcinoma of the head and neck. *Head Neck* **2002**, *24*, 115–126. [CrossRef]
29. Effect of COVID-19 Pandemic Lockdowns on Planned Cancer Surgery for 15 Tumour Types in 61 Countries: An International, Prospective, Cohort Study—The Lancet Oncology. Available online: https://www.thelancet.com/journals/lanonc/article/PIIS1470-2045(21)00493-9/fulltext (accessed on 28 February 2024).
30. Thompson, J.A.; Lubek, J.E.; Amin, N.; Joy, R.; Dyalram, D.; Ord, R.A.; Taylor, R.J.; Wolf, J.S.; Mehra, R.; Cullen, K.J.; et al. Impact of the Novel Coronavirus 2019 (COVID-19) Pandemic on Head and Neck Cancer Care. *Otolaryngol. Head Neck Surg.* **2022**, *166*, 93–100. [CrossRef]

31. Schoonbeek, R.C.; de Jel, D.V.C.; van Dijk, B.A.C.; Willems, S.M.; Bloemena, E.; Hoebers, F.J.P.; van Meerten, E.; Verbist, B.M.; Smeele, L.E.; Halmos, G.B.; et al. Fewer head and neck cancer diagnoses and faster treatment initiation during COVID-19 in 2020: A nationwide population-based analysis. *Radiother. Oncol.* **2022**, *167*, 42–48. [CrossRef]
32. Yao, P.; Cooley, V.; Kuhel, W.; Tassler, A.; Banuchi, V.; Long, S.; Savenkov, O.; Kutler, D.I. Times to Diagnosis, Staging, and Treatment of Head and Neck Cancer Before and During COVID-19. *OTO Open* **2021**, *5*, 2473974X211059429. [CrossRef]
33. Heimes, D.; Müller, L.K.; Schellin, A.; Naujokat, H.; Graetz, C.; Schwendicke, F.; Goedecke, M.; Beck-Broichsitter, B.; Kämmerer, P.W. Consequences of the COVID-19 Pandemic and Governmental Containment Policies on the Detection and Therapy of Oral Malignant Lesions—A Retrospective, Multicenter Cohort Study from Germany. *Cancers* **2021**, *13*, 2892. [CrossRef] [PubMed]
34. Gršić, K.; Blivajs, I.; Pastorčić Grgić, M.; Prgomet, D.; Lukinović, J.; Vugrinec, O.; Matoc, L.; Miličić, B.; Leović, D. The impact of COVID-19 on head and neck cancer treatment delay. *Acta Clin. Croat.* **2022**, *61*, 19–25. [CrossRef] [PubMed]
35. Shaw, R.; COVIDSurg Collaborative. UK Head and neck cancer surgical capacity during the second wave of the COVID-19 pandemic: Have we learned the lessons? COVIDSurg collaborative. *Clin. Otolaryngol.* **2021**, *46*, 729–735. [CrossRef] [PubMed]
36. Escobar, N.; DiMaggio, C.; Pocock, B.; Pescovitz, A.; McCalla, S.; Joseph, K.-A. Effects of COVID-19 on Surgical Delays in Patients with Breast Cancer in NYC Public Hospitals: A Multicenter Study. *Ann. Surg. Oncol.* **2023**, *30*, 23–30. [CrossRef]
37. Mullangi, S.; Aviki, E.M.; Chen, Y.; Robson, M.; Hershman, D.L. Factors Associated With Cancer Treatment Delay Among Patients Diagnosed With COVID-19. *JAMA Netw. Open* **2022**, *5*, e2224296. [CrossRef]
38. AJMC. Vulnerable populations: Who are they? *Am. J. Manag. Care* **2006**, *12*, S348–S352.
39. Romero Starke, K.; Reissig, D.; Petereit-Haack, G.; Schmauder, S.; Nienhaus, A.; Seidler, A. The isolated effect of age on the risk of COVID-19 severe outcomes: A systematic review with meta-analysis. *BMJ Glob. Health* **2021**, *6*, e006434. [CrossRef]
40. Wiemers, E.E.; Abrahams, S.; AlFakhri, M.; Hotz, V.J.; Schoeni, R.F.; Seltzer, J.A. Disparities in Vulnerability to Severe Complications from COVID-19 in the United States. *medRxiv* **2020**, medRxiv:2020.05.28.20115899. [CrossRef]

Journal of
Clinical Medicine

MDPI

Article

Pharyngeal Mucosal Space Abscess: A Special Entity That Merits Special Management—Our Experience in 106 Cases

Charikleia Maiou [1,*], Vasileios A. Lachanas [1], Stergios Nik Doumas [2], Nikolaos Kalogritsas [1], Anna Mpouronikou [1], Jiannis Hajiioannou [1], Efthymia Petinaki [3] and Charalampos E. Skoulakis [1]

1 Department of Otorhinolaryngology, University Hospital of Larissa, Viopolis, 41334 Larissa, Greece
2 Maxillofacial Unit, University Hospital of Larissa, 41334 Larissa, Greece
3 Department of Microbiology, University Hospital of Larissa, 41334 Larissa, Greece
* Correspondence: hara_mai@hotmail.com; Tel.: +30-2413-502825

Abstract: Background: Deep neck infections represent a common but heterogeneous medical condition, as clinical manifestations and outcomes vary, depending, among others, on the infection site. The pharyngeal mucosal space (PMS) represents the most superficial neck space, confined between the pharyngeal mucosa and the pharyngeal constrictor muscles. The collection of pus in the PMS (pharyngeal mucosal abscess (PMA)) is considered rare and is rarely reported in the literature. This study focuses on infections of the pharyngeal mucosal space, aiming to provide an elaborate description of the clinical behavior of this category and reporting its differences from other categories of deep neck infections (DNIs). **Methods:** A retrospective study of 743 cases of deep neck infections was conducted in a single tertiary center. Cases of abscesses, confined in the pharyngomucosal space (PMAs), were studied, reporting demographics, clinical features, imaging, bacteriology, and treatment data, and comparisons with other DNIs were made. **Results:** A total of 106 cases of pharyngomucosal space abscesses (PMAs) were reported, representing 14.3% of deep neck infections (DNIs). Dysphagia, odynophagia, and fever were the most common symptoms. Hospitalization with non-surgical drainage was the treatment of choice, resulting in complete recovery with no complications. **Conclusions:** In conclusion, the frequency of PMAs in our series suggests that they may not be as rare as they are considered to be. Symptoms and clinical findings can be similar to those of other DNIs, especially parapharyngeal abscesses, but, overall, PMAs seem to have a milder clinical behavior, highlighting the need for diagnosis and reporting as a separate, recognizable category.

Keywords: deep neck spaces; deep neck infections; pharyngeal mucosal space; abscess

1. Introduction

Deep neck infections (DNIs) represent a group of relatively common clinical entities but with potentially life-threatening consequences. The advent of antibiotics has led to improved infection outcomes, with wide-spectrum empirical intravenous antibiotics being initiated until culture and sensitivities are reported and targeted therapy is applied [1–3]. Nevertheless, the need for potential surgical intervention always comes into consideration. Clinicians are routinely asked to make a call about surgical drainage, deciding on proper timing and surgical access, evaluating the anatomical position of a potential abscess, based on clinical findings and imaging studies.

Sound knowledge of pertinent surgical anatomy is of paramount importance in order to access all involved neck spaces [1,2]. The pharyngeal mucosal space (PMS) has been described as the most superficial neck space, lying deep in the pharyngeal mucosa, anteromedially to the parapharyngeal space, and directly anterior to the retropharyngeal space. Its clinical significance has not been recognized until recently, through cross-sectional imaging studies. Anatomically, it represents the area of the nasopharynx and oropharynx on the inner side of the buccopharyngeal fascia. It is located between the pharyngeal mucosa (superficially) and the investing layer of the deep cervical fascia (pharyngobasilar fascia) (deep). The latter surrounds the pharyngeal constrictors. It extends from the skull base to the lower cricoid border, involving the naso-oro-hypopharynx. It is bordered by the superior constrictor muscles' aponeurosis superiorly, where it merges with the middle layer of deep cervical fascia (Figure 1). PMS consists of five layers, forming the pharyngeal wall. From the internal to the external layers, they include the following: 1. mucosal membrane; 2. submucosa (containing loose areolar tissue, which facilitates deglutition, lymphoid tissue, and minor salivary glands); 3. dense pharyngobasilar fascia; 4. superior constrictor muscles of the pharynx; and 5. buccopharyngeal fascia (outer lining of the space). Dense connective tissue is present only on the deep surface of this layer (deep cervical fascia) [4–8]. Some studies suggest that the peritonsillar space is virtually part of the PMS [4–6]; however, more recent studies define them as separate spaces [8].

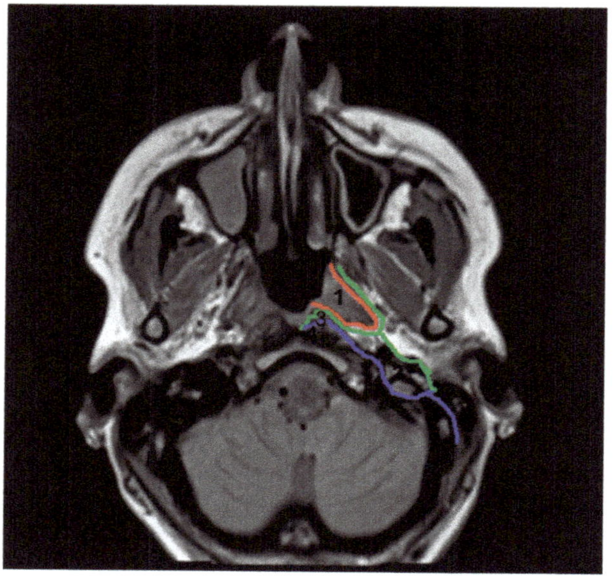

Figure 1. 1. Pharyngomucosal space (PMS), 2. parapharyngeal space (PPS), 3. retropharyngeal space (RPS), and 4. prevertebral space (PVS). Red line: pharyngobasilar fascia; green line: middle layer of deep cervical fascia; and blue line: deep layer of deep cervical fascia.

PMS pathology includes neoplasms and congenital and inflammatory lesions [4–7], while there is a lack of studies on pharyngeal mucosal space abscesses (PMAs) [7]. The isolated collection of pus in the PMS is considered rare; however, the anatomical borders of the PMS suggest a potentially clear clinical distinction between parapharyngeal and peritonsillar abscesses, based on endoscopic and radiologic manifestations (Figure 2) Abscesses confined in the peritonsillar space present with the typical bulging of the peritonsillar space, whereas parapharyngeal abscesses involve neck swelling and diffuse edema of the lateral pharyngeal wall. The observation of inflammation and pus collection, isolated within the lateral pharyngeal wall, has led us to the conclusion that PMAs can be described and treated as a separate category of DNIs.

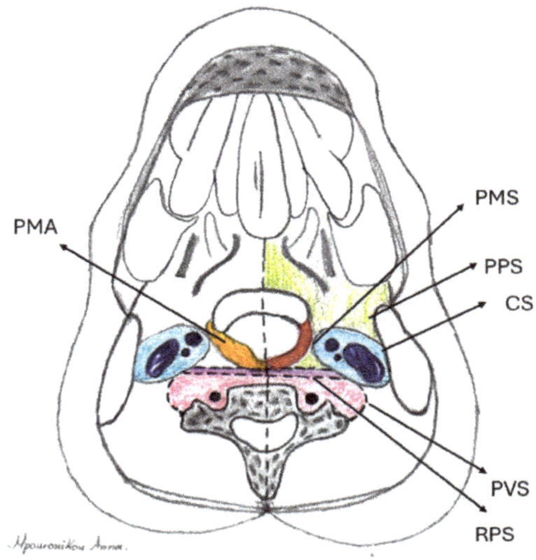

Figure 2. Anatomical relations of pharyngomucosal space (PMS) (red): parapharyngeal space (PPS) (green), carotid space (CS) (blue), prevertebral space (PVS) (purple), and retropharyngeal space (RPS) (pink). Location of pharyngomucosal abscess (PMA) (orange) superficially, in the pharyngeal lumen.

The purpose of this study was to present our experience and highlight the clinical behavior of abscesses constrained in the PMS, in comparison to other DNIs.

2. Materials and Methods

All necessary approvals were obtained, and all participants' data were handled according to the University Hospital of Larissa Scientific Committee's regulations, as well as Helsinki and HIPAA regulations.

A retrospective study of 743 consecutive DNIs treated over the period January 2011–December 2019 was conducted. STROBE guidelines were followed. Diagnosis was suspected based on clinical history and findings and confirmed by imaging. The data of patients with an abscess contained only in the PMS, including their demographics, clinical information, bacteriology, and treatment, were exported and analyzed. PMA cases with pus extension to the peritonsillar or any other neck space were excluded. The means were reported with SDs. X^2 test and t-test were used for comparisons; $p < 0.05$ was considered significant. Data analysis was performed with SPSS 20 software (IBM, Chicago, IL, USA).

3. Results

PMA diagnosis was the second most common diagnosis, following peritonsillar abscesses, involving 106 adults (female/male ratio: 21/85, mean age: 51 ± 14.1 years). (Table 1). Associated comorbidities included hypertension ($n = 22$), dyslipidemia ($n = 20$), heart disease ($n = 8$), thyroid disease ($n = 8$), diabetes mellitus ($n = 7$), asthma ($n = 5$), anemia ($n = 3$), renal insufficiency ($n = 1$), and rheumatoid arthritis ($n = 1$). Eight patients had a history of tonsillectomy. CT scans with contrast were conducted to confirm the diagnosis (Figure 3).

Table 1. Demographics and involved neck spaces of 743 patients with deep neck infections (DNIs).

Space Involved			**Female/Male**	**Mean Age ± SD**
	n **= 743**	**%**	**243/500**	**39.55 ± 17.18**
Peritonsillar	527	70.9	179/348	35.46 ± 14.9
Pharyngomucosal	106	14.3	21/85	51 ±14.1
Submandibular	46	6.2	17/29	45.39 ± 21.3
Parapharyngeal	11	1.5	4/7	43.81 ± 28.37
Retropharyngeal	8	1.1	5/3	45.5 ± 28.3
Ludwig's angina	6	0.8	3/3	64.83 ± 14.91
Masticator	3	0.4	1/2	34.66 ± 6.8
Parotid	3	0.4	1/2	45 ± 19.69
Visceral	1	0.1	1/0	60
Multi-space (>1 of the above)	32	4.3	11/21	52.34 ± 16.57

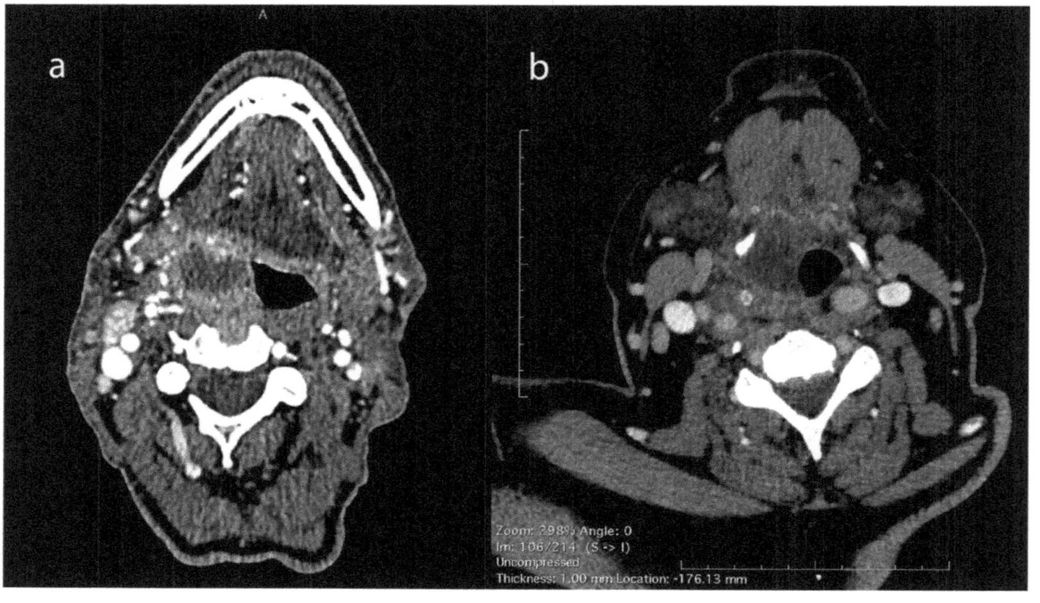

Figure 3. CT scan with contrast of pharyngeal mucosal space abscesses (PMAs). (**a**) Right-side PMA protruding into the pharyngeal lumen, located towards the lateral pharyngeal wall, just under the pharyngeal mucosa and medial to the pharyngeal constrictors, away from the ipsilateral carotid artery and the internal jugular vein. (**b**) Right-side PMA protruding into the pharyngeal lumen and passing medially to the hyoid bone, away from the ipsilateral carotid artery and the internal jugular vein.

The symptoms of patients with PMAs are summarized on Table 2. The most commonly reported symptoms were dysphagia, odynophagia, and fever. The mean onset of symptoms was 3.2 ± 1.7 days prior to admission. Trismus and neck swelling were significantly lower in PMAs compared to non-PMA DNIs ($p < 0.01$), while dysphagia was significantly higher ($p < 0.01$). No association with teeth infections was noted in PMAs.

Table 2. Summary of the patients presenting symptoms with pharyngeal mucosal space abscesses (PMA) versus non-pharyngeal mucosal space deep neck infections (DNIs).

	PMA		Non-PMA DNIs		
Symptoms	n = 106	%	n = 637	%	p
dysphagia	106	100.00	591	92.78	0.004 *
odynophagia/sore throat	63	59.43	348	54.63	0.357
fever	53	50.00	350	54.95	0.344
neck swelling	26	24.53	545	85.56	<0.001 *
trismus	22	20.75	285	44.74	<0.001 *
"hot potato" voice	18	16.98	116	18.21	0.815
drooling	10	9.43	47	7.38	0.462
breathing discomfort	3	2.83	14	2.20	0.604
ear pain	2	1.89	9	1.41	0.708
malaise	1	0.94	31	4.87	0.65
odontalgia	-	-	43	6.75	0.006 *

* Significant difference ($p < 0.05$).

Table 3 tabulates the summary of patients with PMAs' physical examination findings. One-sided lateral pharyngeal wall edema was invariable; pyriform sinus, vallecula, uvula, peritonsillar swelling, and unilaterally enlarged tonsil were noticed in 41%, 27%, 27%, 26%, and 18% of patients, respectively, while nasopharyngeal edema and adenoiditis were found in three patients (Figure 4). Tenderness during palpation of the larynx was noted in all patients. The most common laryngeal endoscopic finding was arytenoid edema (20%), whereas the glottic and subglottic areas were spared. Neck swelling was present in 25% of patients.

Table 3. Summary of physical examination findings upon admission of patients with pharyngeal mucosal space abscesses.

	n = 106	%
Oral Cavity		
odontogenic source of infection	0	0
poor dentition	46	43.4
no clinically noticeable findings	60	56.60
Oropharynx		
lateral pharyngeal wall edema	106	100
vallecula edema	29	27.36
uvula edema	29	27.36
peritonsillar edema	28	26.42
unilaterally enlarged tonsil	19	17.92
soft palate edema	10	9.43
posterior pillar edema	6	5.66
tonsillar exudate	4	3.77
anterior pillar edema	3	2.83

Table 3. *Cont.*

	n = 106	%
Hypopharynx		
pyriform sinus edema	43	40.57
Nasopharynx		
edema/adenoiditis	3	2.83
no clinically noticeable findings	103	97.17
Larynx		
tenderness during palpation	106	100
Supraglottic		
arytenoid cartilage edema	21	19.81
aryepiglottic fold edema	9	8.49
edema of the laryngeal surface of the epiglottis (retention cyst *)	5	4.72
no clinically noticeable findings	81	76.42
Glottic		
true vocal cord edema (Reinke edema *)	2	1.89
no clinically noticeable findings	104	98.11
Subglottic		
no clinically noticeable findings	106	100
Neck		
cervical lymph nodes	26	24.53
- painless	13	12.26
- tenderness	13	12.26
no clinically noticeable findings	80	75.47
Nasal Cavities		
clear secretions	14	13.21
purulent secretions	1	0.94
no clinically noticeable findings	91	85.85
Salivary Glands/Cranial Nerves/Ears		
no clinically noticeable findings	106	100

* Follow-up finding.

The mean WBC count and CRP values upon admission were 14.5 ± 5.11 K/μL (reference range, 4–10.8 K/μL) and 13.4 ± 10.1 (reference range, 0–0.5 mg/dL), respectively. Samples for microbiological analysis were obtained in 61 patients; the remaining 45 samples were not processed due to insufficient purulent material. Cultures yielded 23 positive results (Table 4). All isolated bacteria species were aerobic; the commonest were *Streptococcus pyogenes* (52%) and *Staphylococcus aureus* (30%). None of the positive cultures involved multiple bacterial species. Before admission, 37 patients had been under antibiotics and 6 under steroids based on GP recommendations.

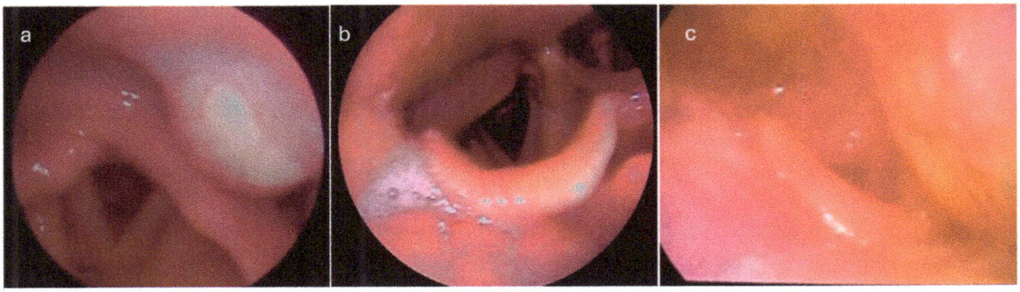

Figure 4. Endoscopic findings in PMA cases. One-sided lateral pharyngeal wall edema (**a–c**) and arytenoid edema (**b**) were the common findings during endoscopy.

Table 4. Distribution of the species isolated from the positive cultures (n = 23) of pharyngeal mucosal space abscesses.

		n	(%)
Aerobic Bacteria			
a.	**Gram-positive**	**21**	**91.3**
1.	*Streptococcus pyogenes*	12	52.2
2.	*Staphylococcus aureus*	7	30.4
3.	*Streptococcus group C*	1	4.3
4.	*Streptococcus anginosus*	1	4.3
b.	**Gram-negative**	**2**	**8.7**
1.	*Pseudomonas aeruginosa*	2	8.7

In-hospital empirical therapy included IV ampicillin–sulbactam combined with metronidazole or clindamycin. Spontaneous drainage was noted in 52 (49%) patients, transoral drainage under local anesthetic in 47 (44%), and aspiration in 7 (7%). The mean time until spontaneous drainage was 1.8 ± 0.8 days from admission. No further surgical intervention was required, and no major adverse event was noted in any patient, while the mean hospital stay was 4.2 ± 1.8 days.

4. Discussion

Up until now, there has been little evidence in the literature about the definition and management of PMA infections. We found only one study (PubMed search) reporting four PMA cases [7]. The term "pharyngeal wall abscess" has also been sporadically used in the literature [9]; thus, no specific description is available. Another study reports four cases of "inferior pole peritonsilar abscesses", the description of which falls within the spectrum of PMAs [10]. However, in our series, PMAs represent 14,3% of DNIs, suggesting that they are not uncommon, and in "real-world" practice, they may be underdiagnosed or misdiagnosed as parapharyngeal abscesses. Although clinical findings can be similar, major differences were reported in our study concerning etiology, severity of symptoms, and progression of the disease.

PMAs are supposed to be mainly associated with pharyngeal mucosa infections, while infections of the teeth, major salivary glands, or other foci lateral to pharyngeal constrictors rarely result in the formation of PMAs [7]. Our results support this, since none of our cases had an odontogenic or salivary source of infection. As for the clinical features, symptoms of PMAs are overall similar to those of DNIs. Dysphagia was reported consistently by all patients, followed by odynophagia and sore throat. Skoulakis et al. [7] did not report trismus and neck swelling in their cases. In our series, mild trismus was noticed in 21% of patients, but this finding was significantly lower than other DNIs. Neck swelling, secondary to neck lymphadenitis, even though significantly lower than other DNIs, was recorded in 25% of patients. The rest of PMA symptoms were not significantly different from other DNIs, however milder in severity. Fever was reported in half of our patients, whilst the mean WBC and CRP values were raised.

Lateral pharyngeal wall edema was a consistent endoscopic finding in all cases, while, in some of them, edema in other oropharyngeal parts coexisted. In 43 (41%) patients with abscess extension to the hypopharyngeal part of the PMA, edema was extended to the pyriform sinus, while in those where pus reached the most inferior part of the PMS, arytenoid or aryepiglottic fold edema coexisted. No other findings from laryngeal endoscopy were recorded, while follow-up of the five cases with epiglottic edema and the two cases with true vocal cord edema revealed the presence of epiglottic retention cysts and Reinke edema, respectively. Tenderness during palpation of the larynx (bilateral movement) was also a constant finding in all patients. Similar findings were reported by Skoulakis et al. [7].

Although clinical findings are of the greatest importance in the suspicion of a PMA, a CT scan with contrast is the "gold standard" to set the diagnosis [7] (Figures 3 and 5). Abscess protrusion into the pharyngeal lumen may give the false impression of a parapharyngeal abscess; however, the PMS is located in the lateral pharyngeal wall, between the pharyngeal mucosa and the pharyngeal constrictors, extending under the hyoid bone and passing medially to it. On the contrary, other spaces extend laterally to the hyoid bone (e.g., carotid space), whereas, for others (e.g., parapharyngeal space), it represents their lower border. Ultrasonography cannot identify the PMS adequately, while MRI may also be of use in selected cases [7]. The high diagnostic accuracy of MRI can be utilized in order to specify the anatomic relation of the abscess with the pharyngeal constrictors, differentiating between PMAs and deeper-extending abscesses [11]. However, the practical need for imaging and the cost-effectiveness can be controversial, as a significant number of cases can resolve rapidly. Nevertheless, unless strongly contraindicated, imaging is highly recommended, so that deeper counterpart involvement may be excluded, especially in cases with severe symptoms and clinical findings.

Streptococcus pyogenes and *Staphylococcus aureus* were the most common bacteria species in our series. The microbiology of PMAs seems to be similar to other DNIs and strongly correlated to pharyngeal microflora [3,7]. However, we only had a small number of positive cultures, so, on these grounds, safe and generalized conclusions cannot be made. Empirical therapy with IV-ampicillin–sulbactam combined with metronidazole or clindamycin proved to be effective in our practice.

Skoulakis et al. suggest that "*the abscess, as a rule, is drained spontaneously*" [7]. This clinical feature is of major importance, differentiating significantly the clinical behavior of PMAs from other deep neck infections. In our series, spontaneous drainage was noted in 49% of patients, and the mean time until spontaneous drainage was 1.8 ± 0.8 days from admission. In all instances, the spontaneous pharyngeal mucosa opening was small, and the flow of pus was slow, often allowing the patient to swallow it. We believe that this was the main reason why no complications related to tracheobronchial pus aspiration were noted in any of these patients. The PMS lies just deep to the pharyngeal mucosa, while dense connective tissue is present only at its deeper border, hence hindering infection from spreading towards deeper spaces and facilitating pus drainage of potential abscesses intraluminally, by virtue of least resistance. Furthermore, the pharyngeal constrictors' pressure on the abscess during the pharyngeal peristaltic wave facilitates spontaneous drainage through the "vulnerable" mucosa. Transoral drainage under local anesthesia or aspiration may also be considered, in order to speed up recovery and shorten hospital-stay. The lack of established guidelines in the literature, concerning algorithms on the management of DNIs, is possibly due to the heterogeneity of clinical manifestations. However, the basic principle remains the need for hospitalization and surgical drainage, taking into account risk factors for major complications [12]. Thus, the clinical importance of recognizing a PMA can affect the decision-making process when surgery comes into question and can predict the duration of in-hospital treatment, as minimal interventions seem to be adequately effective.

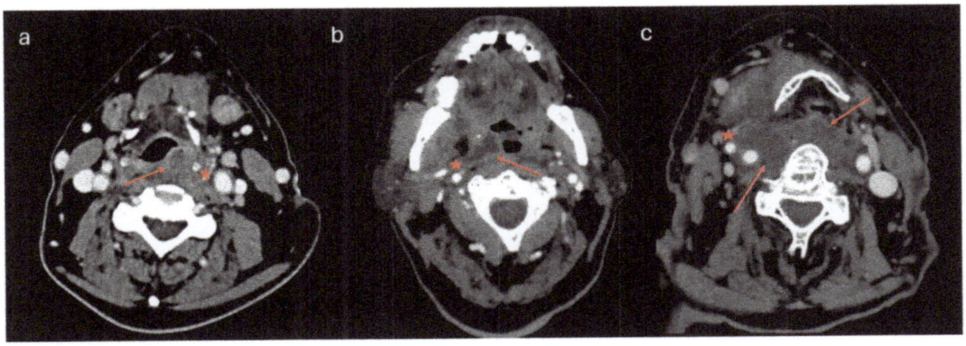

Figure 5. CT images of different categories of DNIs: (**a**) left-side PMA protruding into the pharyngeal lumen, passing medially to the hyoid bone; (**b**) right-side peritonsillar abscess, extending to the parapharyngeal space towards the right carotid artery and jugular vein; and (**c**) extended right-side parapharyngeal and retropharyngeal abscess. Arrows and stars indicate the margins of the abscess.

In our series, all PMAs were managed conservatively, with minimal intervention, no major adverse events were noted, and no further surgical interventions were needed. Parapharyngeal abscesses, however, and multi-space abscesses (involving more than one space; the majority including the parapharyngeal space) were treated surgically (63%, 66%, respectively). Additionally, the mean hospital stay in the PMA group was significantly lower (Table 5). Major complications of other DNIs, such as mediastinitis and airway obstruction, are unlikely to occur because of the superficial location of the PMS in the pharyngeal lumen. A dense deep border, constricting the PMS from spreading into the deep layer of the deep cervical fascia, together with spontaneous drainage may be the reason why abscesses constrained in PMS fare better than parapharyngeal and retropharyngeal abscesses, which are associated with high rates of major complications and the need for, sometimes multiple, surgical interventions [13].

Table 5. Surgical treatment and duration of hospital stay.

Space Involved	Total	Surgical Drainage		Mean Hospital Stay ± SD
		n	%	
Pharyngomucosal	106	0	0	4.2 ± 1.8
Parapharyngeal	11	7	63.6	9.88 ± 4.51 ($p < 0.0001$ *)
Multi-space (incl. parapharyngeal, submandibular, retropharyngeal, peritonsillar, masticator, visceral)	32	21	65.6	12 ± 8.8 ($p < 0.0001$ **)

* Unpaired *t*-test, t = 8.2473, df = 115, ** Unpaired *t*-test, t = 8.6141, df = 136.

Limitations

Even though our data were withdrawn from a prospectively collected database, the retrospective nature of our study represents its main limitation, along with the fact that the data had been collected at a single center. However, the relatively large number of cases minimizes the bias and provides meaningful results. The existing literature gap regarding this topic limits the theoretical foundations of our study, therefore highlighting the need for further research. Potential multi-center observational studies are required to confirm our results and assess the description of PMAs in the future.

5. Conclusions

Our study suggests that PMAs are not as rare as they are considered to be; however, there is a lack of research on abscesses in this space. PMAs have much in common with other DNIs: PMAs' symptoms and clinical findings are similar to those of other DNIs; however, trismus and neck swelling seem to be significantly lower in PMAs. Projection of the lateral pharyngeal wall represents the most consistent finding, calling for differential diagnosis, mainly between parapharyngeal and PMS abscesses.

Imaging studies can confirm the diagnosis, with CT with contrast being the modality of choice. Overall, PMAs seem to be less dangerous than their deep-seated counterparts, since their superficial location renders them amenable to spontaneous drainage, aspiration, incision, and intraoral drainage, obviating expansion into deeper structures.

In conclusion, we believe that lesions of the pharyngeal mucosal space represent a group of cervical lesions with special clinical and radiological characteristics that require diverse methods of treatment. Familiarization with the anatomy of the pharyngeal mucosal space and the clinical course of its inflammatory lesions can lead to optimal management of these not-so-rare cases, potentially sparing patients from unnecessary imaging and surgical intervention. Our assessment is that, as a rule, the diversity of this space is not adequately acknowledged by clinicians; thus, more data reporting and further research are required in order to ensure that all cases of inflammations of this space are recognized and treated correctly.

Author Contributions: Conceptualization, C.E.S.; methodology, V.A.L. and S.N.D.; software, V.A.L.; validation, E.P., J.H. and C.E.S.; formal analysis C.M. and V.A.L.; investigation, C.M. and N.K.; resources, E.P.; data curation, C.M., S.N.D., N.K. and A.M.; writing—original draft preparation, C.M. and V.A.L.; writing—review and editing, C.M. and V.A.L.; visualization, C.M., V.A.L. and A.M.; supervision, C.E.S., E.P. and J.H.; project administration, C.E.S. All authors have read and agreed to the published version of the manuscript.

Funding: This research received no external funding.

Institutional Review Board Statement: The study was conducted in accordance with the Declaration of Helsinki, and approved by the Internal Ethics Committee of the Department of Medicine of the University of Thessaly, Greece (protocol code: 1755, date of approval: 11 May 2021).

Informed Consent Statement: Informed consent was obtained from all subjects involved in the study.

Data Availability Statement: The data presented in this study are available on request from the corresponding author due to privacy reasons.

Conflicts of Interest: The authors declare no conflicts of interest.

References

1. Christian, J.M.; Goddard, A.C.; Gillespie, M.B. Deep Neck and Odontogenic Infections. In *Cummings Otolaryngology—Head and Neck Surgery*, 6th ed.; Elsevier: Amsterdam, The Netherlands, 2015; pp. 164–175.
2. Chan, Y.; Goddard, J.C. Neck Spaces and Fascial Planes. In *KJ Lee's Essential Otolaryngology*, 11th ed.; McGraw Hill: New York, NY, USA, 2016; pp. 585–605.
3. Beka, D.; Lachanas, V.A.; Doumas, S.; Xytsas, S.; Kanatas, A.; Petinaki, E.; Skoulakis, C. Microorganisms involved in deep neck infection (DNIs) in Greece: Detection, identification and susceptibility to antimicrobials. *BMC Infect. Dis.* **2019**, *19*, 850. [CrossRef] [PubMed]
4. Parker, G.D.; Harnsberger, H.R.; Jacobs, J.M. The pharyngeal mucosal space. *Semin. Ultrasound CT MR* **1990**, *11*, 460–475.
5. Harnsberger, H.R. The parapharyngeal and pharyngeal mucosal space. In *Handbook of Head and Neck Imaging*; Harnsberger, H.R., Ed.; Mosby-Year Book: St. Louis, MO, USA, 1995; pp. 29–45.
6. Mafee, M.F.; Valvasorri, G.E.; Becker, M. *Imaging of the Head and Neck*, 2nd ed.; Thieme: New York, NY, USA, 1995; p. 15.
7. Skoulakis, C.E.; Papadakis, C.E.; Bizakis, J.G.; Nikolidakis, A.A.; Manios, A.G.; Helidonis, E.S. Abscess of the pharyngeal mucosal space—An unusual location. *J. Otolaryngol.* **2003**, *32*, 121–124. [CrossRef]
8. Warshafsky, D.; Goldenberg, D.; Kanekar, S.G. Imaging anatomy of deep neck spaces. *Otolaryngol. Clin. N. Am.* **2012**, *45*, 1203–1221. [CrossRef] [PubMed]
9. Khoury, M.; Dong, S.X.; Alsaffar, H.; Johnson-Obaseki, S.; Caulley, L. Isolated oropharyngeal abscess with hypopharyngeal extension recurring 12 years after initial surgical management: A case report and review of the literature. *SAGE Open Med. Case Rep.* **2022**, *10*, 2050313X221089119. [CrossRef] [PubMed]
10. Licameli, G.R.; Grillone, G.A. Inferior pole peritonsillar abscess. *Otolaryngol. Head Neck Surg.* **1998**, *118*, 95–99. [CrossRef] [PubMed]
11. Vierula, J.P.; Nurminen, J.; Jussila, V.; Nyman, M.; Heikkinen, J.; Pape, B.; Sorvettula, K.; Mattila, K.; Hirvonen, J. Diagnostic performance of short noncontrast biparametric 3-T MRI for tonsillar infections: Comparison with a full protocol including contrast-enhanced sequences. *Eur. Radiol. Exp.* **2023**, *7*, 65. [CrossRef] [PubMed]
12. Sheikh, Z.; Yu, B.; Heywood, E.; Quraishi, N.; Quraishi, S. The assessment and management of deep neck space infections in adults: A systematic review and qualitative evidence synthesis. *Clin. Otolaryngol.* **2023**, *48*, 540–562. [CrossRef] [PubMed]
13. Loperfido, A.; Stasolla, A.; Giorgione, C.; Mammarella, F.; Celebrini, A.; Acquaviva, G.; Bellocchi, G. Management of Deep Neck Space Infections: A Large Tertiary Center Experience. *Cureus* **2023**, *15*, e34974. [CrossRef] [PubMed]

Journal of
Clinical Medicine

MDPI

Protocol

Parachute Technique: A New Endoscopic Method for Closing Recurrent Oronasal Fistulas in Cleft Palate Patients

Aleksander Zwierz, Oskar Komisarek * and Paweł Burduk

Department of Otolaryngology, Audiology and Phoniatrics, Collegium Medicum, Nicolaus Copernicus University in Torun, Jagiellońska 13-15, 85-067 Bydgoszcz, Poland; aleksanderzwierz@gmail.com (A.Z.); pburduk@cm.umk.pl (P.B.)
* Correspondence: oskarkomisarek@cm.umk.pl

Abstract: Objective: To present an innovative endoscopic method, the "Parachute Technique," for effectively closing recurrent oronasal fistulas in cleft palate patients using autologous tissue. **Summary Background Data**: Oronasal fistulas are common complications after cleft palate repair, often leading to impaired quality of life due to difficulties with speech, eating, and an increased risk of infections. Current surgical methods exhibit high recurrence rates, especially in cases involving significant scarring or large defects. Therefore, there is a need for new techniques that improve outcomes and reduce recurrence. **Methods**: The study introduced the "Parachute Technique," which uses autologous tissue from the inferior nasal turbinate to create a mucosal flap. This flap is transposed through the fistula using a guidewire under endoscopic guidance. The endoscopic approach minimized trauma to the surrounding tissues and allowed for precise manipulation during the procedure. **Results**: The "Parachute Technique" successfully closed recurrent oronasal fistulas, particularly in cases where conventional surgical methods had failed. The use of autologous tissue reduced the immunological risks, while the minimally invasive nature of the endoscopic procedure decreased the postoperative morbidity and improved the healing outcomes. **Conclusions**: The "Parachute Technique" offers a promising alternative for the treatment of recurrent oronasal fistulas in cleft palate patients, providing a minimally invasive, effective solution that can be easily adopted by specialists across multiple surgical disciplines.

Keywords: oronasal fistula; cleft palate; parachute technique; endoscopic repair; inferior nasal turbinate flap

1. Introduction

Oronasal fistulas are common complications following primary cleft palate repair, significantly affecting patients' quality of life by impairing speech and eating functions and increasing the risk of respiratory infections [1]. The development of these fistulas results from a combination of anatomical and procedural factors. The primary causes of fistula formation include the type and extent of the cleft, surgical technique and operator experience, and biological factors.

Patients with complete cleft palates, classified as Veau classifications III and IV, and those with concurrent cleft lip are more prone to fistula development [2]. A wider cleft increases the tension at the closure site, potentially leading to wound dehiscence [3].

Additionally, the choice of closure method and the surgeon's skill are crucial [4]. Less experienced surgeons may inadequately assess the tissue tension or improperly prepare flaps, increasing the risk of complications [5]. Biological factors such as insufficient vascularization of tissues, the presence of scars from previous surgeries, and infections can adversely affect the healing process, promoting fistula formation [6].

Various surgical methods are employed to close oronasal fistulas. Local mucoperiosteal flaps utilize adjacent tissues to cover the defect. While suitable for smaller fistulas, they may have a high recurrence rate in cases of large defects or scarred tissues [7]. Tongue flaps involve the use of well-vascularized flaps from the tongue to close large fistulas. Although effective, they can cause patient discomfort and require a longer healing period [8]. Tissue grafts, such as fascia lata or dermal fat grafts, allow for the closure of defects when local tissues are insufficient [9]. Alloplastic materials and biomaterials, including collagen membranes, titanium meshes, or bone substitutes, can support tissue regeneration and provide additional structural support [10]. Microvascular and endoscopic techniques represent modern methods that enable the precise closure of fistulas with minimal invasiveness; an example is endoscope-assisted repair using a graft from the inferior turbinate [11].

Despite the availability of numerous methods, the recurrence rate of fistulas remains significant, reaching up to 68% in some adult patient groups [1]. Factors contributing to recurrences include tension at the closure site, insufficient vascularization, the presence of scars and previous surgeries, and postoperative infections [12]. Excessive tension can lead to wound edge separation, while poor blood supply limits the healing capacity [13]. Scar tissue can hinder tissue mobilization and affect elasticity, and a wound infection can cause dehiscence and the formation of new fistulas [14].

There is a clear need for developing new, more effective methods for closing oronasal fistulas that minimize the risk of recurrence and improve both the functional and aesthetic outcomes. In response to these challenges, we present an innovative endoscopic technique for closing recurrent oronasal fistulas in cleft patients termed the "Parachute Technique". The aim of this method is to enhance the treatment efficacy through a novel surgical approach that minimizes invasiveness and supports natural healing processes.

2. Procedure Description

Below is a detailed description of the Parachute Technique, an endoscopic method developed for closing recurrent oronasal fistulas in cleft palate patients. A video recording of the entire procedure is provided, and each step is illustrated with intraoperative figures (Figure 1).

1. Identification of the Oronasal Fistula

The procedure begins by inserting a sterile probe through the oral cavity into the oronasal fistula to precisely determine its location and size. Simultaneously, a 0-degree or 30-degree rigid endoscope is introduced into the nasal cavity. Using the endoscope, the surgeon locates the tip of the probe protruding through the fistula, allowing visualization of the defect from both sides.

2. Preparation of the Nasal Cavity

The area around the fistula in the nasal cavity is thoroughly cleaned using saline irrigation to remove mucus, debris, and any crusts. Granulation or scar tissue around the edges of the fistula is gently removed using a microdebrider under endoscopic control. Local vasoconstrictive agents, such as adrenaline-soaked tampons, or electrocautery are applied to minimize bleeding during the procedure.

3. Excision of the Inferior Nasal Turbinate

Under endoscopic guidance, the inferior nasal turbinate on the side of the fistula is identified.

Optionally, the inferior turbinate on the contralateral side may be selected if it is larger and more suitable for reconstruction. Using microsurgical instruments, the inferior nasal turbinate is excised at its base, separating it from the lateral wall of the nasal cavity. The excised turbinate is carefully removed through the anterior nostril and placed on the operating table outside the nasal cavity for further preparation.

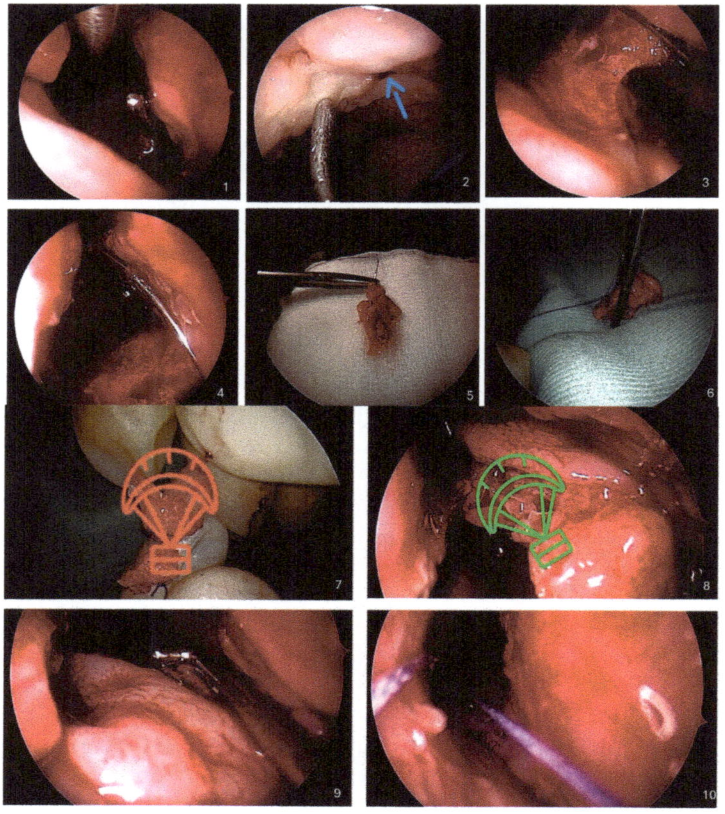

Figure 1. A step-by-step illustration of the "Parachute Technique" for closing a recurrent oronasal fistula in patients with cleft palate, comprising ten sequential images: (**1**,**2**) Identification of the oronasal fistula: The introduction of a sterile probe through the oral cavity into the oronasal fistula to precisely determine its location and size. Simultaneously, an endoscope is inserted into the nasal cavity to visualize the tip of the probe protruding through the fistula from both sides. (**3**) Preparation of the nasal cavity: Thorough cleaning of the area around the fistula in the nasal cavity using saline irrigation to remove mucus, debris, and any crusts. Granulation or scar tissue around the edges of the fistula is gently removed under endoscopic control. (**4**) Passing the needle: Insertion of a sterile needle through the fistula from the oral cavity into the nasal cavity using a guidewire. The needle is advanced through the nasal cavity and exited through the anterior nostril. (**5**–**7**) Preparation of the flap from the inferior nasal turbinate: The identification and excision of the inferior nasal turbinate under endoscopic guidance. The excised turbinate is prepared by partially separating the mucous membrane from its bony part without complete detachment, allowing it to be unfolded into a "parachute" shape. The needle is passed through the excised turbinate, piercing it to half its thickness. (**8**,**9**) Placement and securing of the flap: The needle is carefully withdrawn back through the anterior nostril, nasal cavity, and fistula into the oral cavity, pulling the prepared flap along with it. Under endoscopic control, the flap is positioned to provide full and even coverage of the fistula edges, with the mucosal surface facing the nasal cavity. The flap is secured in place and a guide suture is fixed to the oral cavity. (**10**) Application of a silicone dressing: A thin layer of medical-grade silicone or a silicone stent is applied to the nasal side of the flap to protect it, stabilize it, and prevent the formation of adhesions in the nasal cavity.

4. Preparation of the Flap from the Inferior Nasal Turbinate

Using a guidewire, a sterile needle is inserted through the fistula from the oral cavity into the nasal cavity. The needle is then advanced through the nasal cavity and exited through the anterior nostril. The needle is passed through the excised inferior nasal turbinate, piercing it to half its thickness. Without completely detaching it, the mucous membrane of the inferior nasal turbinate is gently partially separated from its bony part. This partial separation allows the mucous membrane to be unfolded, forming a "parachute" shape.

5. Transposition of the Flap Through the Fistula

The needle is carefully withdrawn back through the anterior nostril, nasal cavity, and fistula into the oral cavity, pulling the flap of the inferior nasal turbinate along with it. In this way, the flap is transposed through the fistula from the nasal cavity into the oral cavity. The surgeon ensures that the mucosal 'parachute' is properly positioned, with the mucosal surface facing the nasal cavity, while the bony parts of the inferior turbinate effectively plug the fistula channel.

6. Securing the Flap

Under endoscopic guidance, the flap position is carefully adjusted to ensure complete and uniform coverage of the fistula margins. Any folds or creases that could impede the healing process are meticulously avoided. The flap is anchored in place by fixing an absorbable guiding suture of the parachute flap to the mucosa of the oral cavity near the fistula's ostium. Ensuring the flap is tension-free is essential for adequate vascularization and optimal healing.

7. Application of Silicone Dressing

A thin layer of medical-grade silicone or a silicone stent is placed on the nasal aspect of the flap. This dressing serves to protect and stabilize the flap while preventing adhesion formation within the nasal cavity. The silicone dressing is carefully shaped to conform to the nasal anatomy without obstructing the airflow and is anchored with nonabsorbable sutures at the base of the nasal vestibule. If necessary, gentle packing is also applied to further support the structure.

8. Postoperative Management

The patient is instructed to gently cleanse the nasal cavity with saline sprays or irrigations to maintain moisture and prevent crusting. A soft diet is recommended, and activities that could increase nasal pressure, such as nose blowing or strenuous physical exertion, should be avoided. Prophylactic antibiotics are prescribed to minimize the risk of infection, and analgesics are provided as needed for pain management. Regular follow-up appointments are scheduled to monitor the healing progress and evaluate the success of the procedure. The silicone stent is removed after 14 days, with endoscopic examinations performed as necessary.

Remarks

The procedure is performed under general anesthesia with endotracheal intubation, ensuring patient safety and optimal surgical conditions. Strict aseptic conditions are maintained throughout the procedure to minimize the risk of infection. Gentle handling of the mucous membrane and bony tissue is crucial to preserve their integrity and viability. This technique is particularly useful for patients with recurrent fistulas where previous methods have failed and there is a need for an alternative approach.

3. Discussion

Closing recurrent oronasal fistulas in patients with cleft palate presents a significant surgical challenge due to scar tissue formation, the limited availability of healthy tissues, and a high risk of recurrence [9]. The introduction of the Parachute Technique offers a novel approach to addressing these difficult cases. This method involves utilizing the excised inferior nasal turbinate to create a mucosal flap shaped like a "parachute," which is then transposed through the fistula using a guidewire and needle. By employing the patient's own tissues, this technique allows for a multilayered closure of the defect, promoting better healing and integration with surrounding structures.

One of the primary advantages of the Parachute Technique is the use of autologous tissues. Employing the patient's own mucosal and bony tissues eliminates the risk of immunological reactions and rejection, which can enhance the healing process and improve the long-term success of the repair [8]. Additionally, the technique is minimally invasive due to the use of endoscopic guidance. This allows for precise manipulation within a confined surgical field, minimizing damage to adjacent tissues and reducing postoperative morbidity [11].

The effectiveness of this method is particularly notable in difficult cases where traditional techniques have failed. Patients with recurrent fistulas, especially those complicated by scar tissue from previous surgeries, may benefit significantly from this approach. The technique avoids the need to harvest tissues from distant donor sites, thereby reducing additional trauma and potential complications in other areas of the body. Furthermore, the multilayered closure provided by the Parachute Technique promotes faster tissue regeneration and decreases the risk of residual fistula formation, potentially leading to improved patient outcomes. An additional advantage of the Parachute Technique is its role in preventing ascending infections of the nasal cavity and paranasal sinuses. By effectively sealing the oronasal communication, the technique limits the transfer of oral flora, food debris, and liquids into the nasal passages. This is particularly relevant in patients with a profoundly altered oral ecosystem, which is often observed in individuals with long-standing or recurrent fistulas. In such cases, chronic exposure of the nasal cavity to microbial and enzymatic agents originating from the oral environment significantly increases the risk of local inflammation and secondary infection. By restoring anatomical separation between the oral and nasal compartments, the technique helps re-establish the local microbiological balance and promotes long-term mucosal health.

However, several limitations and drawbacks of the Parachute Technique should be considered. This procedure demands advanced endoscopic skills and proficiency in instrument manipulation within a confined surgical field, requiring a level of expertise that may not be available in all centers, thereby potentially limiting its widespread adoption. Collaboration between specialists from various fields, such as maxillofacial surgery, plastic surgery, and ENT, could help address this challenge. Furthermore, the precision and delicacy required during the procedure can extend the operation time compared with traditional techniques, increasing the overall burden on both the patient and the surgical team.

Anatomical variations or previous surgical interventions may also pose challenges. In some patients, the inferior nasal turbinate may not be suitable for excision or use as a flap, limiting the applicability of the technique [15]. Additionally, although the inferior nasal turbinate is not considered a critical structure, its removal can lead to nasal function disorders, such as mucosal dryness, epistaxis, or alterations in nasal airflow patterns [16]. These potential complications necessitate careful patient selection and thorough preoperative evaluation.

The requirement for specialized equipment is another consideration. The necessity of using an endoscope and specific surgical instruments may present challenges in facilities with limited access to modern medical technology [14]. This factor could impede the implementation of the Parachute Technique in resource-constrained settings, where traditional methods might remain the standard of care.

In conclusion, the Parachute Technique represents a promising alternative for the treatment of recurrent oronasal fistulas in patients with a cleft palate. Its main advantages include the utilization of autologous tissues, minimal invasiveness, and effectiveness in challenging cases where other methods have failed. Nevertheless, to facilitate the broader adoption of this technique, it is essential to acknowledge and address its limitations. These include the need for advanced endoscopic skills, potential complications associated with the removal of the inferior nasal turbinate, and the requirement for specialized equipment. Ongoing research, along with targeted training programs for surgeons, may help optimize the technique and expand its applicability in clinical practice. By carefully weighing the benefits against the drawbacks, clinicians can make informed decisions about incorporating the Parachute Technique into their surgical repertoire for the management of recurrent oronasal fistulas.

4. Conclusions

In conclusion, the Parachute Technique offers a promising alternative for the treatment of recurrent oronasal fistulas in cleft palate patients. By addressing many of the challenges associated with traditional surgical methods, it aims to enhance the treatment efficacy, reduce the recurrence rates, and improve both the functional and aesthetic outcomes. With further research and training, this technique has the potential to become a valuable addition to clinical practice, contributing to better patient outcomes and satisfaction.

Author Contributions: Conceptualization, A.Z., O.K. and P.B.; methodology, A.Z., O.K. and P.B.; validation, A.Z., O.K. and P.B.; formal analysis, O.K.; investigation, A.Z. and P.B.; resources, A.Z. and P.B.; writing—original draft preparation, O.K.; writing—review and editing, O.K , A.Z. and P.B.; visualization, O.K.; supervision, P.B.; project administration, A.Z. All authors have read and agreed to the published version of the manuscript.

Funding: This research received no external funding.

Institutional Review Board Statement: Ethical review and approval were waived for this study due to the fact that it does not constitute a research study involving human subjects, but rather describes a surgical technique applied during a standard therapeutic procedure in an individual patient.

Informed Consent Statement: Written informed consent has been obtained from the patient.

Data Availability Statement: No new data were created or analyzed in this study. Data sharing is not applicable to this article.

Acknowledgments: A complete visual presentation of the Parachute Technique, including intraoperative video and illustrations, is available from the corresponding author upon reasonable request.

Conflicts of Interest: The authors declare no conflicts of interest.

References

1. Cohen, S.R.; Kalinowski, J.; LaRossa, D.; Randall, P. Cleft palate fistulas: A multivariate statistical analysis of prevalence, etiology, and surgical management. *Plast. Reconstr. Surg.* **1991**, *87*, 1041–1047. [CrossRef] [PubMed]
2. Murrell, G.L.; Requena, R.; Karakla, D.W. Oronasal Fistula Repair with Three Layers. *Plast. Reconstr. Surg.* **2001**, *107*, 143–147. [CrossRef] [PubMed]
3. Parwaz, M.A.; Sharma, R.K.; Parashar, A.; Nanda, V.; Biswas, G.; Makkar, S. Width of cleft palate and postoperative palatal fistula–do they correlate? *J. Plast. Reconstr. Aesthetic Surg.* **2009**, *62*, 1559–1563. [CrossRef] [PubMed]

4. Muzaffar, A.R.; Byrd, S.H.; Rohrich, R.J.; Johns, D.F.; LeBlanc, D.; Beran, S.J.; Anderson, C.; Papaioannou, A. Incidence of Cleft Palate Fistula: An Institutional Experience with Two-Stage Palatal Repair. *Plast. Reconstr. Surg.* **2001**, *108*, 1515–1518. [CrossRef] [PubMed]
5. Gamble, C.; Persson, C.; Willadsen, E.; Albery, L.; Andersen, H.S.; Antoneli, M.Z.; Appelqvist, M.; Aukner, R.; Bodling, P.; Bowden, M. Timing of Primary Surgery for Cleft Palate. *N. Engl. J. Med.* **2023**, *389*, 795–807. [CrossRef] [PubMed]
6. Honnebier, M.B.O.M.; Johnson, D.S.; Parsa, A.A.; Dorian, A.; Parsa, F.D. Closure of Palatal Fistula with a Local Mucoperiosteal Flap Lined with Buccal Mucosal Graft. *Cleft Palate Craniofacial J.* **2000**, *37*, 127–129. [CrossRef] [PubMed]
7. Posnick, J.C.; Getz, S.B. Surgical closure of end-stage palatal fistulas using anteriorly-based dorsal tongue flaps. *J. Oral. Maxillofac. Surg.* **1987**, *45*, 907–912. [CrossRef] [PubMed]
8. Diah, E.; Lo, L.J.; Yun, C.; Wang, R.; Wahyuni, L.K.; Chen, Y.R. Cleft oronasal fistula: A review of treatment results and a surgical management algorithm proposal. *Change Gung Med. J.* **2007**, *30*, 529–537.
9. Sadhu, P. Oronasal fistula in cleft palate surgery. *Indian J. Plast. Surg.* **2009**, *42* (Suppl. 1), S123–S128. [CrossRef]
10. Cole, P.; Horn, T.W.; Thaller, S. Use Decellularized Dermal Grafting (AlloDerm) Persistent Oro-Nasal Fistulas After Tert. Cleft Palate Repair. *J. Craniofacial Surg.* **2006**, *17*, 636–641. [CrossRef]
11. Kim, B.Y.; Seo, B.F. Endoscope-Assisted Multilayered Repair in Oronasal Fistula. *Ear Nose Throat J.* **2023**, *102*, 268–271. [CrossRef]
12. Pinborough-Zimmerman, J.; Canady, C.; Yamashiro, D.K.; Morales, L. Articulation and Nasality Changes Resulting from Sustained Palatal Fistula Obturation. *Cleft Palate Craniofacial J.* **1998**, *35*, 81–87. [CrossRef]
13. Bajaj, A.K.; Wongworawat, A.A.; Punjabi, A. Management of Alveolar Clefts. *J. Craniofacial Surg.* **2003**, *14*, 840–846. [CrossRef]
14. Khojasteh, A.; Kheiri, L.; Motamedian, S.R.; Nadjmi, N. Regenerative medicine in the treatment of alveolar cleft defect: A systematic review of the literature. *J. Cranio-Maxillofac. Surg.* **2015**, *43*, 1608–1613. [CrossRef] [PubMed]
15. Borba, A.M.; Borges, A.H.; Da Silva, C.S.V.; Brozoski, M.A.; Naclério-Homem, M.D.G.; Miloro, M. Predictors of complication for alveolar cleft bone graft. *Br. J. Oral Maxillofac. Surg.* **2014**, *52*, 174–178. [CrossRef] [PubMed]
16. Bittermann, G.K.P.; Van Es, R.J.J.; De Ruiter, A.P.; Frank, M.H.; Bittermann, A.J.N.; van der Molen, A.B.M.; Koole, R.; Rosenberg, A.J.W.P. Incidence of complications in secondary alveolar bone grafting of bilateral clefts with premaxillary osteotomy: A retrospective cohort study. *Clin. Oral Investig.* **2020**, *24*, 915–925. [CrossRef] [PubMed]

Journal of
Clinical Medicine

MDPI

Article

Evaluation of GDF15 Significance as a Biomarker in Laryngeal Squamous Cell Carcinoma

Aleksandra Romanowicz [1], Oskar Komisarek [1,2,*], Anna Klimaszewska-Wiśniewska [3], Paulina Antosik [3], Kacper Naglik [3], Joanna Czech [1], Witold Wrzesiński [1], Marta Kodzik [1,2], Magdalena Bodnar [4], Dariusz Grzanka [3] and Paweł Burduk [1,2]

1 Department of Otolaryngology, Laryngological Oncology and Maxillofacial Surgery, University Hospital, 85-168 Bydgoszcz, Poland; romanowicz.aleks@gmail.com (A.R.); otolaryngologia@biziel.pl (J.C.); wiwrz@tlen.pl (W.W.); kodzik@poczta.onet.eu (M.K.); pburduk@wp.pl (P.B.)
2 Department of Otolaryngology, Phoniatrics and Audiology, Faculty of Medicine, Collegium Medicum, Nicolaus Copernicus University in Toruń, 87-100 Toruń, Poland
3 Department of Clinical Pathomorphology, Collegium Medicum in Bydgoszcz, Nicolaus Copernicus University in Toruń, 87-100 Toruń, Poland; ania.klimaszewska@op.pl (A.K.-W.); paulina.antosik@cm.umk.pl (P.A.); kapi.n@wp.pl (K.N.); d_grzanka@cm.umk.pl (D.G.)
4 Department of Obstetrics, Women's Diseases and Gynaecological Oncology, Collegium Medicum in Bydgoszcz, Nicolaus Copernicus University in Toruń, 87-100 Toruń, Poland; magdalena.bodnar@cm.umk.pl
* Correspondence: oskar.komisarek@cm.umk.pl

Simple Summary: Laryngeal squamous cell carcinoma (LSCC) is a common head and neck cancer with limited survival rates despite advances in treatment options. Identifying reliable biomarkers could improve early diagnosis and treatment outcomes. In this study, we investigated the growth differentiation factor 15 (GDF15), a protein with roles in various cancers, to determine its significance in LSCC. By analyzing tissue samples from patients and public datasets, we assessed whether GDF15 expression correlated with clinical factors and survival outcomes. Our findings suggest that GDF15 may serve as a prognostic biomarker for LSCC, potentially aiding in patient stratification and treatment planning. This research contributes to a better understanding of GDF15's role in cancer and highlights its potential utility in improving LSCC management. Future studies could build on these insights to explore GDF15's role as a therapeutic target.

Abstract: Background/Objectives: Laryngeal squamous cell carcinoma (LSCC) is a common malignancy with unsatisfactory survival rates, highlighting the need for reliable biomarkers to improve its diagnosis and prognosis. Growth differentiation factor 15 (GDF15), a protein implicated in various cancers, has not been thoroughly investigated in LSCC. This study aimed to evaluate the significance of GDF15 expression in LSCC by integrating immunohistochemical analysis of archival tissue samples with RNA sequencing data from public databases (TCGA and GEO) to provide comprehensive clinical insights. **Methods**: We analyzed archival tissue samples from 65 patients with LSCC using immunohistochemistry and evaluated GDF15 expression profiles from The Cancer Genome Atlas (TCGA) and Gene Expression Omnibus (GEO) datasets. Statistical analyses included Kaplan–Meier survival analysis and Cox proportional hazards regression to assess the correlation between GDF15 expression, clinicopathological variables, and survival outcomes. **Results**: GDF15 expression did not significantly differ between tumor and adjacent normal tissues. However, in the tissue macroarray (TMA) cohort, high GDF15 expression was significantly associated with a lower TNM stage and less advanced pT status. Kaplan–Meier analysis revealed that high GDF15 expression correlated with reduced overall survival in the TMA cohort, suggesting its utility in risk stratification. Multivariate analysis identified GDF15 as an independent prognostic factor for disease-free survival in

LSCC. **Conclusions**: Our findings suggest that GDF15 may serve as a prognostic biomarker for LSCC, particularly in early-stage disease. Elevated GDF15 levels, which are associated with poorer overall survival, could be integrated into diagnostic panels to enhance risk stratification and inform treatment decisions. Furthermore, GDF15 may be a promising target for therapeutic intervention. Further research is warranted to validate these results and explore their potential in clinical practice.

Keywords: laryngeal squamous cell carcinoma; GDF15; tissue macroarrays; immunohistochemistry

1. Introduction

Laryngeal carcinoma is the second most common malignancy of the aerodigestive tract, comprising approximately 20% of head and neck cancers. It occurs nearly five times more frequently in men than in women. The vast majority of cases are squamous cell carcinomas (LSCC), with tobacco and alcohol consumption being the most significant risk factors [1–5]. Patients are frequently diagnosed at an advanced stage, and the 5-year survival rate remains around 65% [3]. Despite the availability of radiotherapy and systemic treatments, surgery continues to be a cornerstone of management, depending on the disease stage and local extension.

Due to the still unsatisfactory prognosis, there is a pressing need to identify novel and reliable biomarkers to improve risk stratification and guide therapeutic decisions. Currently used biomarkers, such as p16, EGFR, and HPV status, often lack sensitivity and specificity. Growth differentiation factor 15 (GDF15), a divergent member of the TGF-β superfamily, has emerged as a potential candidate biomarker because of its involvement in inflammation, cellular stress response, and tumor progression [6–8].

GDF15, also known as MIC-1, PLAB, or PDF, is encoded on chromosome 19p12–13 and plays a pleiotropic role in multiple tissues, including the placenta, liver, kidney, and macrophages. It exerts both pro- and anti-tumorigenic effects, depending on the cancer type and tumor microenvironment [8,9]. Mechanistically, GDF15 engages multiple signaling pathways, including ERK, PI3K/AKT, and MAPK, and is a transcriptional target of p53 [8]. Overexpression of this gene has been observed in several cancers, including breast, cervix, prostate, colon, and oral cavity cancers, and is often associated with poor prognosis [10–19].

However, the role of GDF15 in laryngeal squamous cell carcinoma remains unexplored. This study aimed to comprehensively evaluate the clinical significance of this association in LSCC. By integrating immunohistochemical analyses of tumor tissue with transcriptomic data from TCGA and GEO, we aimed to assess the diagnostic and prognostic potential of GDF15 in this type of cancer. The rationale for selecting GDF15 stems from its emerging role in tumor progression, immune modulation, and cancer-related systemic effects such as cachexia. While GDF15 has been implicated in various malignancies, including prostate, pancreatic, and gastric cancers, its role in LSCC remains unexplored. Our study is the first to systematically evaluate GDF15 expression in LSCC using both protein and mRNA-level analyses, addressing a significant knowledge gap in biomarker research for this cancer type.

2. Materials and Methods

2.1. Patients and Tissue Material

The study was conducted using archival formalin-fixed, paraffin-embedded (FFPE) tissue samples obtained between 2016 and 2020 from patients diagnosed with laryngeal squamous cell carcinoma (LSCC) at the Department of Otolaryngology, Oncological Laryngology, and Maxillofacial Surgery, University Hospital No. 2, Bydgoszcz, and the Department of Clinical Pathomorphology, Collegium Medicum in Bydgoszcz, Nicolaus Copernicus University, Toruń, Poland. The diagnosis was confirmed by two independent pathologists using hematoxylin and eosin (H&E)-stained sections.

A total of 85 patients were initially screened. Twenty patients were excluded: 10 due to prior oncologic treatment, 5 due to the presence of carcinoma in situ or a second primary tumor, and 5 due to the absence of tumor cells on immunohistochemical staining. This resulted in a final study cohort of 65 patients, referred to as the tissue macroarray (TMA) cohort.

Tumor samples were reclassified according to the AJCC 8th edition TNM criteria to ensure consistency. Adjacent non-tumorous tissues (NATs) were collected from all surgical specimens; however, only 21 NAT samples met the predefined quality thresholds ($\geq$70% epithelial cellularity and preserved morphology). Samples that failed to meet these criteria were excluded due to tissue degradation, fragmentation, or insufficient epithelial content. All NATs included in the final analysis were histologically confirmed to be free of malignant cells.

The clinicopathological data of the 65 patients are presented in Table 1. The study protocol was approved by the Bioethics Committee of Collegium Medicum in Bydgoszcz of Nicolaus Copernicus University in Toruń (KB 58/2022) and was conducted in accordance with the Declaration of Helsinki.

Table 1. Association of GDF15 with clinicopathological variables in the TMA cohort.

Variable	*n* (%)	GDF15 Low	GDF15 High	*p*-Value
Demographic variables				
Age (years) $\leq$ 60	17 (26.15)	7 (41.18)	10 (58.82)	>0.999
Age (years) > 60	48 (73.85)	21 (43.75)	27 (56.25)	>0.999
Gender: Male	55 (84.62)	22 (40.00)	33 (60.00)	0.306
Gender: Female	10 (15.38)	6 (60.00)	4 (40.00)	0.306
Tumor characteristics				
Tumor grade G1	16 (24.62)	6 (37.50)	10 (62.50)	0.854
Tumor grade G2	45 (69.23)	20 (44.44)	25 (55.56)	0.854
Tumor grade G3	4 (6.15)	2 (50.00)	2 (50.00)	0.854
pT status T1	32 (49.23)	8 (25.00)	24 (75.00)	0.020
pT status T2	23 (35.39)	14 (60.87)	9 (39.13)	0.020
pT status T3–T4	10 (15.38)	6 (60.00)	4 (40.00)	0.020
pN status N0	52 (80.00)	20 (38.46)	32 (61.54)	0.210
pN status N1–N2	13 (20.00)	8 (61.54)	5 (38.46)	0.210
Resection margin: negative	50 (76.92)	23 (46.00)	27 (54.00)	0.554
Resection margin: positive	15 (23.08)	5 (33.33)	10 (66.67)	

2.2. Survival Definitions

Overall survival (OS) was defined as the time from the date of curative surgery to death from any cause. Disease-free survival (DFS) was defined as the time from the date of curative surgery to the time of relapse or death. OS and DFS data were censored for patients who were alive at the last follow-up (11 January 2023). The median follow-up time, calculated using the reverse Kaplan–Meier method, was 49 months for OS and 46 months for DFS.

2.3. Tissue Macroarray Construction and Immunohistochemistry

Formalin-fixed, paraffin-embedded (FFPE) tissue samples were used to construct tissue macroarrays (TMA). Representative tumor areas with $\geq$80% tumor cell content were identified on hematoxylin and eosin (H&E) stained slides. Tissue cores were extracted and inserted into recipient blocks, which were sectioned at 3 μm using a rotary microtome and placed on high-adhesive, glass slides.

Immunohistochemical (IHC) staining was performed using an automated BenchMark® Ultra platform (Roche Diagnostics/Ventana Medical Systems, Tucson, AZ, USA) and the UltraView DAB detection system. The sections were incubated with a rabbit polyclonal anti-GDF15 antibody (HPA011191, Sigma-Aldrich, St. Louis, MO, USA) at 1:150 dilution for 32 min. Positive and negative controls were also included.

Two independent pathologists evaluated GDF15 protein expression using a modified immunoreactive score (IRS), which was calculated by multiplying the staining intensity (0–3) by the percentage of positive cells (0–4). The average of three randomly selected fields at 20× magnification was used. Expression was dichotomized into low (IRS < 4) and high (IRS ≥ 4) groups based on the Evaluate Cutpoints software.

2.4. Extraction of RNA Sequencing TCGA Data and Clinical Information

RNA sequencing data (DESeq2 normalized counts) for GDF15 expression in 116 LSCC tissues and 12 adjacent tissues were downloaded from The Cancer Genome Atlas (TCGA) using the University of California Santa Cruz (UCSC) Xena Browser (https://xenabrowser.net/, accessed on 10 February 2023), whereas corresponding clinical information was retrieved from cBioPortal (https://www.cbioportal.org, accessed on 10 February 2023). The clinical endpoints were OS and DFS. The former was defined as the time from the date of curative surgery to the time of death from any cause, while the latter was defined as the time from the date of curative surgery to the time of recurrence or progression. Overall survival and DFS data were available for 116 (100%) and 87 (75%) patients. GDF15 expression levels were categorized into low- and high-level groups based on the optimal cut-off values determined using the Evaluate Cutpoints software [20]. The cut-off values for OS and DFS were 9.731 (<9.731, low expression; ≥9.731, high expression) and 7.217 (<7.217, low expression; ≥7.217, high expression), respectively. The median OS and DFS in the TCGA cohort were 65 and 76 months, respectively. Due to methodological and technical differences between datasets, different cut-off values were applied to define high versus low GDF15 expression in each cohort. In the TMA cohort, protein expression was dichotomized using Evaluate Cutpoints software based on IRS values to maximize prognostic discrimination. In the TCGA cohort, two separate optimal thresholds were generated using the same software: 9.731 for overall survival (OS) and 7.217 for disease-free survival (DFS). These values reflect differences in the expression distribution and survival-specific risk stratification.

In the GEO microarray datasets, which contained normalized gene expression values with distinct dynamic ranges, median expression values were used as cut-offs for dichotomization. Although this introduces variability, each cut-off was statistically validated within its respective dataset. As the datasets differ in platform (IHC vs. RNA-Seq vs. microarray) and data structure, internal validation was deemed most appropriate to preserve prognostic value while avoiding artificial harmonization across biologically distinct data types.

2.5. GEO Data Collection

The expression levels of GDF15 were extracted from the Gene Expression Omnibus (GEO) database through the ShinyGEO web-based application (http://gdancik.github.io/shinyGEO/, accessed on 13 March 2023) [20]. Five GEO datasets for LSCC: GSE25727 [21], GSE27020 [22], GSE59102 [23], GSE117973 [24,25], and GSE51985 [26] were included. If several probes were mapped to GDF15, the mean value was used as the final expression of this gene. In addition, GEO data were used as an independent validation of our GDF15 expression results. Due to the limited number of clinical samples available in our study (65 LSCC cases and only 21 NAT samples), integrating publicly available GEO datasets allowed us to extend our analysis and compare our findings with those from independent cohorts. This approach enabled a more comprehensive evaluation of the relationship between GDF15 expression and clinical parameters, thereby strengthening the overall interpretation of our results.

2.6. Statistical Analysis

All statistical analyses were performed using GraphPad Prism (version 8.0, GraphPad Software, San Diego, CA, USA), SPSS (version 28.0, IBM Corporation, Armonk, NY, USA), or RStudio (version 1.3.1093) software packages. GraphPad Prism was used for descriptive statistics, normality testing (Shapiro–Wilk test), and group comparisons (Mann–Whitney U test and chi-squared test). SPSS was used for univariable and multivariable Cox proportional hazards regression analyses, including the backward elimination method and multiple imputation of missing data. Kaplan–Meier survival curves and log-rank tests were generated using SPSS. RStudio was used for additional data visualization and handling. The optimal expression thresholds for GDF15 were determined using the Evaluate Cutpoints software. Data distribution was determined using the Shapiro–Wilk test, and appropriate parametric or nonparametric statistical tests were applied. Overall survival (OS) was defined as the time from the date of curative surgery to death from any cause. Disease-free survival (DFS) was defined as the time from the date of curative surgery to the time of relapse or death. Patients who were alive at the last follow-up (11 January 2023) were censored. The median follow-up times, calculated using the reverse Kaplan–Meier method, were 49 months for OS and 46 months for DFS. The Kaplan–Meier method and log-rank test were used to depict and compare unadjusted survival curves for OS and DFS. Univariable and multivariable Cox proportional hazards regression analyses were conducted to explore the predictors of survival by estimating the hazard ratios (HR) and 95% confidence intervals (CI). A backward elimination procedure was used to build all multivariable models, with a significance level of $p < 0.2$ to enter the model and $p \leq 0.05$ to stay. The proportional hazard assumption was verified by testing for significant interactions when each variable was entered as a time-based covariate. In the TCGA cohort, multiple imputation of missing variables for the Cox proportional hazards models was used to adjust for the bias of missing data; however, variables with amounts of missing data over 20% were not considered for the model. It was assumed that the missing data for the predictor variables occurred randomly. Combined estimates were obtained from 10 imputed datasets. To enhance clarity and underscore the methodological innovation of our study, we added a schematic overview (Figure 1) that illustrates the integrative design of our approach. This schematic outlines the parallel analysis of protein-level data (IHC from the TMA cohort) and transcriptomic-level data (RNA sequencing from TCGA and microarray from GEO), demonstrating how these independent sources complement each other to reinforce the validity and robustness of our findings. By integrating immunohistochemical profiling with large-scale public datasets, our design enabled cross-platform validation and highlighted the clinical relevance of GDF15 expression in LSCC from multiple analytical perspectives. Associations were considered statistically significant if the two-sided p-value was <0.05.

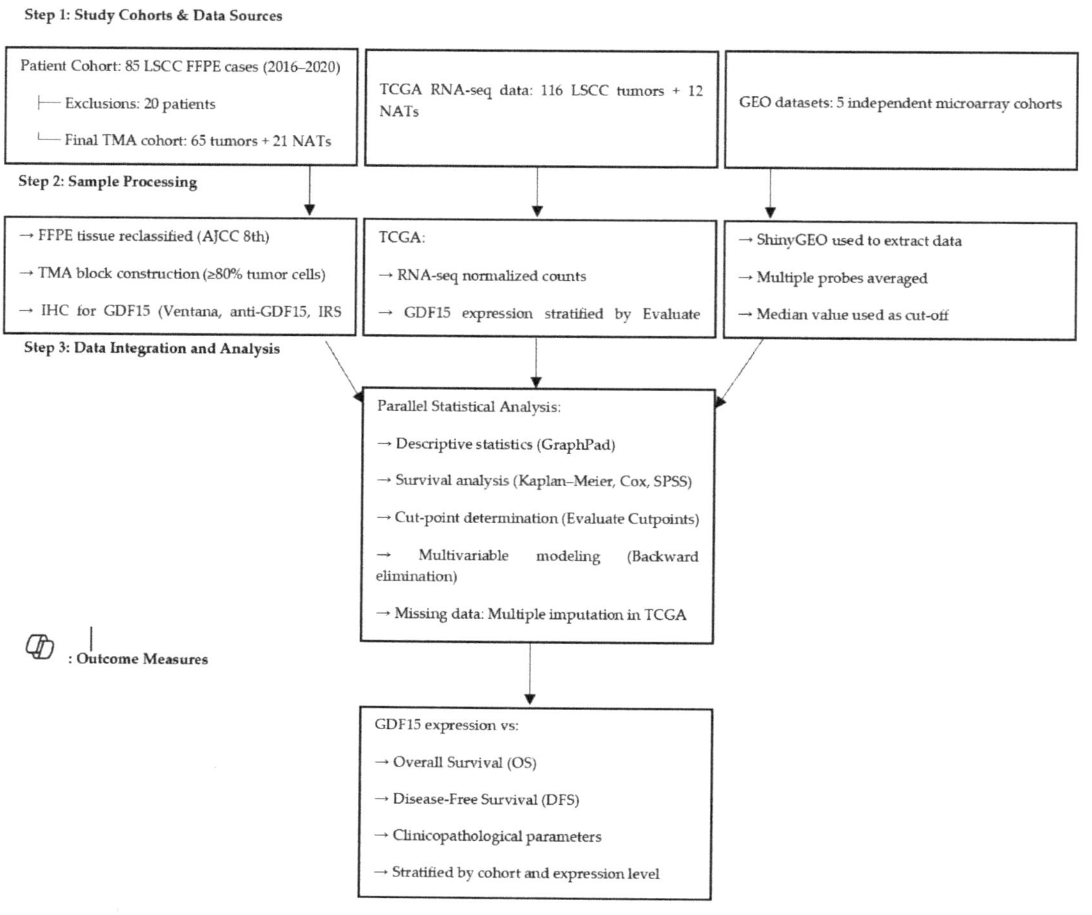

Figure 1. Schematic representation of the study design. The workflow integrates immunohistochemistry (IHC) data from the TMA cohort (n = 65 tumor samples, n = 21 normal adjacent tissues) with transcriptomic datasets from TCGA (RNA sequencing) and GEO (microarray). This multi-platform approach was used to evaluate the prognostic significance of GDF15 in laryngeal squamous cell carcinoma (LSCC), allowing for cross-cohort and cross-platform validation.

3. Results

3.1. *Immunohistochemical Analysis of GDF15 Expression Comparing Tumor Tissue with Adjacent Normal Tissue*

At the protein level, GDF15 expression, assessed by immunohistochemistry (IHC), revealed primarily cytoplasmic staining at any level of expression intensity in tumor tissues and non-tumor tissues adjacent to the tumor. Representative IHC images demonstrated the variation in GDF15 staining intensity between the tumor tissues (Figure 2). However, tumor tissues showed a more heterogeneous and often stronger staining pattern than adjacent normal tissues. Additionally, the staining pattern observed in the tumor tissues exhibited significant heterogeneity, with variations in the intensity across different regions of the same sample. Although representative IHC images (Figure 2) demonstrated a stronger and more heterogeneous GDF15 staining pattern in tumor tissues than in adjacent normal tissues, the difference was not statistically significant. This discrepancy may be attributed to the relatively small number of high-quality NAT samples (n = 21), which limits the statistical power. Moreover, the semi-quantitative IRS scoring system used in this study, although standardized and widely applied, may not fully capture subtle differences in staining intensity and distribution across heterogeneous tumor regions. Finally, interindividual variability in baseline GDF15 expression among non-neoplastic tissues could further dilute the overall statistical differences between groups.

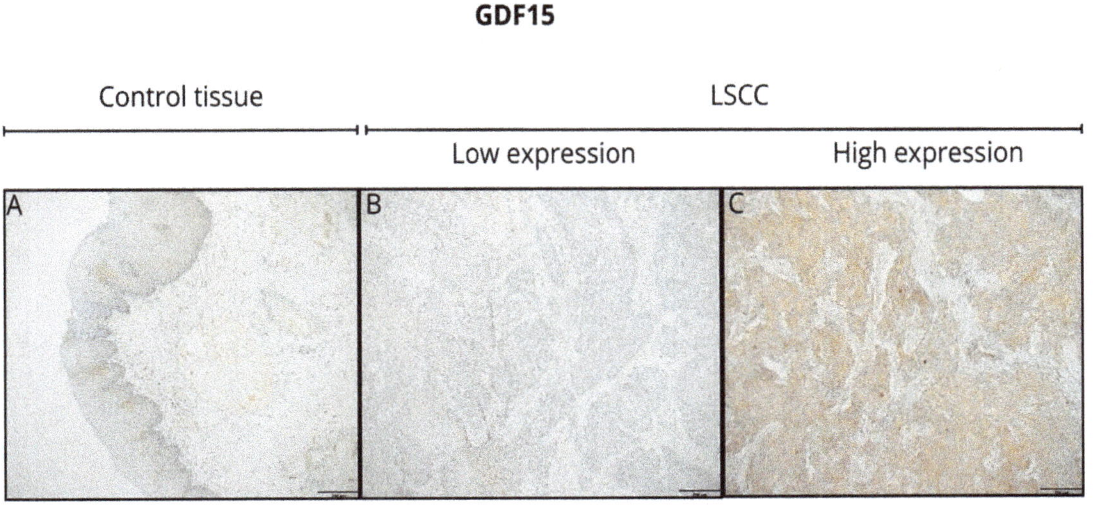

Figure 2. Representative images of immunohistochemical expression of GDF15 in laryngeal squamous cell carcinoma (LSCC) (**B**,**C**) and histologically normal tissue adjacent to the tumor (control tissue) (**A**). Original magnification: 10×. Scale bar = 200 µm.

3.2. Comparison of GDF15 Expression Between Tumor Tissue and Non-Tumor Tissue in TMA and Publicly Available Cohorts

There was no statistically significant difference in GDF15 expression between tumor and non-tumor tissues at either the protein or mRNA expression levels (Figure 3). Boxplot graphs in Figure 2 illustrate GDF15 expression levels in tumor tissue versus histologically normal tissue across various cohorts, including the institutional TMA, TCGA, and GEO datasets.

3.3. Stratified Analysis by Clinical and Lifestyle Variables

To assess the potential impact of key clinical and lifestyle factors on GDF15 expression, we performed subgroup analyses stratifying the data by sex, smoking status, and alcohol consumption status. These analyses did not reveal any statistically significant differences in GDF15 expression between subgroups ($p > 0.05$). Based on these findings, we combined the groups for further analyses. This result confirmed that the influence of these factors on GDF15 expression in our cohort was negligible.

3.4. Association Between GDF15 Expression and Clinicopathological Variables in TMA and TCGA Cohorts

After data dichotomization according to the established cut-off values, the TMA cohort included 28 (43.08%) samples with low and 37 (56.92%) samples with high GDF15 expression, and the TCGA cohort included 89 (76.72%) samples with low and 27 (23.28%) samples with high gene expression.

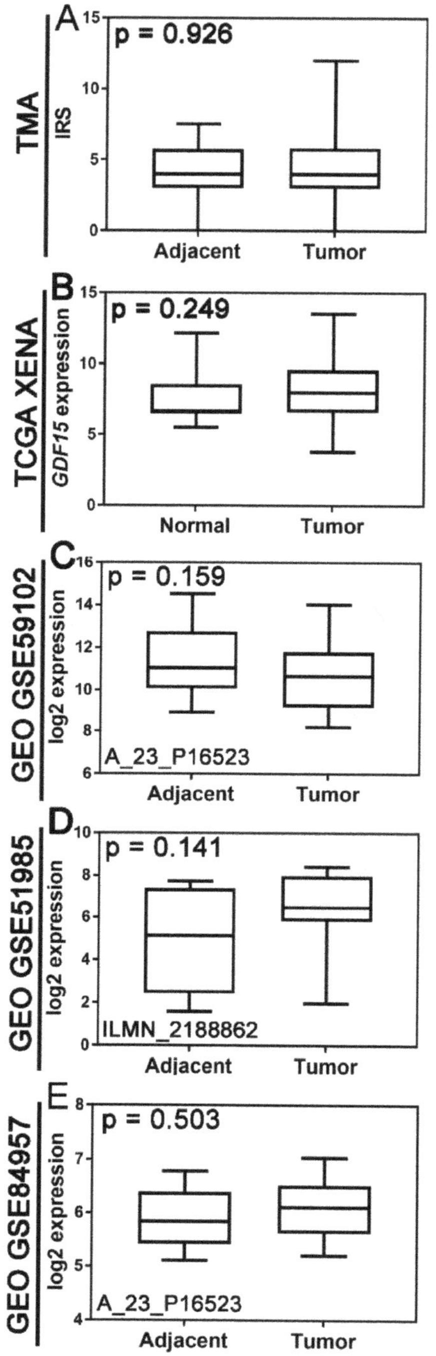

Figure 3. Expression of GDF15 in laryngeal squamous cell carcinoma compared to non-cancerous control tissue. Boxplot graphs of (**A**) GDF15 expression in tumor tissue (n = 65) and histologically normal tissue adjacent to the tumor (n = 21) of the institutional tissue microarray (TMA) cohort based on immunohistochemistry (IHC); (**B**) GDF15 expression levels in tumor tissue (n = 116) and normal solid tissue (n = 11) based on RNA-seq data from The Cancer Genome Atlas (TCGA) and Genotype-

Tissue Expression (GTEx) databases, respectively, downloaded from the UCSC Xena Browser. **(C)** GDF15 expression in tumor tissue (n = 29) and histologically normal tissue adjacent to the tumor (n = 13) based on gene chip data derived from the Gene Expression Omnibus (GEO) database using the ShinyGEO web-based tool. The GSE number and probe information are provided. **(D)** GDF15 expression in tumor tissue (n = 10) and corresponding adjacent non-neoplastic tissue (n = 10) based on gene chip data derived from the Gene Expression Omnibus (GEO) database using the ShinyGEO web-based tool. The GSE number and probe information are provided. **(E)** GDF15 expression in tumor tissue (n = 9) and corresponding adjacent non-neoplastic tissue (n = 9) based on gene chip data derived from the Gene Expression Omnibus (GEO) database using the ShinyGEO web-based tool. The GSE number and probe information are provided.

In the TMA LSCC cohort (Table 1), high GDF15 expression was significantly associated with less advanced pT stages (p = 0.02). Moreover, high GDF15 expression was significantly associated with a lower TNM stage (p = 0.019). A statistically significant relationship was also observed between GDF15 expression and the location of the primary tumor.

In the TCGA cohort, there were no statistically significant differences in clinicopathological variables depending on the GDF15 expression status (Table 2). However, the association between GDF15 expression and N status was of borderline statistical significance (p = 0.047; Table 2).

Table 2. Association of GDF15 with clinicopathological variables in the TCGA cohort.

Variable	*n* (%)	GDF15 Low	GDF15 High	*p*-Value
Demographic variables				
Age < 60	40 (34.48)	33 (82.50)	7 (17.50)	0.358
Age ≥ 60	76 (65.52)	56 (73.68)	20 (26.32)	
Male	96 (82.76)	74 (77.08)	22 (22.92)	0.780
Female	20 (17.24)	15 (75.00)	5 (25.00)	
Tumor grade				
G1	8 (6.90)	7 (87.50)	1 (12.50)	0.111
G2	71 (61.21)	50 (70.42)	21 (29.58)	
G3–G4	33 (28.45)	29 (87.88)	4 (12.12)	
N/A	4 (3.45)	–	–	
T status				
T1	7 (6.03)	5 (71.43)	2 (28.57)	0.966
T2	20 (17.24)	15 (75.00)	5 (25.00)	
T3	33 (28.45)	25 (75.76)	8 (24.24)	
T4	56 (48.28)	44 (78.57)	12 (21.43)	
N status				
N0	52 (44.83)	35 (67.31)	17 (32.69)	**0.047**
N1–N2	63 (54.31)	53 (84.13)	10 (15.87)	
N/A	1 (0.86)	–	–	
TNM stage				
I–II	15 (12.93)	10 (66.67)	5 (33.33)	0.327
III	19 (16.38)	13 (68.42)	6 (31.58)	
IV	82 (70.69)	66 (80.49)	16 (19.51)	
Lymphovascular invasion				
No	42 (36.21)	33 (78.57)	9 (21.43)	>0.999
Yes	36 (31.03)	28 (77.78)	8 (22.22)	
N/A	38 (32.76)	–	–	
Alcohol consumption				
No	39 (33.62)	33 (84.62)	6 (15.38)	0.240
Yes	75 (64.66)	55 (73.33)	20 (26.67)	
N/A	2 (1.72)	–	–	

3.5. Relationships to Survival

In Kaplan–Meier survival analysis of the TMA cohort, high GDF15 expression was significantly associated with reduced overall survival (OS) compared with low GDF15 expression (median OS: not reached vs. not reached; log-rank p = 0.004; Figure 4A), although there was no significant difference in disease-free survival (DFS) (median DFS: not reached vs. not reached; log-rank p = 0.188; Figure 4B). Furthermore, in the TCGA Xena and GEO cohorts, high GDF15 expression was not significantly associated with worse OS or DFS (Figure 4C–F). In the GEO cohort (Figure 4F), no significant association was observed between GDF15 expression and survival (p = 0.231).

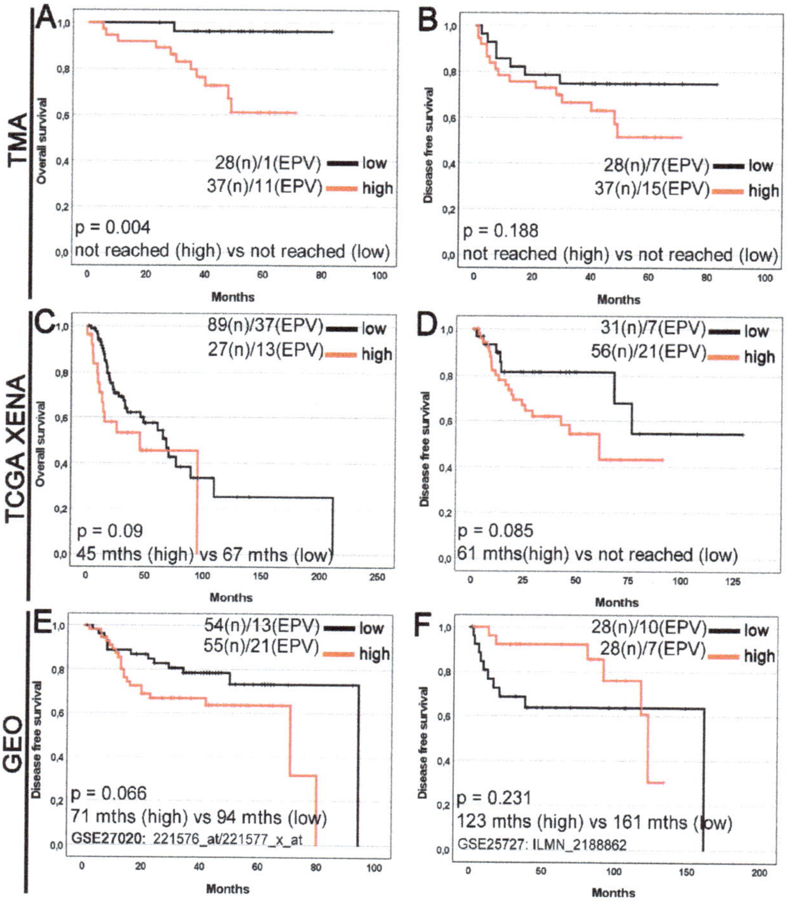

Figure 4. Kaplan–Meier curves for the overall survival (**A**,**C**) and disease-free survival (**B**,**D**–**F**) of laryngeal squamous cell carcinoma patients stratified by GDF15 expression. The survival curves were plotted based on the (**A**,**B**) immunohistochemistry data for the tissue microarray (TMA) cohort; gene expression levels for (**C**,**D**) The Cancer Genome Atlas (TCGA) dataset downloaded from the UCSC Xena Browser; (**E**,**F**) the Gene Expression Omnibus (GEO) datasets downloaded from the ShinyGEO web-based tool (the GSE number and probe information are shown). The cases were divided into two expression groups (low and high) according to (**A**–**D**) the optimal cut-off point determined by the Evaluate Cutpoints software and (**E**,**F**) the median expression. The results are shown with median OS or DFS (in months; abbreviated as mths) for high and low expression groups, as well as the p-value from the log-rank test. The number of cases (n) and events (EPV) in the low- and high-expression groups are displayed.

The area under the prognostic ROC curve for GDF15 as a prognostic marker for OS in the TMA cohort was 0.71, with an asymptotic p-value of 0.004 (Figure 5).

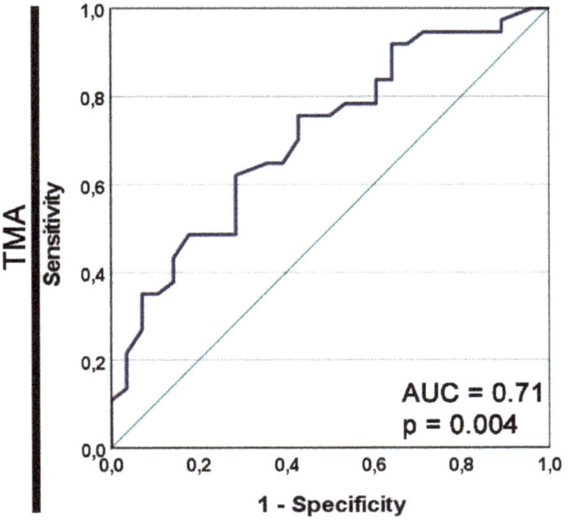

Figure 5. Receiver operating characteristic (ROC) curve for GDF15 as a prognostic marker for overall survival in the tissue microarray (TMA) cohort. The asymptotic p-value of the ROC curve is shown. AUC, area under the ROC curve.

As presented in Table 3, a univariate analysis of DFS in the TMA cohort indicated statistically significant univariable hazard ratios (HRs) for positive resection margins (HR 2.52, 95% CI 1.05–6.04, $p = 0.038$) and pT2 stage (HR 2.65, 95% CI 1.03–6.86, $p = 0.044$). In the multivariate Cox regression model, high GDF15 expression remained an independent predictor of disease-free survival (HR 2.98; 95% CI 1.16–7.65; $p = 0.023$). This suggests that elevated GDF15 levels may identify patients at an increased risk of recurrence, regardless of the tumor stage.

Table 3. Univariable and Multivariable Cox Regression Analyses for Disease-Free Survival in TMA Cohort.

Variable	*n*/EPV	Univariable HR	95% CI	*p*	Multivariable HR	95% CI	*p*
			Lower–Upper			Lower–Upper	
GDF15 (high vs. low)	37/15–28/7	1.81	0.74–4.43	0.197	**2.98**	**1.16–7.65**	**0.023**
TNM stage							
I (reference)	30/6	REF.	–	–	REF.	–	–
II vs. I	17/8	2.92	1.01–8.43	0.048	**4.64**	**1.53–14.13**	**0.007**
III–IV vs. I	18/8	2.23	0.77–6.44	0.138	**3.13**	**1.06–9.27**	**0.040**

Abbreviations: HR—hazard ratio; CI—confidence interval; EPV—events per variable; REF.—reference category; GDF15—growth differentiation factor 15; TNM—tumor-node-metastasis.

Additionally, TNM stage II (HR 4.64; 95% CI 1.53–14.13; $p = 0.007$) and stages III–IV (HR 3.13; 95% CI 1.06–9.27; $p = 0.04$) were also significantly associated with reduced DFS, confirming the expected clinical progression patterns. Notably, other variables included in the model were eliminated during backward selection due to a lack of statistical significance and were therefore excluded from the final model.

In the TCGA cohort, multivariate analysis revealed that sex (HR 0.30; 95% CI 0.15–0.59; $p = 0.0006$) and tumor grade G2 (HR 4.83; 95% CI 1.14–20.43; $p = 0.032$) were independent predictors of overall survival. Female patients and those with lower-grade tumors exhibited better prognoses, in line with established clinical expectations (Table 4).

Table 4. Univariable and multivariable Cox analyses of overall survival (n = 116) and disease-free survival (n = 87) in the TCGA cohort.

Outcome	Variable	Multivariable HR	95% CI	p
Overall Survival				
Sex (male vs. female)		0.30	0.15–0.59	0.0006
Tumor grade (G2 vs. G1)		4.83	1.14–20.43	0.032
	G3–G4 vs. G1	2.13	0.47–9.70	0.326
Disease-Free Survival				
N stage (N1–N3 vs. N0)		2.69	1.14–6.35	0.024

Abbreviations: HR—hazard ratio; CI—confidence interval.

The only independent predictor of disease-free survival was lymph node status. Patients with N1–N3 disease had significantly worse DFS (HR 2.69; 95% CI 1.14–6.35; p = 0.024), underscoring the prognostic importance of nodal involvement in LSCC.

4. Discussion

Growth differentiation factor 15 (GDF15) is a peptide hormone belonging to the transforming growth factor beta (TGFβ) superfamily that exhibits diverse physiological and pathological effects across multiple contexts. Under physiological conditions, GDF15 is present in various human tissues, including the placenta, liver, prostate, bladder, kidneys, colon, and endometrium, although in small quantities. Elevated serum concentrations of GDF15 have been associated with various malignancies, indicating its potential utility as a diagnostic biomarker for neoplastic diseases [7,25]. The pleiotropic effects of this protein have spurred extensive research into its role in the formation and progression of malignant tumors, as well as its involvement in cancer metastasis. Previous studies evaluating GDF15 as a marker for malignant tumors and metastasis diagnosis prompted us to investigate its expression in patients with laryngeal squamous cell carcinoma (LSCC). To our knowledge, this is the first study to evaluate GDF15 expression in LSCC, and our findings further support its potential as a prognostic biomarker.

In our study, we demonstrated that the lack of a statistically significant difference in GDF15 expression between tumor tissue and normal tissue adjacent to the tumor may suggest similar levels of activity of this protein in both types of tissue. However, it is important to consider the potential differences in cellular composition and microenvironment present in these two types of tissues, which could influence the interpretation of the results. The associations between GDF15 expression and clinical variables, such as T feature and TNM stage, exhibited variations between the tissue microarray (TMA) and The Cancer Genome Atlas (TCGA) cohorts, as indicated by the data dichotomization and analysis presented earlier. The TMA cohort assessed protein expression levels, whereas the TCGA and GEO cohorts measured molecular levels, that is, gene/mRNA expression levels. In the TMA cohort, consisting of 28 samples with low gene expression and 37 samples with high gene expression, the frequency of high and low GDF15 protein expression significantly differed in relation to the T feature according to the pT status and TNM stage. Notably, patients with stage I disease demonstrated a higher prevalence of high GDF15 protein expression than low expression levels. Conversely, no statistically significant differences in clinicopathological variables were observed in the TCGA cohort. The significant association between high GDF15 expression and poorer overall survival in patients with laryngeal squamous cell carcinoma, predominantly observed in the tissue microarray (TMA) dataset, may suggest the potential prognostic value of this protein. Third, methodological differences between the assessment of protein expression in the TMA cohort and mRNA expression in the TCGA and GEO datasets could also contribute to these discrepant findings. Finally, the relatively small sample size of our cohort may limit the statistical power, thereby affecting the interpretation of survival outcomes. However, the lack of significant differences in disease-free survival across all datasets necessitates further analysis, considering additional prognostic factors. The absence of a statistically significant difference in GDF15 expression between tumors and adjacent normal tissues does not negate its prognostic utility. This suggests that the prognostic relevance of GDF15 may stem from its functional role in the tumor microenvironment and systemic signaling, rather than its differential abundance alone. This pattern has also been observed for other biomarkers, where clinical outcomes are more tightly associated with systemic or functional effects than with absolute expression differences. The trends approaching statistical significance in DFS and overall survival observed in the TCGA and GEO datasets suggest the potential broader significance of GDF15 expression in cancer prognosis. Analysis of these trends indicates that higher levels of GDF15 may be associated with worse survival outcomes, which could have significant clinical implications. However, it is important to note that the significant association between high GDF15 expression and reduced overall survival was observed exclusively in the TMA cohort and not replicated in the TCGA or GEO datasets. This lack of validation across independent cohorts limits the generalizability of our findings and suggests that the prognostic value of GDF15 may be context-dependent or influenced by methodological factors, such as protein-level versus transcript-level assessment, cohort size, or clinical heterogeneity.

Moreover, the TMA cohort revealed a paradoxical pattern in which high GDF15 expression was associated with less advanced TNM and pT stages—typically linked to better prognosis—yet correlated with worse overall survival. This apparent contradiction may reflect the pleiotropic nature of GDF15, which not only marks local tumor behavior but may also indicate systemic effects, such as inflammation, cachexia, or immune modulation, that contribute to poorer outcomes independently of tumor stage.

These findings underscore the complex interplay of GDF15 in laryngeal squamous cell carcinoma and highlight the need for comprehensive investigations. Future studies with larger cohorts and robust event data are necessary to confirm these results, precisely delineate the prognostic role of GDF15, and explore its potential application in clinical practice.

Clinical studies have indicated its involvement in promoting metastasis [6,27]. Moreover, GDF15 expression is correlated with decreased survival in cancer patients, particularly in laryngeal squamous cell carcinoma, highlighting its potential prognostic value [6]. Additionally, the concentration of this marker has been shown to be significant in colorectal [28,29], gastric [30,31], pancreatic [32,33], breast [34,35], and prostate cancers [36,37]. However, to better understand the role of GDF15 as a prognostic biomarker, further research is needed, considering methodological limitations and other prognostic factors. Despite these limitations, our results suggest that GDF15 could be an important prognostic factor in various types of cancer, with significant clinical implications for cancer treatment and patient care.

The paradoxical observation that high GDF15 expression in the TMA cohort is associated with less advanced TNM and pT stages yet correlates with poorer overall survival, may also reflect the systemic effects of GDF15 that are not directly captured by local tumor characteristics. GDF15 acts as a stress-response cytokine and has been implicated in tumor-induced metabolic dysregulation, particularly anorexia and cachexia. Elevated circulating levels of GDF15 have been shown to contribute to weight loss, muscle wasting, and impaired tolerance to treatment, all of which may negatively affect overall survival, independent of tumor burden [38–42]. Thus, it is possible that increased GDF15 expression reflects an aggressive tumor phenotype associated with systemic catabolic effects, which could partly explain the discrepancy between the lower TNM stage and poor prognosis in our cohort.

This study had several limitations that must be acknowledged. First, the cohort size was very small, which reduced the statistical power and generalizability of our findings. Second, the low number of events per variable precluded us from performing Cox proportional hazards analysis in relation to overall survival time. These limitations underscore the need for caution when drawing definitive conclusions. Future studies with larger cohorts and more robust event data are necessary to validate our findings and provide more comprehensive insights into the role of GDF15 as a prognostic biomarker for laryngeal squamous cell carcinoma.

Our findings provide novel prognostic insights beyond the currently used LSCC biomarkers, such as EGFR, p16, and HPV status, which often lack consistency across cohorts. In contrast, GDF15 was independently associated with disease-free survival in multivariable models. This suggests that GDF15 may capture unique biological processes potentially related to tumor-induced systemic effects that are not reflected by traditional histopathological or molecular markers. Based on our findings, GDF15 shows potential as a prognostic biomarker in LSCC, as its elevated expression correlates with poor overall survival. Its integration into diagnostic panels could facilitate more accurate risk stratification and early detection of aggressive disease phenotypes when combined with other established markers. Furthermore, given its involvement in tumor progression and systemic effects, such as cachexia and metabolic dysregulation, targeting GDF15 or its downstream pathways may offer a novel therapeutic strategy. Future studies are warranted to evaluate the feasibility and clinical efficacy of incorporating GDF15 into routine diagnostic workflows and as a potential target for therapeutic intervention in LSCC.

We refined our study parameters, rationale, and methods to enhance the clarity and robustness of our findings. Detailed justifications for the sample selection, data analysis, and clinical relevance of GDF15 are provided throughout the manuscript, thereby strengthening the validity of our results and the overall solidity of the study.

5. Conclusions

The study results showed no significant difference in GDF15 expression between the tumor and adjacent normal tissues. However, variability in GDF15 expression was observed in relation to clinical variables exclusively in the TMA cohort. Although elevated GDF15 levels were significantly associated with poorer overall survival in the TMA cohort, this finding was not consistently replicated in the TCGA and GEO datasets. Therefore, although GDF15 may have prognostic potential, its utility as a robust biomarker requires further validation in larger, independent, and clinically diverse populations.

Author Contributions: Conceptualization: A.R., O.K., and P.A.; Methodology: A.R. and P.A.; Validation: P.A.; Formal analysis: A.K.-W.; Investigation: J.C., M.K., W.W., K.N., M.B. and D.G.; Resources: A.R., J.C., M.K., P.B., and W.W.; Data curation: K.N.; Writing—original draft: O.K., A.R.; Writing—review & editing: O.K., A.R. and P.A.; Visualization: P.A., K.N. and J.C.; Project administration: A.R.; Supervision: P.B. and M.B.; Funding acquisition: D.G. All authors have read and agreed to the published version of the manuscript.

Funding: This research received no external funding.

Institutional Review Board Statement: The study was conducted in accordance with the Declaration of Helsinki and approved by the Institutional Review Board of the Nicolaus Copernicus University in Toruń, Collegium Medicum in Bydgoszcz (protocol code KB 58/2022, approved on 18 January 2022, valid until the end of 2025).

Informed Consent Statement: This study did not involve identifiable human participants, and therefore, written informed consent for publication was not required.

Data Availability Statement: Data supporting the reported results are available from the corresponding author upon reasonable request.

Acknowledgments: The authors thank the Department of Pathomorphology for providing materials and laboratory assistance.

Conflicts of Interest: The authors declare no conflicts of interest.

Abbreviations

The following abbreviations are used in this manuscript:

AJCC	American Joint Committee on Cancer
DFS	Disease-Free Survival
FFPE	Formalin-Fixed, Paraffin-Embedded
GDF15	Growth Differentiation Factor 15
GEO	Gene Expression Omnibus
GTEx	Genotype-Tissue Expression
HR	Hazard Ratio
IHC	Immunohistochemistry
IRS	Immunoreactive Score
LSCC	Laryngeal Squamous Cell Carcinoma
N/A	Not Available
OS	Overall Survival
ROC	Receiver Operating Characteristic
TCGA	The Cancer Genome Atlas
TGF-β	Transforming Growth Factor Beta
TMA	Tissue Macroarray

References

1. Hoffman, H.T.; Karnell, L.H.; Funk, G.F.; Robinson, R.A.; Menck, H.R. The National Cancer Data Base Report on Cancer of the Head and Neck. *Arch. Otolaryngol. Neck Surg.* **1998**, *124*, 951. [CrossRef]
2. Chu, E.A.; Kim, Y.J. Laryngeal Cancer: Diagnosis and Preoperative Work-Up. *Otolaryngol. Clin. N. Am.* **2008**, *41*, 673–695. [CrossRef]
3. Steuer, C.E.; El-Deiry, M.; Parks, J.R.; Higgins, K.A.; Saba, N.F. An Update on Larynx Cancer. *CA Cancer J. Clin.* **2017**, *67*, 31–50. [CrossRef] [PubMed]
4. Wang, X.; Bi, Y.; Liu, G.; Wang, W.; Cui, H. Smoking and Alcohol Consumption with the Risk of 11 Common Otolaryngological Diseases: A Bidirectional Mendelian Randomization. *Eur. Arch. Otorhinolaryngol.* **2023**, *280*, 5615–5623. [CrossRef]
5. Saad, M.A.; Kuo, S.Z.; Rahimy, E.; Zou, A.E.; Korrapati, A.; Rahimy, M.; Kim, E.; Zheng, H.; Yu, M.A.; Wang-Rodriguez, J.; et al. Alcohol-Dysregulated miR-30a and miR-934 in Head and Neck Squamous Cell Carcinoma. *Mol. Cancer* **2015**, *14*, 181. [CrossRef] [PubMed]
6. Li, Y.-L.; Chang, J.T.; Lee, L.-Y.; Fan, K.-H.; Lu, Y.-C.; Li, Y.-C.; Chiang, C.-H.; You, G.-R.; Chen, H.-Y.; Cheng, A.-J. GDF15 Contributes to Radioresistance and Cancer Stemness of Head and Neck Cancer by Regulating Cellular Reactive Oxygen Species via a SMAD-Associated Signaling Pathway. *Oncotarget* **2017**, *8*, 1508–1528. [CrossRef]
7. Ahmed, D.S.; Isnard, S.; Lin, J.; Routy, B.; Routy, J.-P. GDF15/GFRAL Pathway as a Metabolic Signature for Cachexia in Patients with Cancer. *J. Cancer* **2021**, *12*, 1125–1132. [CrossRef]
8. Corre, J.; Hébraud, B.; Bourin, P. Concise Review: Growth Differentiation Factor 15 in Pathology: A Clinical Role? *Stem Cells Transl. Med.* **2013**, *2*, 946–952. [CrossRef]
9. Adela, R.; Banerjee, S.K. GDF-15 as a Target and Biomarker for Diabetes and Cardiovascular Diseases: A Translational Prospective. *J. Diabetes Res.* **2015**, *2015*, 490842. [CrossRef]
10. Mullican, S.E.; Lin-Schmidt, X.; Chin, C.-N.; Chavez, J.A.; Furman, J.L.; Armstrong, A.A.; Beck, S.C.; South, V.J.; Dinh, T.Q.; Cash-Mason, T.D.; et al. GFRAL Is the Receptor for GDF15 and the Ligand Promotes Weight Loss in Mice and Nonhuman Primates. *Nat. Med.* **2017**, *23*, 1150–1157. [CrossRef]
11. Wischhusen, J.; Melero, I.; Fridman, W.H. Growth/Differentiation Factor-15 (GDF-15): From Biomarker to Novel Targetable Immune Checkpoint. *Front. Immunol.* **2020**, *11*, 951. [CrossRef]

12. Au Yeung, S.L.; Luo, S.; Schooling, C.M. The Impact of GDF-15, a Biomarker for Metformin, on the Risk of Coronary Artery Disease, Breast and Colorectal Cancer, and Type 2 Diabetes and Metabolic Traits: A Mendelian Randomisation Study. *Diabetologia* **2019**, *62*, 1638–1646. [CrossRef] [PubMed]
13. Li, L.; Zhang, R.; Yang, H.; Zhang, D.; Liu, J.; Li, J.; Guo, B. GDF15 Knockdown Suppresses Cervical Cancer Cell Migration In Vitro Through the TGF-β/Smad2/3/Snail1 Pathway. *FEBS Open Bio* **2020**, *10*, 2750–2760. [CrossRef] [PubMed]
14. Sadasivan, S.M.; Chen, Y.; Gupta, N.S.; Han, X.; Bobbitt, K.R.; Chitale, D.A.; Williamson, S.R.; Rundle, A.G.; Tang, D.; Rybicki, B.A. The Interplay of Growth Differentiation Factor 15 (GDF15) Expression and M2 Macrophages during Prostate Carcinogenesis. *Carcinogenesis* **2020**, *41*, 1074–1082. [CrossRef]
15. Ma, J.; Tang, X.; Sun, W.; Liu, Y.; Tan, Y.; Ma, H.; Zhu, D.; Wang, M.; Wang, L.; Li, J.; et al. Mutant GDF15 Presents a Poor Prognostic Outcome for Patients with Oral Squamous Cell Carcinoma. *Oncotarget* **2016**, *7*, 2113–2122. [CrossRef]
16. Klimaszewska-Wiśniewska, A.; Neska-Długosz, I.; Buchholz, K.; Durślewicz, J.; Grzanka, D.; Kasperska, A.; Antosik, P.; Zabrzyński, J.; Grzanka, A.; Gagat, M. Prognostic Significance of KIF11 and KIF14 Expression in Pancreatic Adenocarcinoma. *Cancers* **2021**, *13*, 3017. [CrossRef]
17. Buchholz, K.; Antosik, P.; Grzanka, D.; Gagat, M.; Smolińska, M.; Grzanka, A.; Gzil, A.; Kasperska, A.; Klimaszewska-Wiśniewska, A. Expression of the Body-Weight Signaling Players: GDF15, GFRAL and RET and Their Clinical Relevance in Gastric Cancer. *J. Cancer* **2021**, *12*, 4698–4709. [CrossRef]
18. Remmele, W.; Stegner, H.E. Recommendation for uniform definition of an immunoreactive score (IRS) for immunohistochemical estrogen receptor detection (ER-ICA) in breast cancer tissue. *Pathologe* **1987**, *8*, 138–140.
19. Ogłuszka, M.; Orzechowska, M.; Jędroszka, D.; Witas, P.; Bednarek, A.K. Evaluate Cutpoints: Adaptable Continuous Data Distribution System for Determining Survival in Kaplan-Meier Estimator. *Comput. Methods Programs Biomed.* **2019**, *177*, 133–139. [CrossRef]
20. Dumas, J.; Gargano, M.A.; Dancik, G.M. *shinyGEO*: A Web-Based Application for Analyzing Gene Expression Omnibus Datasets. *Bioinformatics* **2016**, *32*, 3679–3681. [CrossRef]
21. Fountzilas, E.; Markou, K.; Vlachtsis, K.; Nikolaou, A.; Arapantoni-Dadioti, P.; Ntoula, E.; Tassopoulos, G.; Bobos, M.; Konstantinopoulos, P.; Fountzilas, G.; et al. Identification and Validation of Gene Expression Models That Predict Clinical Outcome in Patients with Early-Stage Laryngeal Cancer. *Ann. Oncol.* **2012**, *23*, 2146–2153. [CrossRef]
22. Fountzilas, E.; Kotoula, V.; Angouridakis, N.; Karasmanis, I.; Wirtz, R.M.; Eleftheraki, A.G.; Veltrup, E.; Markou, K.; Nikolaou, A.; Pectasides, D.; et al. Identification and Validation of a Multigene Predictor of Recurrence in Primary Laryngeal Cancer. *PLoS ONE* **2013**, *8*, e70429. [CrossRef]
23. Plaça, J.R.; Bueno, R.D.B.E.L.; Pinheiro, D.G.; Panepucci, R.A.; De Araújo, L.F.; Mamede, R.C.M.; Figueiredo, D.L.A.; Silva, W.A. Gene Expression Analysis of Laryngeal Squamous Cell Carcinoma. *Genom. Data* **2015**, *5*, 9–12. [CrossRef] [PubMed]
24. Mock, A.; Plath, M.; Moratin, J.; Tapken, M.J.; Jäger, D.; Krauss, J.; Fröhling, S.; Hess, J.; Zaoui, K. EGFR and PI3K Pathway Activities Might Guide Drug Repurposing in HPV-Negative Head and Neck Cancers. *Front. Oncol.* **2021**, *11*, 678966. [CrossRef]
25. Metzger, K.; Moratin, J.; Freier, K.; Hoffmann, J.; Zaoui, K.; Plath, M.; Stögbauer, F.; Freudlsperger, C.; Hess, J.; Horn, D. A Six-Gene Expression Signature Related to Angiolymphatic Invasion Is Associated with Poor Survival in Laryngeal Squamous Cell Carcinoma. *Eur. Arch. Otorhinolaryngol.* **2021**, *278*, 1199–1207. [CrossRef]
26. Lian, M.; Fang, J.; Han, D.; Ma, H.; Feng, L.; Wang, R.; Yang, F. Microarray Gene Expression Analysis of Tumorigenesis and Regional Lymph Node Metastasis in Laryngeal Squamous Cell Carcinoma. *PLoS ONE* **2013**, *8*, e84854. [CrossRef]
27. Siddiqui, J.A.; Pothuraju, R.; Khan, P.; Sharma, G.; Muniyan, S.; Seshacharyulu, P.; Jain, M.; Nasser, M.W.; Batra, S.K. Pathophysiological Role of Growth Differentiation Factor 15 (GDF15) in Obesity, Cancer, and Cachexia. *Cytokine Growth Factor Rev.* **2022**, *64*, 71–83. [CrossRef]
28. Zhang, Y.; Wang, X.; Zhang, M.; Zhang, Z.; Jiang, L.; Li, L. GDF15 Promotes Epithelial-to-Mesenchymal Transition in Colorectal [Corrected]. *Artif. Cells Nanomed. Biotechnol.* **2018**, *46*, 652–658. [CrossRef]
29. Mehta, R.S.; Chong, D.Q.; Song, M.; Meyerhardt, J.A.; Ng, K.; Nishihara, R.; Qian, Z.; Morikawa, T.; Wu, K.; Giovannucci, E.L.; et al. Association Between Plasma Levels of Macrophage Inhibitory Cytokine-1 Before Diagnosis of Colorectal Cancer and Mortality. *Gastroenterology* **2015**, *149*, 614–622. [CrossRef]
30. Han, M.; Dai, D.; Yousafzai, N.A.; Wang, F.; Wang, H.; Zhou, Q.; Lu, H.; Xu, W.; Feng, L.; Jin, H.; et al. CXXC4 Activates Apoptosis through Up-Regulating GDF15 in Gastric Cancer. *Oncotarget* **2017**, *8*, 103557–103567. [CrossRef]
31. Guo, J.; Bian, Y.; Wang, Y.; Chen, L.; Yu, A.; Sun, X. S100A4 Influences Cancer Stem Cell-like Properties of MGC803 Gastric Cancer Cells by Regulating GDF15 Expression. *Int. J. Oncol.* **2016**, *49*, 559–568. [CrossRef] [PubMed]
32. Kaur, S.; Chakraborty, S.; Baine, M.J.; Mallya, K.; Smith, L.M.; Sasson, A.; Brand, R.; Guha, S.; Jain, M.; Wittel, U.; et al. Potentials of Plasma NGAL and MIC-1 as Biomarker(s) in the Diagnosis of Lethal Pancreatic Cancer. *PLoS ONE* **2013**, *8*, e55171. [CrossRef]
33. Yang, Y.; Yan, S.; Tian, H.; Bao, Y. Macrophage Inhibitory Cytokine-1 versus Carbohydrate Antigen 19-9 as a Biomarker for Diagnosis of Pancreatic Cancer: A PRISMA-Compliant Meta-Analysis of Diagnostic Accuracy Studies. *Medicine* **2018**, *97*, e9994. [CrossRef] [PubMed]

34. Peake, B.F.; Eze, S.M.; Yang, L.; Castellino, R.C.; Nahta, R. Growth Differentiation Factor 15 Mediates Epithelial Mesenchymal Transition and Invasion of Breast Cancers through IGF-1R-FoxM1 Signaling. *Oncotarget* **2017**, *8*, 94393–94406. [CrossRef]
35. Gkretsi, V.; Stylianou, A.; Kalli, M.; Louca, M.; Voutouri, C.; Zaravinos, A.; Stylianopoulos, T. Silencing of Growth Differentiation Factor-15 Promotes Breast Cancer Cell Invasion by Down-Regulating Focal Adhesion Genes. *Anticancer Res.* **2020**, *40*, 1375–1385. [CrossRef]
36. Zhao, L.; Lee, B.Y.; Brown, D.A.; Molloy, M.P.; Marx, G.M.; Pavlakis, N.; Boyer, M.J.; Stockler, M.R.; Kaplan, W.; Breit, S.N.; et al. Identification of Candidate Biomarkers of Therapeutic Response to Docetaxel by Proteomic Profiling. *Cancer Res.* **2009**, *69*, 7696–7703. [CrossRef]
37. Li, J.; Veltri, R.W.; Yuan, Z.; Christudass, C.S.; Mandecki, W. Macrophage Inhibitory Cytokine 1 Biomarker Serum Immunoassay in Combination with PSA Is a More Specific Diagnostic Tool for Detection of Prostate Cancer. *PLoS ONE* **2015**, *10*, e0122249. [CrossRef]
38. Lerner, L.; Hayes, T.G.; Tao, N.; Krieger, B.; Feng, B.; Wu, Z.; Nicoletti, R.; Chiu, M.I.; Gyuris, J.; Garcia, J.M. Plasma Growth Differentiation Factor 15 Is Associated with Weight Loss and Mortality in Cancer Patients. *J. Cachexia Sarcopenia Muscle* **2015**, *6*, 317–324. [CrossRef]
39. Baek, S.J.; Okazaki, R.; Lee, S.-H.; Martinez, J.; Kim, J.-S.; Yamaguchi, K.; Mishina, Y.; Martin, D.W.; Shoieb, A.; McEntee, M.F.; et al. Nonsteroidal Anti-Inflammatory Drug-Activated Gene-1 over Expression in Transgenic Mice Suppresses Intestinal Neoplasia. *Gastroenterology* **2006**, *131*, 1553–1560. [CrossRef]
40. Johnen, H.; Lin, S.; Kuffner, T.; Brown, D.A.; Tsai, V.W.-W.; Bauskin, A.R.; Wu, L.; Pankhurst, G.; Jiang, L.; Junankar, S.; et al. Tumor-Induced Anorexia and Weight Loss Are Mediated by the TGF-Beta Superfamily Cytokine MIC-1. *Nat. Med.* **2007**, *13*, 1333–1340. [CrossRef]
41. Ost, M.; Igual Gil, C.; Coleman, V.; Keipert, S.; Efstathiou, S.; Vidic, V.; Weyers, M.; Klaus, S. Muscle-Derived GDF15 Drives Diurnal Anorexia and Systemic Metabolic Remodeling during Mitochondrial Stress. *EMBO Rep.* **2020**, *21*, e48804. [CrossRef]
42. Breen, D.M.; Jagarlapudi, S.; Patel, A.; Zou, C.; Joaquim, S.; Li, X.; Kang, L.; Pang, J.; Hales, K.; Ziso-Qejvanaj, E.; et al. Growth Differentiation Factor 15 Neutralization Does Not Impact Anorexia or Survival in Lipopolysaccharide-Induced Inflammation. *iScience* **2021**, *24*, 102554. [CrossRef]

Journal of
Clinical Medicine

MDPI

Article

Maxillary Sinus Puncture: A Traditional Procedure in Decline—Insights from SHIP

Fabian Paperlein [1,*], Johanna Klinger-König [2], Chia-Jung Busch [1], Christian Scharf [1] and Achim Georg Beule [1,3]

[1] Department of Otorhinolaryngology, Head and Neck Surgery, University Medicine Greifswald, 17475 Greifswald, Germany
[2] Department of Psychiatry and Psychotherapy, University Medicine Greifswald, 17475 Greifswald, Germany
[3] Department of Otorhinolaryngology, Head and Neck Surgery, University Hospital Münster, 48149 Münster, Germany
* Correspondence: fabian.paperlein@med.uni-greifswald.de

Abstract: Background: Maxillary sinus puncture (MSP), once a cornerstone for diagnosing and treating acute rhinosinusitis (ARS), has declined with the rise in less invasive techniques. This study explores MSP trends, its association with age, and long-term effects on quality of life using data from the Study of Health in Pomerania (SHIP). **Methods:** Data from SHIP-START-2 (n = 2332), SHIP-START-3 (n = 1717), and SHIP-TREND-0 (n = 4420) cohorts were analyzed to assess MSP prevalence, demographic correlations, and quality- of-life impacts using SNOT-20-D, EQ-5D-3L, and SF-12. **Results:** MSP prevalence was higher in older SHIP-START cohorts (11.2% in START-2) compared to SHIP-TREND-0 (9.5%), reflecting its historical decline. The procedure was more frequently reported by participants aged > 60 years (e.g., 14.0% in START-2) than by younger groups (<40 years: 3.5% in START-2). MSP was associated with increased SNOT-20-D scores across cohorts (e.g., +0.28 in START-2, $p < 0.001$) and minor reductions in EQ-5D-3L and SF-12 mental health scores, indicating greater symptom burden but limited general health impact. The age- and time-related decline in MSP highlights its diminishing role in modern practice. **Conclusions:** While MSP offers diagnostic insights and serves as an indicator for ARS, its modest impact on long-term quality-of-life underscores the need for alternative, minimally invasive techniques for sinonasal conditions.

Keywords: maxillary sinus puncture; rhinosinusitis; sinonasal quality of life; SNOT-20-D; historical medical practice; population-based study; SHIP; otorhinolaryngology

1. Introduction

Maxillary sinus puncture (MSP) was long considered the gold standard for diagnosing and treating acute rhinosinusitis (ARS), particularly in the late 20th century [1,2]. Historically used both diagnostically and therapeutically through irrigation, MSP has largely been replaced by endoscopic middle meatal cultures (EDMMs), which are less invasive, more accessible, and associated with reduced patient discomfort and risk [1]. While MSP remains in use in some countries undergoing procedural refinement [3], contemporary European and national guidelines now recognize it only as a secondary option, typically for microbiological sampling in more severe ARS cases managed in secondary or tertiary care settings [4,5].

Despite this decline, MSP use may have persisted longer in rural or resource-limited settings, such as those formerly in East Germany, due to historical practice patterns and

https://doi.org/10.3390/jcm14155578

systemic differences in healthcare infrastructure. We hypothesize that MSP was more prevalent in these regions and age groups with limited access to newer diagnostic techniques, and may serve as a retrospective proxy marker for severe ARS episodes. To explore this hypothesis, we analyzed data from the Study of Health in Pomerania (SHIP), a large-scale, longitudinal, and population-based health study in northeastern Germany. The SHIP was established to investigate the prevalence of chronic diseases, risk factors, and their interactions in the general adult population. The assessments include standardized face-to-face interviews, self-report questionnaires, physical examinations, and various biospecimens. It comprises several cohorts [6,7]:

- **SHIP-START**: The original cohort with baseline data collected between 1997 and 2001, followed by START-2 (2008–2012) and START-3 (2014–2016);
- **SHIP-TREND**: An independent cohort established in 2008 (TREND-0: 2008–2012) to refresh the population sample;
- **SHIP-NEXT**: Launched in 2021 but excluded from this analysis due to ongoing data collection.

Participants were randomly selected from regional registries and underwent standardized clinical assessments, interviews, and validated questionnaires, including the Sinonasal Outcome Test—German version (SNOT-20-D), the EuroQol 5-Dimension 3-Level questionnaire (EQ-5D-3L), and the 12-Item Short Form Survey (SF-12).

Objective

This study aims to assess age- and time-related trends in MSP use across SHIP cohorts and to evaluate its long-term association with sinonasal symptom burden and quality of life. Our findings offer insights into the historical role of MSP in ARS management and its potential utility as an epidemiological indicator in population health research.

2. Materials and Methods

2.1. Study Design and Population

The analyses used data from the Study of Health in Pomerania (SHIP), a population-based cohort study conducted in northeastern Germany to examine the prevalence of chronic diseases, risk factors, and healthcare utilization in the general adult population [7]. We included participants from two distinct SHIP cohorts:

- **SHIP-START**, the first cohort, with baseline data collected in 1997–2001 (START-0; n = 4308). We used follow-up data from START-2 (2008–2012; n = 2333) and START-3 (2014–2016; n = 1717);
- **SHIP-TREND-0**, the baseline data of an independent second cohort recruited in the same region (2008–2012; n = 4420).

The START and TREND cohorts were drawn from the same geographic area but included non-overlapping participants. Data from START-3 were used only for longitudinal consistency analysis and excluded from cross-sectional analyses to avoid repeated- measurement bias. Ethics approval was obtained for all cohorts and waves, and participants provided written informed consent. Access to the dataset was granted through formal application to the SHIP data committee.

2.2. Assessment of Sinonasal History and Interventions

In SHIP-START-2 and START-3, participants completed a 20-item sinus-specific questionnaire designed to capture sinonasal symptoms, structural abnormalities, surgical history, and interventions. For the present study, we selected six items focusing on procedural history—namely, maxillary sinus puncture (MSP), septoplasty, and paranasal sinus surgery—which directly align with our study objectives.

The timing of each reported procedure was recorded via open-ended responses, allowing participants to indicate either the year or age at which the intervention occurred. Other questionnaire items, although relevant to broader rhinologic phenotyping, were excluded to maintain a clear focus on intervention trends and quality-of-life outcomes.

In SHIP-TREND-0, only two of the six procedural questions—those concerning MSP and paranasal sinus surgery—were included, due to financial constraints limiting questionnaire length.

The six selected items were as follows:

1. Have you ever had your nasal septum straightened? (0 = no, 1 = yes);
2. If yes, when? (open-ended response);
3. Have you ever undergone a maxillary sinus puncture?* (0 = no, 1 = yes);
4. If yes, when? (open-ended response);
5. Have you ever had surgery on the paranasal sinuses?* (0 = no, 1 = yes);
6. If yes, when? (open-ended response).

Only the questions marked with an asterisk (*) were included in SHIP-TREND-0. All six items were included in SHIP-START-2 and SHIP-START-3.

2.3. *Quality-of-Life Instruments*

Quality of life was assessed using three validated tools:

- **SNOT-20-D:** This 20-item questionnaire evaluates symptom burden and quality-of-life impact in individuals with sinonasal complaints. It includes items on nasal obstruction, facial pressure, and olfactory function. The German version (SNOT-20-D) is a standardized translation of the original SNOT-20 developed by Piccirillo et al. [8] and was the best-available tool at the time of SHIP-START for sinonasal health assessment in a German-speaking population. Higher scores indicate greater symptom severity; a mean score of ≥ 0.8 was defined as the minimal clinically important difference (MCID);
- **EQ-5D-3L:** This is a standardized measure of general health across five domains: mobility, self-care, usual activities, pain/discomfort, and anxiety/depression. Index scores were calculated using German-specific value sets [9,10], with higher values indicating better health. The EQ-5D is validated for use in CRS research and general populations [11];
- **SF-12:** This a concise, validated tool for assessing subjective physical and mental health. It produces two summary scores (physical and mental component summaries). Higher scores reflect better perceived health status [12].

2.4. *Use of AI Tools*

OpenAI's ChatGPT-4 was used to support language refinement and formatting during manuscript preparation. No data analysis or scientific interpretation was performed using AI tools.

2.5. *Statistical Analysis*

All analyses were performed using R version 4.2.1. Descriptive statistics are presented as means (M) with standard deviations (SDs) for continuous variables, and counts (n) with percentages (%) for categorical variables.

Linear regression models were used to evaluate the association between MSP and quality-of-life outcomes (SNOT-20-D, EQ-5D-3L, and SF-12). Models were adjusted for age, sex, smoking status, and allergy history. The main exposure variable was intervention status (MSP vs. no intervention), with the latter used as the reference group.

To explore the effect of the timing of the intervention, we performed additional linear regressions using the following:

- Years since MSP;
- Age at MSP;
- Interaction: years since × age at MSP;
- Interaction: age at MSP × sex.

Timing analyses were restricted to SHIP-START-2, as TREND-0 did not include timing data. For descriptive purposes, we also examined the distribution of interventions by age and calendar year and assessed the consistency of MSP reporting between START-2 and START-3 in overlapping participants.

3. Results

3.1. Cohort Characteristics and MSP Prevalence

In START-2, 2306 out of 2332 participants provided valid data on MSP use in earlier decades, of whom 258 (11.2%) reported undergoing the procedure. In TREND-0, 4235 out of 4420 participants provided valid data, with 401 (9.5%) reporting MSP. The mean age was higher in START-2 (57.4 years) compared to TREND-0 (52.0 years), consistent with START-2 being a follow-up cohort and TREND-0 being a baseline population. The gender distribution was comparable across cohorts (53.0% women in START-2; 51.5% in TREND-0).

Figure 1 visualizes the age-related distribution of sinonasal procedures across both cohorts. MSP shows a clear increase with age, peaking in the >60 group (14.0% in START-2 and 13.8% in TREND-0), while being rare among participants < 40 years (3.5% in START-2, 3.3% in TREND-0). In contrast, septoplasty (STP) and endoscopic sinus surgery (ESS) are more evenly distributed across age groups, with STP slightly more common among younger individuals. These age patterns reflect historical shifts in clinical practice, where MSP was more common in prior decades. Self-reported allergy prevalence was substantially higher in TREND-0 (29.3%) than in START-2 (9.4%). Smoking was also more common in TREND-0 (26.9%) than in START-2 (20.8%), particularly among younger participants.

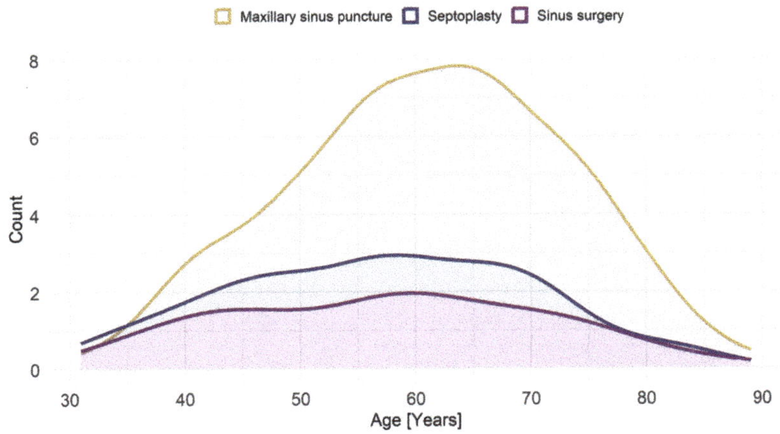

Figure 1. Age distribution of sinonasal procedures. Procedures include MSP (maxillary sinus puncture), STP (septoplasty), and ESS (endoscopic sinus surgery). The graph shows MSP being most frequently performed in older age groups, peaking around 60–70 years, while STP and ESS exhibit a more balanced distribution across ages, with slightly higher prevalence in middle-aged individuals.

Quality-of-life measures showed only minor cohort differences. EQ-5D-3L index scores averaged 0.9 in both cohorts. SNOT-20-D mean scores were 0.7, with higher values in women and younger participants. SF-12 general and mental health scores were similar across cohorts, with slightly lower physical scores in older participants. These baseline characteristics are summarized in Table 1.

Table 1. Descriptive statistics for START-2 and TREND-0 cohorts by demographic groups.

			START-2				
Variable	**N**	**Overall**	**Men**	**Women**	**<40 Years**	**40–60 Years**	**>60 Years**
Sex [women]	2332	1235 (53.0)	–	–	148 (57.4)	581 (54.4)	506 (50.3)
Age [years]	2332	57.4 (13.7)	58.3 (13.8)	56.5 (13.5)	35.8 (2.5)	50.2 (6.1)	70.5 (6.8)
Allergies [yes]	2309	217 (9.4)	73 (6.7)	144 (11.8)	24 (9.3)	105 (9.9)	88 (8.9)
Current smoking [yes]	2323	484 (20.8)	232 (21.2)	252 (20.5)	81 (31.4)	309 (29.0)	94 (9.4)
EQ-5D-3L index	2301	0.9 (0.2)	0.9 (0.1)	0.9 (0.2)	0.9 (0.1)	0.9 (0.1)	0.9 (0.2)
SF12 general health	2318	3.0 (0.7)	3.0 (0.7)	3.0 (0.7)	3.4 (0.7)	3.1 (0.7)	2.9 (0.6)
SF12 physical health	2262	47.0 (9.1)	46.9 (9.3)	47.1 (8.9)	50.7 (7.0)	48.5 (8.3)	44.4 (9.7)
SF12 mental health	2262	52.5 (8.7)	54.0 (7.7)	51.2 (9.3)	51.7 (8.6)	51.9 (8.7)	53.4 (8.6)
SNOT-20-D summary score	1247	13.1 (12.2)	11.0 (10.5)	15.1 (13.4)	15.1 (12.8)	14.0 (12.8)	11.2 (10.8)
SNOT-20-D mean score	1247	0.7 (0.6)	0.6 (0.5)	0.8 (0.7)	0.8 (0.6)	0.7 (0.6)	0.6 (0.5)
SNOT-20-D MCID [yes]	1247	407 (32.6)	161 (26.3)	246 (38.7)	66 (43.7)	226 (34.9)	115 (25.7)
Maxillary sinus puncture [yes]	2306	258 (11.2)	116 (10.7)	142 (11.6)	9 (3.5)	111 (10.5)	138 (14.0)
Age at puncture [years]	218	35.7 (15.8)	37.7 (17.9)	34.2 (13.6)	26.8 (5.4)	30.7 (12.1)	40.2 (17.3)
Time since puncture [years]	218	25.1 (15.2)	25.7 (16.7)	24.6 (14.0)	9.1 (5.2)	20.7 (12.5)	29.7 (15.9)
			TREND-0				
Variable	**N**	**Overall**	**Men**	**Women**	**< 40 years**	**40–60 years**	**> 60 years**
Sex [women]	4420	2275 (51.5)	–	–	582 (53.8)	990 (52.1)	703 (48.9)
Age [years]	4420	52.0 (15.5)	52.6 (15.7)	51.3 (15.2)	31.4 (5.1)	50.3 (6.1)	69.6 (5.7)
Allergies [yes]	4248	1245 (29.3)	443 (21.4)	802 (36.8)	372 (34.8)	557 (29.8)	316 (24.1)
Current smoking [yes]	4398	1183 (26.9)	624 (29.3)	559 (24.7)	458 (42.5)	593 (31.2)	132 (9.3)
EQ-5D-3L index	4369	0.9 (0.1)	0.9 (0.1)	0.9 (0.2)	0.9 (0.1)	0.9 (0.1)	0.9 (0.2)
SF12 general health	4404	3.1 (0.7)	3.1 (0.7)	3.0 (0.7)	3.4 (0.7)	3.1 (0.7)	2.8 (0.6)
SF12 physical health	4310	47.3 (8.8)	47.6 (8.7)	47.0 (9.0)	51.4 (6.1)	47.6 (8.6)	43.7 (9.4)
SF12 mental health	4310	52.4 (8.6)	53.8 (7.9)	51.2 (9.1)	51.5 (7.8)	52.0 (9.0)	53.8 (8.6)
SNOT-20-D summary score	2422	13.8 (12.0)	12.3 (11.3)	15.4 (12.4)	14.2 (12.0)	14.3 (12.5)	12.8 (10.9)
SNOT-20-D mean score	2422	0.7 (0.6)	0.6 (0.6)	0.8 (0.6)	0.7 (0.6)	0.7 (0.6)	0.6 (0.5)
SNOT-20-D MCID [yes]	2422	853 (35.2)	359 (29.5)	494 (41.0)	220 (36.7)	422 (36.0)	211 (32.5)
Maxillary sinus puncture [yes]	4235	401 (9.5)	182 (8.8)	219 (10.1)	35 (3.3)	186 (10.0)	180 (13.8)

3.2. Longitudinal Consistency and MSP Timing

Longitudinal data from 1596 participants who provided MSP information in both START-2 and START-3 revealed that 181 individuals reported MSP consistently. Of these, 72 provided timing data in both waves, with 26.4% reporting the exact same year and another 26.4% differing by only one year. An additional 33 participants reported MSP in START-3 but not in START-2, and most dated their procedures before 2008, suggesting recall limitations rather than actual new interventions.

The distribution of MSP by year shows a clear historical peak in the mid to late 20th century, with most interventions dated before 2000. This decline is visualized in Figure 2.

As illustrated in Figure 1, cross-sectional age distributions mirror these longitudinal patterns. Older adults, who likely underwent MSP in earlier decades, show the highest prevalence, reinforcing the age–procedure relationship.

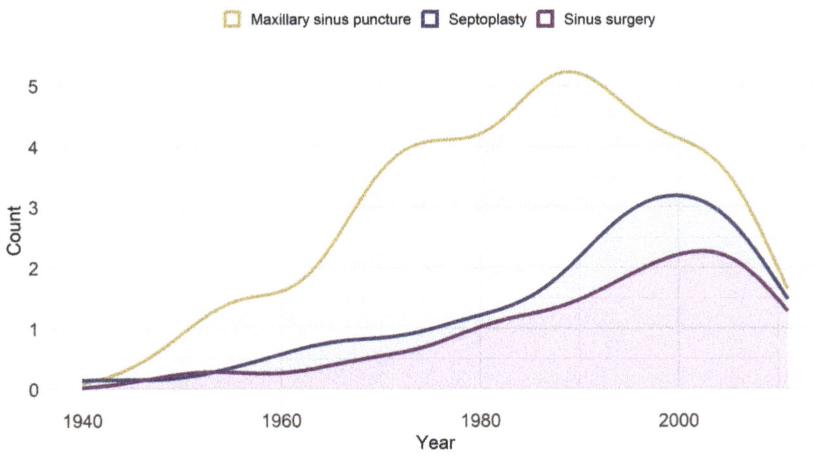

Figure 2. Trends in sinonasal procedures, including MSP, STP, and ESS, from 1940 to 2012. The graph illustrates the peak usage of MSP in the late 20th century, followed by a decline in recent years, alongside more gradual trends in STP and ESS.

3.3. Impact of MSP on Quality of Life

MSP was consistently associated with a greater sinonasal symptom burden. In START-2, MSP participants had a mean SNOT-20-D score 0.28 points higher than non-MSP participants ($p < 0.001$); in TREND-0, the difference was 0.17 points ($p < 0.001$). Moreover, MSP participants were significantly more likely to meet or exceed the minimal clinically important difference (MCID) threshold of ≥ 0.8, with odds ratios of 2.41 (95% CI: 1.62–3.57) in START-2 and 1.56 (95% CI: 1.18–2.07) in TREND-0 (Table 2).

Table 2. Associations between maxillary sinus puncture (MSP) and quality-of-life outcomes, adjusted for age, sex, smoking status, and allergy history. Significant associations ($p < 0.05$) are highlighted in **bold**. Continuous outcomes are shown as regression coefficients (β) with 95% confidence intervals (CIs); binary outcomes are shown as odds ratios (ORs). The reference group comprises participants without MSP.

Outcome	Cohort	N (No MSP)	N (MSP)	Estimate [95% CI]	p-Value
EQ-5D-3L index (β)	START-2	1919	238	**−0.02 [−0.04; −0.001]**	**0.042**
	TREND-0	3692	397	0.01 [−0.01; 0.02]	0.324
SF-12 general health (β)	START-2	1932	241	−0.06 [−0.14; 0.03]	0.193
	TREND-0	3721	400	−0.05 [−0.11; 0.02]	0.178
SF-12 physical health (β)	START-2	1883	237	−0.94 [−2.10; 0.22]	0.112
	TREND-0	3650	392	−0.81 [−1.66; 0.04]	0.060
SF-12 mental health (β)	START-2	1883	237	**−1.24 [−2.41; −0.07]**	**0.039**
	TREND-0	3650	392	−0.36 [−1.25; 0.52]	0.423
SNOT-20-D mean score (β)	START-2	1051	119	**0.28 [0.17; 0.39]**	**8.9×10^{-7}**
	TREND-0	2117	231	**0.17 [0.09; 0.25]**	**5.6×10^{-5}**
SNOT-20-D MCID (OR)	START-2	1051	119	**2.41 [1.62; 3.57]**	**1.3×10^{-5}**
	TREND-0	2117	231	**1.56 [1.18; 2.07]**	**5.4×10^{-6}**

General health measures were less affected. EQ-5D-3L scores were marginally lower in START-2 MSP participants ($\beta = -0.02$, $p = 0.042$), while SF-12 mental health scores also declined slightly ($\beta = -1.24$, $p = 0.039$). No significant associations were observed for general or physical health scores in TREND-0.

The combined impact of MSP across different health domains is visualized in Figure 3. Here, standardized regression coefficients (z-scores) allow for comparison across scales. SNOT-20-D scores show the strongest deviation, clearly indicating increased symptom burden in MSP participants. Effects on general health and mental health were more modest, though directionally consistent.

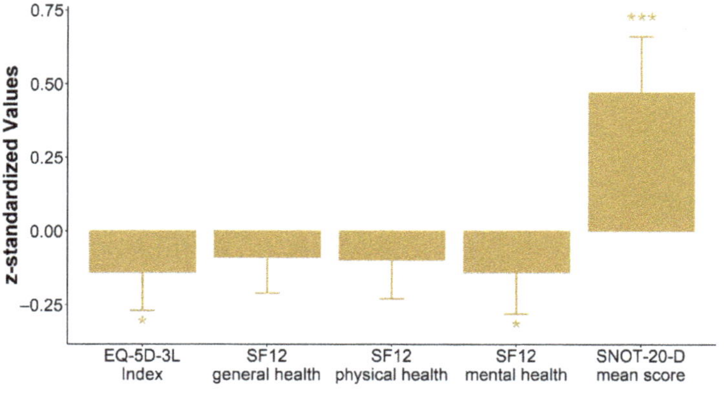

Figure 3. Impact of maxillary sinus puncture (MSP) on quality of life: comparison across multiple domains. Results are presented as standardized coefficients (z-scores) for the EQ-5D-3L index, SF-12 (general health, physical health, and mental health), and SNOT-20-D mean score to enable direct comparability between the scores. For the EQ-5D-3L and SF-12, positive values indicate better quality of life/subjective health, whereas for the SNOT-20-D, negative values indicate fewer symptoms. Changes are presented relative to no intervention. Significant differences are denoted by * $p < 0.05$ and *** $p < 0.001$.

Further exploratory analyses in START-2 assessed whether age at intervention or time since MSP affected outcomes. Table 3 shows a borderline association between age at intervention and EQ-5D-3L scores ($p = 0.053$), but no robust patterns across other measures.

Table 3. Impact of demographics and time since intervention on quality-of-life measures of START-2: Results are stratified by intervention (maxillary sinus puncture), with F-values and p-values indicating the statistical significance of the associations.

Outcome	Statistic	Time Since Intervention	Age at Intervention	Time × Age Interaction	Age × Sex Interaction
EQ-5D-3L index	N	216	216	216	216
	F-value	2.81	2.60	0.20	1.61
	p-value	0.041	0.053	0.994	0.188
SF-12 general health	N	218	218	218	218
	F-value	0.80	2.10	0.64	0.90
	p-value	0.497	0.101	0.766	0.444
SF-12 physical health	N	213	213	213	213
	F-value	1.24	1.51	1.18	3.05
	p-value	0.296	0.214	0.309	0.030
SF-12 mental health	N	213	213	213	213
	F-value	0.92	1.52	1.05	0.24
	p-value	0.432	0.209	0.403	0.869
SNOT-20-D summary score	N	106	106	106	106
	F-value	0.64	1.43	0.66	0.63
	p-value	0.593	0.239	0.740	0.594

4. Discussion

4.1. Significance of the Study

This study is one of the first to investigate maxillary sinus puncture (MSP) using a large, population-based epidemiological dataset with longitudinal data. Our analysis of over 6700 participants across two major German cohorts (SHIP-START-2 and SHIP-TREND-0) reveals both historical and age-related trends in MSP use, and provides rare insights into its long-term association with sinonasal and general quality of life.

We demonstrate that MSP, although now rarely used and largely reserved for selected or recalcitrant cases, may serve as a proxy marker for prior episodes of severe acute rhinosinusitis (ARS). Our findings suggest that MSP is associated with a small but consistent long-term reduction in sinonasal quality of life, even decades after the procedure.

4.2. Historical Trends and Age Distribution

A central finding of this study is the temporal decline in MSP, both in national inpatient data and within our population sample. Figures 2 and 4 show a sharp reduction in MSP procedures in Germany—from 2927 in 2005 to just 321 in 2023. This trend reflects updates in clinical guidelines and a broader shift toward minimally invasive alternatives such as endoscopic sinus surgery (ESS) and endoscopically directed middle meatal cultures (EDMMs) [4,5,13–15].

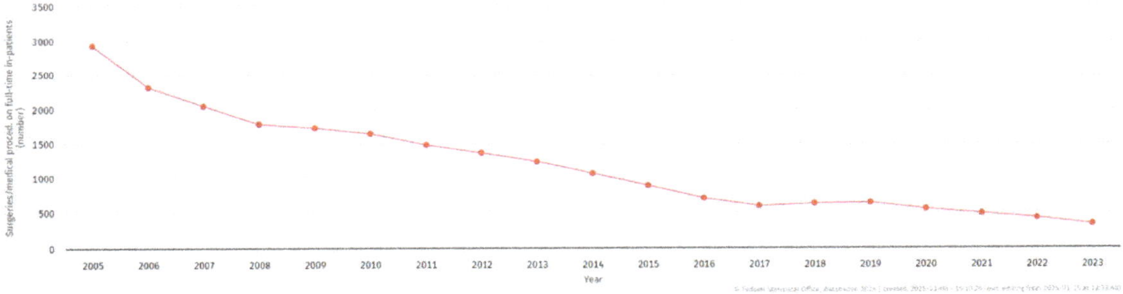

Figure 4. Trend in maxillary sinus puncture (MSP) performed on inpatients in Germany (2005–2023). The data, categorized by surgical and procedural codes (1–4-digit hierarchy), were sourced from case-based hospital statistics (DRG). © Federal Statistical Office of Germany (Destatis), 2024. Status: 8 January 2025, 15:10:26.

Despite its decline, MSP remains in use in specific clinical contexts, including intensive care units [16], for young children under general anesthesia [17], and in some Eastern European countries where refinement continues [3]. Globally, MSP has been largely replaced by less invasive techniques such as endoscopic sinus surgery, and published data on its trends remain limited. Neto et al. [16] observed that while MSP was historically important for managing hospital-acquired rhinosinusitis, its role has diminished as newer approaches became available. In Brazil, national health data (DATASUS) from 2008 to 2025 recorded no procedures under its specific code, likely reflecting replacement by endonasal interventions or reclassification under broader sinonasal codes. These contrasting patterns underscore MSP's role as a marker of changing medical practice, shaped by guidelines, infrastructure, and training.

As shown in Figure 1, MSP was disproportionately more common in older adults, particularly those aged 60 years and above. This reflects its widespread use in earlier decades [18], prior to the adoption of ESS as standard practice. In contrast, procedures like septoplasty (STP) and sinus surgery (SS) show a more balanced age distribution.

4.3. Reliability of Self-Reported MSP and Recall Bias

Longitudinal data from participants who completed both START-2 and START-3 suggest a moderate level of recall accuracy. Among those reporting MSP at both time points, approximately 40% recalled the same or nearly the same year of intervention. This level of consistency is notable given the average time lag of 26 years since the procedure.

Reporting discrepancies—seen at a consistency rate of 52.78%—highlight typical challenges in long-term recall. Factors such as the perceived importance of MSP, its outpatient nature, and cognitive decline with age may influence accuracy [19]. The inability to cross-validate responses with medical records due to German privacy law further limits validation, although this is a common challenge in population-based research.

4.4. Impact on Quality of Life

Our findings show a statistically significant association between MSP and reduced sinonasal quality of life, measured by SNOT-20-D. Participants with a history of MSP reported higher symptom scores and were more likely to exceed the clinically important difference threshold (see Table 2).

This association persisted across both cohorts and was evident years after the procedure, indicating a long-term burden. Although general health measures (EQ-5D-3L, SF-12) showed more modest changes, slight reductions in physical and mental health scores were observed in MSP groups (see Figure 3).

Given MSP being primarily used for severe ARS, these results suggest that ARS may have lasting effects, possibly contributing to or overlapping with chronic rhinosinusitis (CRS). Our findings align with previous studies reporting long-term quality-of-life burdens from sinonasal disease [20,21], but extend this knowledge by showing such effects long after intervention.

These findings support the hypothesis that severe ARS—often treated with MSP—may contribute to or accelerate CRS development, a pathway not well characterized in epidemiologic studies [5].

Similarly, general quality of life showed a limited but consistent decline in MSP patients across EQ-5D-3L and SF-12 domains. While most QoL studies measure short-term outcomes (e.g., within 2 weeks post-intervention), our long-term design offers unique value. For instance, Stjärne et al. [22] reported residual EQ-5D burden in ARS patients weeks after onset, and Sathananthar et al. [23] observed symptom relief 20 months after canine fossa puncture (CFP), especially in cases of severe maxillary sinus disease.

QoL tools such as SNOT-16 and EQ-5D have shown acceptable sensitivity but were not developed for long-term ARS tracking [24,25]. Al-Asadi et al. [26] further showed elevated SNOT-22 in recurrent ARS cases. Our findings, using SNOT-20-D, expand this evidence base by linking MSP to persistent symptom burden in a population setting.

This supports MSP as a retrospective marker of past severe ARS and suggests a potential link to CRS evolution, meriting further longitudinal study.

4.5. Confounding Variables

In our cohorts, allergy prevalence increased over time—from 9.4% in START-2 to 29.3% in TREND-0—which may reflect both a true rise in incidence and improved diagnostic awareness, consistent with global trends [27]. Smoking rates also differed by age and cohort, with younger participants in TREND-0 reporting a higher smoking prevalence (26.9%) compared to START-2 (20.8%). These patterns align with broader public health data: in 1995, smoking was most prevalent among individuals aged 30–49 [28], while recent CDC data from 2022 show the highest cigarette use among adults aged 45–64, and e-cigarette use was concentrated among those aged 18–24 [29].

Given the known associations between allergies, smoking, and sinonasal symptom burden, we adjusted for both variables in all regression models. While they may contribute to the baseline variation in quality-of-life scores, their inclusion as covariates reduces the likelihood of residual confounding.

4.6. Limitations

This study has several limitations: First, recall bias may have affected self-reported procedural data, though the relatively high agreement between START-2 and START-3 lends support to the reliability of these reports. Second, selection bias may have occurred if patients recently operated on were not yet captured in follow-up rounds. Third, the lack of validation with clinical records is a recognized constraint in German cohort studies due to decentralized health data systems. Additionally, MSP cases were relatively few compared to the total sample, which limits the power to detect small subgroup effects. The dataset also lacked details on sinus surgery types, which likely ranged from minimally invasive techniques (e.g., FESS) to more extensive procedures performed in earlier decades. Finally, quality-of-life instruments like SNOT-20-D were originally validated for CRS, not ARS, though they remain widely used due to the lack of ARS-specific long-term tools.

5. Conclusions

This study confirms that MSP—a declining but historically important procedure—remains detectable in population surveys and correlates with reduced sinonasal quality of life years later. Approximately 40% of participants accurately recalled the procedure timing decades after the event, offering a promising benchmark for memory-dependent epidemiologic work.

As one of the first large-scale studies to examine long-term quality-of-life effects following MSP, our results support its use as a retrospective proxy for severe ARS. These findings underline the need for more longitudinal studies to understand how acute infections may evolve into chronic conditions and affect general health outcomes over time.

Author Contributions: Conceptualization, F.P. and A.G.B.; methodology, F.P. and J.K.-K.; formal analysis, J.K.-K.; investigation, F.P.; data curation, F.P.; writing—original draft preparation, F.P.; writing—review and editing, J.K.-K., C.-J.B., C.S. and A.G.B.; supervision, A.G.B. All authors have read and agreed to the published version of the manuscript.

Funding: This study was funded by the Deutsche Forschungsgemeinschaft (DFG, German Research Foundation)—Project Number 493623784 and the Gerhard Domagk Nachwuchsförderprogramm (Clinician Scientist Program Rural_Age Scholarship to F.S.). The Study of Health in Pomerania (SHIP) is part of the Community Medicine Research Network of the University Medicine Greifswald, which is supported by the German Federal Ministry of Education and Research (BMBF), the Ministry of Cultural Affairs of the State of Mecklenburg–Western Pomerania, and the 'Greifswald Approach to Individualized Medicine (GANI_MED)' network. Data access was granted through a formal application to the SHIP data committee.

Institutional Review Board Statement: The SHIP was approved by the Ethics Committee of the University Medicine Greifswald. The study was conducted according to the guidelines of the Declaration of Helsinki, and approved by the Institutional Review Board (Ethics Committee) of Ernst-Moritz-Arndt University, Faculty of Medicine, Ethics Committee, Institute for Pharmacology, Friedrich-Löffler Strasse 23d, 17481 Greifswald, Germany (protocol codes: S2 = BB 80/09, date of approval: 2 October 2009; S3 = BB 122/13, date of approval: 5 November 2013; T0 = BB 39/08, date of approval: 19 June 2008; T1 = BB 174/15, date of approval: 22 December 2015).

Informed Consent Statement: All SHIP participants provided written informed consent at the time of data collection.

Data Availability Statement: The data used in this study are part of the SHIP project and are available upon reasonable request from the SHIP data access committee.

Acknowledgments: The authors would like to thank the Study of Health in Pomerania (SHIP) research team and participants for their valuable contributions to this study. We acknowledge the use of ChatGPT-4 (OpenAI, 2023) to support language refinement and formatting during the manuscript preparation. No data analysis, scientific interpretation, or content generation was performed using AI tools.

Conflicts of Interest: The authors declare no conflicts of interest.

Abbreviations

The following abbreviations are used in this manuscript:

MSP	Maxillary Sinus Puncture
ARS	Acute Rhinosinusitis
CRS	Chronic Rhinosinusitis
SNOT-20-D	Sinonasal Outcome Test (20-item, German version)
EQ-5D-3L	EuroQol 5-Dimension, 3-Level
SF-12	12-Item Short Form Health Survey
MCID	Minimal Clinically Important Difference
SHIP	Study of Health in Pomerania
ESS	Endoscopic Sinus Surgery
EDMM	Endoscopically Directed Middle Meatal Culture
QoL	Quality of Life
CI	Confidence Interval
OR	Odds Ratio
DFG	Deutsche Forschungsgemeinschaft
BMBF	Federal Ministry of Education and Research (Germany)

References

1. Benninger, M.S.; Payne, S.C.; Ferguson, B.J.; Hadley, J.A.; Ahmad, N. Endoscopically directed middle meatal cultures versus maxillary sinus taps in acute bacterial maxillary rhinosinusitis: A meta-analysis. *Otolaryngol. Neck Surg.* **2006**, *134*, 3–9. [CrossRef] [PubMed]
2. Mees, K. (Ed.) *Die Unspezifische Rhino-Sinusitis: Aktuelle Aspekte zur Konservativen und Operativen Wiederherstellung der Mukoziliaren Clearance*; Springer: Berlin/Heidelberg, Germany, 1996.
3. Kryukov, A.; Tovmasyan, A.; Lapchenko, A.; Bolgar, A.; Kishinevskii, A.; Timofeeva, M.; Artemyeva-Karelova, A.; Ogorodnikov, D. Optimizatsiya metoda punktsionnogo lecheniya ostrogo bakterial'nogo verkhnechelyustnogo sinusita. *Vestn. Otorinolaringol.* **2024**, *89*, 15–20. [CrossRef] [PubMed]
4. Stuck, B.A.; Beule, A.; Jobst, D.; Klimek, L.; Laudien, M.; Lell, M.; Vogl, T.J.; Popert, U. Leitlinie "Rhinosinusitis"—Langfassung: S2k-Leitlinie der Deutschen Gesellschaft für Allgemeinmedizin und Familienmedizin und der Deutschen Gesellschaft für Hals-Nasen-Ohren-Heilkunde, Kopf- undHals-Chirurgie e. V. *HNO* **2018**, *66*, 38–74. [CrossRef] [PubMed]
5. Fokkens, W.; Lund, V.; Hopkins, C.; Hellings, P.; Kern, R.; Reitsma, S.; Toppila-Salmi, S.; Bernal-Sprekelsen, M.; Mullol, J. Executive summary of EPOS 2020 including integrated care pathways. *Rhinology* **2020**, *58*, 82–111. [CrossRef]
6. Völzke, H. Größte Gesundheitsstudie SHIP Startet mit Dritter Basisgruppe und Betritt Neuland in der Bevölkerungs-Forschung. 2021. Available online: https://www2.medizin.uni-greifswald.de/cm/fv/fileadmin/user_upload/ship/dokumente/PI-23-2021-Universitaetsmedizin-Greifswald.pdf (accessed on 10 January 2025).
7. Völzke, H.; Schössow, J.; Schmidt, C.O.; Jürgens, C.; Richter, A.; Werner, A.; Werner, N.; Radke, D.; Teumer, A.; Ittermann, T.; et al. Cohort Profile Update: The Study of Health in Pomerania (SHIP). *Int. J. Epidemiol.* **2022**, *51*, e372–e383. [CrossRef]
8. Piccirillo, J.; Merritt, M.; Richards, M. Psychometric and clinimetric validity of the 20-Item Sino-Nasal Outcome Test (SNOT-20). *Otolaryngol.–Head Neck Surg.* **2002**, *126*, 41–47. [CrossRef]
9. Greiner, W.; Claes, C.; Busschbach, J.; Graf von der Schulenburg, J.M. Validating the EQ-5D with time trade off for the German population. *Eur. J. Health Econ.* **2005**, *6*, 124–130. [CrossRef]
10. Konerding, U.; Elkhuizen, S.G.; Faubel, R.; Forte, P.; Malmström, T.; Pavi, E.; Janssen, M.B. The validity of the EQ-5D-3L items: An investigation with type 2 diabetes patients from six European countries. *Health Qual. Life Outcomes* **2014**, *12*, 181. [CrossRef]

11. Lange, B.; Holst, R.; Thilsing, T.; Baelum, J.; Kjeldsen, A. Quality of life and associated factors in persons with chronic rhinosinusitis in the general population: A prospective questionnaire and clinical cross-sectional study. *Clin. Otolaryngol.* **2013**, *38*, 474–480. [CrossRef]
12. Bullinger, M.; Kirchberger, I.; Ware, J. Der deutsche SF-36 Health Survey. *J. Public Health* **1995**, *3*, 21–36. [CrossRef]
13. Orlandi, R.R.; Kingdom, T.T.; Smith, T.L.; Bleier, B.; DeConde, A.; Luong, A.U.; Poetker, D.M.; Soler, Z.; Welch, K.C.; Wise, S.K.; et al. International consensus statement on allergy and rhinology: Rhinosinusitis 2021. *Int. Forum Allergy Rhinol.* **2021**, *11*, 213–739. [CrossRef]
14. Joniau, S.; Vlaminck, S.; van Landuyt, H.; Kuhweide, R.; Dick, C. Microbiology of sinus puncture versus middle meatal aspiration in acute bacterial maxillary sinusitis. *Am. J. Rhinol.* **2005**, *19*, 135–140. [CrossRef]
15. Kim, D.H.; Kim, S.W.; Basurrah, M.A.; Hwang, S.H. Diagnostic Value of Middle Meatal Cultures versus Maxillary Sinus Culture in Acute and Chronic Sinusitis: A Systematic Review and Meta-Analysis. *J. Clin. Med.* **2022**, *11*, 6069. [CrossRef]
16. Mendes Neto, J.; Guerreiro, V.; Hirai, E.; Kosugi, E.; Santos, R.; Gregório, L. The role of maxillary sinus puncture on the diagnosis and treatment of patients with hospital-acquired rhinosinusitis. *Braz. J. Otorhinolaryngol.* **2012**, *78*, 35–41. [CrossRef]
17. Hsin, C.-H.; Tsao, C.-H.; Su, M.-C.; Chou, M.-C.; Liu, C.-M. Comparison of maxillary sinus puncture with endoscopic middle meatal culture in pediatric rhinosinusitis. *Am. J. Rhinol.* **2008**, *22*, 280–284. [CrossRef] [PubMed]
18. Benninger, M.; Sedory Holzer, S.; Lau, J. Diagnosis and treatment of uncomplicated acute bacterial rhinosinusitis: Summary of the Agency for Health Care Policy and Research evidence-based report. *Otolaryngol.–Head Neck Surg.* **2000**, *122*, 1–7. [CrossRef] [PubMed]
19. Hosemann, W.; Loew, T.; Forster, M.; Kühnel, T.; Beule, A. Perioperative Schmerzen und Ängste bei endoskopischen Nasennebenhöhleneingriffen mit konventioneller Nasentamponade. *Laryngo-Rhino-Otol.* **2011**, *90*, 476–480. [CrossRef]
20. Erskine, S.; Hopkins, C.; Kumar, N.; Wilson, J.; Clark, A.; Robertson, A.; Kara, N.; Sunkaraneni, V.; Anari, S.; Philpott, C. A cross sectional analysis of a case-control study about quality of life in CRS in the UK; a comparison between CRS subtypes. *Rhinol. J.* **2016**, *54*, 311–315. [CrossRef] [PubMed]
21. Plath, M.; Sand, M.; Cavaliere, C.; Plinkert, P.; Baumann, I.; Zaoui, K. Normative data for interpreting the SNOT-22. *Acta Otorhinolaryngol. Ital.* **2023**, *43*, 390–399. [CrossRef]
22. Stjärne, P.; Odebäck, P.; Ställberg, B.; Lundberg, J.; Olsson, P. High costs and burden of illness in acute rhinosinusitis: Real-life treatment patterns and outcomes in Swedish primary care. *Prim. Care Respir. J.* **2012**, *21*, 174–179. [CrossRef]
23. Sathananthar, S.; Nagaonkar, S.; Paleri, V.; Le, T.; Robinson, S.; Wormald, P.J. Canine fossa puncture and clearance of the maxillary sinus for the severely diseased maxillary sinus. *Laryngoscope* **2005**, *115*, 1026–1029. [CrossRef]
24. Garbutt, J.; Spitznagel, E.; Piccirillo, J. Use of the modified SNOT-16 in primary care patients with clinically diagnosed acute rhinosinusitis. *Arch. Otolaryngol.–Head Neck Surg.* **2011**, *137*, 792–797. [CrossRef]
25. Quadri, N.; Lloyd, A.; Keating, K.; Nafees, B.; Piccirillo, J.; Wild, D. Psychometric evaluation of the Sinonasal Outcome Test-16 and activity impairment assessment in acute bacterial sinusitis. *Otolaryngol.–Head Neck Surg.* **2013**, *149*, 161–167. [CrossRef]
26. Al-Asadi, Z.; Cui, R.; Lombardo, D.; Dewey, J.; Ramadan, H.; Makary, C. Impact of recurrent acute rhinosinusitis on quality of life. *Int. Forum Allergy Rhinol.* **2024**, *14*, 732–734. [CrossRef] [PubMed]
27. Shin, Y.H.; Hwang, J.; Kwon, R.; Lee, S.W.; Kim, M.S.; GBD 2019 Allergic Disorders Collaborators; Shin, J.I.; Yon, D.K. Global, regional, and national burden of allergic disorders and their risk factors in 204 countries and territories, from 1990 to 2019: A systematic analysis for the Global Burden of Disease Study 2019. *Allergy* **2023**, *78*, 2232–2254. [CrossRef] [PubMed]
28. Jha, P.; Ranson, M.; Nguyen, S.; Yach, D. Estimates of global and regional smoking prevalence in 1995, by age and sex. *Am. J. Public Health* **2002**, *92*, 1002–1006. [CrossRef] [PubMed]
29. Centers for Disease Control and Prevention. Tobacco Product Use Among Adults—United States. 2022. Available online: https://www.cdc.gov/tobacco/php/data-statistics/adult-data-cigarettes/index.html (accessed on 14 January 2025).

MDPI AG
Grosspeteranlage 5
4052 Basel
Switzerland
Tel.: +41 61 683 77 34

Journal of Clinical Medicine Editorial Office
E-mail: jcm@mdpi.com
www.mdpi.com/journal/jcm

www.ingramcontent.com/pod-product-compliance
Lightning Source LLC
Chambersburg PA
CBHW061453210926
51850CB00008B/1704
9783725873142